Aditi Lahiri and Sandra Kotzor (Eds.)
The Speech Processing Lexicon

Phonology and Phonetics

Editor
Aditi Lahiri

Volume 22

The Speech Processing Lexicon

Neurocognitive and Behavioural Approaches

Edited by
Aditi Lahiri and Sandra Kotzor

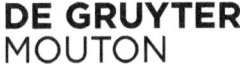

ISBN 978-3-11-063492-1
e-ISBN (PDF) 978-3-11-042265-8
e-ISBN (EPUB) 978-3-11-042277-1
ISSN 1861–4191

Library of Congress Cataloging-in-Publication Data
A CIP catalog record for this book has been applied for at the Library of Congress.

Bibliografische Information der Deutschen Nationalbibliothek
The Deutsche Nationalbibliothek lists this publication in the Deutschen Nationalbibliografie;
detailed bibliographic data are available on the internet http://dnb.dnb.de.

© 2018 Walter de Gruyter GmbH, Berlin/Boston
This volume is text- and page-identical with the hardback published in 2017.
Typesetting: Kovertus, Haarlem
Printing and binding: CPI books GmbH, Leck

♾ Printed on acid-free paper
Printed in Germany

www.degruyter.com

In acknowledgement of her continuing achievements and with deep gratitude for her inspiration—

To one of the contributors, the rest would like to dedicate this book:

Sheila Blumstein

Table of Contents

Allard Jongman and Aditi Lahiri
Introduction —— 1

Sheila E. Blumstein
Phonetic categories and phonological features: Evidence from the cognitive neuroscience of language —— 4

Allard Jongman and Bob McMurray
On invariance: Acoustic input meets listener expectations —— 21

Emily Myers, Alexis R. Johns, F. Sayako Earle and Xin Xie
The invariance problem in the acquisition of non-native phonetic contrasts: From instances to categories —— 52

Sandra Kotzor, Allison Wetterlin and Aditi Lahiri
Symmetry or asymmetry: Evidence for underspecification in the mental lexicon —— 85

Julia R. Drouin, Nicholas R. Monto and Rachel M. Theodore
Talker-specificity effects in spoken language processing: Now you see them, now you don't —— 107

Chao-Yang Lee
Processing acoustic variability in lexical tone perception —— 129

Sara Guediche
Flexible and adaptive processes in speech perception —— 155

Jack Ryalls and Rosalie Perkins
Foreign accent syndrome: Phonology or phonetics? —— 187

Joan A. Sereno
How category learning occurs in adults and children —— 193

Vipul Arora and Henning Reetz
Automatic speech recognition: What phonology can offer —— 211

Eiling Yee
Fluid semantics: Semantic knowledge is experience-based and dynamic —— 236

Subject index —— 256

Allard Jongman and Aditi Lahiri
Introduction

This special volume celebrates Sheila Blumstein's many and sustained contributions to our understanding of language, and in particular, phonological processing. Professor Blumstein has devoted her career to understanding how speech is produced, perceived, and represented in the brain. Working with the legendary Roman Jakobson at Harvard University, she obtained her doctorate in Linguistics in 1970 with a ground-breaking dissertation that investigated the phonology of speech patterns in aphasic patients. This work was based on observations of sound substitutions and errors in patient interviews. Published as a book by Mouton in 1973, *A Phonological Investigation of Aphasic Speech* clearly indicated the focus of her research: the representation of speech and language in the brain.

Within a few years, Professor Blumstein extended her interests to the acoustics and perception of speech, beginning a long-time collaboration with Ken Stevens at MIT. This turned into a very fruitful partnership, leading to seminal work on the theory of acoustic invariance. This research showed that the mapping between acoustic properties and perceived phonetic categories is richer, and more consistent and invariant, than previously thought, a finding which necessitated a new conception of the relation between the production and perception of speech. It is important to note that at the time that Professor Blumstein started investigating the speech signal in the 1970s, the prevalent scientific opinion was that there was no simple mapping between acoustic signal and perceived phonemes because the speech signal was too variable. Acoustic properties were strongly affected by contextual factors such as variations in speaker, speaking rate, and phonetic environment. Careful consideration of Fant's acoustic theory of speech production led her to the hypothesis that invariant acoustic properties could be found in the speech signal. In contrast to previous research that was heavily dependent on the speech spectrograph and its representation of consonant release bursts and vocalic formant transitions as distinct acoustic events, Professor Blumstein focused more on global acoustic properties such as the overall shape of the spectrum at the release of the stop consonant. Through careful and detailed acoustic analysis and subsequent perceptual verification, she uncovered stable invariant acoustic properties that consistently signaled important linguistic features such as place and manner of articulation. Professor Blumstein supported these claims by investigating a variety of speech sound classes (including stop consonants,

Allard Jongman, Department of Linguistics, University of Kansas
Aditi Lahiri, Faculty of Linguistics, Philology and Phonetics, University of Oxford

fricatives, and approximants) in a variety of languages because she fully appreciated that conclusions drawn on the basis of one language can be misleading and universal generalizations can only be made after crosslinguistic comparisons. Professor Blumstein's work on acoustic features resulted in a series of pivotal and influential publications, co-authored with Ken Stevens and her students.

Professor Blumstein subsequently expanded her investigation to understand the processes involved in the recognition of words rather than individual speech sounds. Her research in this domain called for reconsideration of the then dominant view that lexical access proceeds on the basis of categorical phonemes rather than more fine-grained continuous acoustic information. The fact that subtle yet systematic acoustic differences can affect activation of word candidates in the mental lexicon indicated that acoustic information not directly relevant for phoneme identification is not discarded but is retained and plays a critical role in word comprehension. This finding provides a crucial piece of evidence in the ongoing debate about the structure of the mental lexicon.

In parallel to her seminal work on speech acoustics and perception, Professor Blumstein continued her investigation of language and speech processing impairments in brain-damaged patients which she had started with her dissertation. She initially collaborated with Harold Goodglass at the Boston VA Medical Center, who had been a member of her dissertation committee. Goodglass and colleagues were the first to apply experimental and quantitative methods to the study of the syntax of agrammatics. Professor Blumstein subsequently focused on speech processing deficits in aphasics and practically single-handedly launched this field of research which thrives today. Prior to her research in the 1970s, our understanding of the manner in which speech production and perception breaks down subsequent to focal brain damage was based solely on perceptual judgments and phonetic transcription – both quite unreliable. She applied her knowledge of acoustics to speech processing in neurologically-impaired populations, affording us an entirely new perspective not only on what is going wrong in these individuals, but providing insights into component processes of the normal system.

Throughout her career, Professor Blumstein was the principal investigator on simultaneous long-term grants for her work on acoustics and for her work on aphasia. In addition to that, she also served as Dean, Interim Provost, and even Interim President at Brown. However, at heart, Professor Blumstein has continued to predominantly be a researcher. After her term as Interim President, she spent a sabbatical leave to master newly developed brain-imaging techniques which allowed her to answer questions that were previously impossible to tackle. Her most recent acoustic research uses fMRI to investigate cortical regions involved in the perception of phonetic category invariance as well as neural systems underlying lexical competition.

Professor Blumstein is co-founder of Brown University's Barus Speech Lab where she has taught, supervised, and mentored hundreds of undergraduates, graduates, and postdocs. This lab is one of the world's leading research centers for the study of speech at all levels: acoustics, psycholinguistic processing, and neurolinguistic processing. The chapters in this Festschrift are all inspired by her work. While they show a remarkable range in topics, they all stay true to Professor Blumstein's original goal: to understand how speech and language are represented and processed in the brain. The chapters cover a wide range of topics reflecting her interests. They vary in their specificity of representation covering a wide range of models, from a more episodic approach considering talker specificity in Drouin et al. to an underspecified representation in Lahiri & Kotzor. The invariance and categorisation of phonological features is touched upon from different perspectives by Professor Blumstein herself as well as in chapters by Jongman & McMurray, Myers et al., Sereno, and Lahiri & Kotzor. Arora & Reetz provide further evidence for the invariance of phonological features (rather than segments) via machine learning. Equally broad is the coverage of phonological units that play a role in the invariance problem: variability in segmental features, duration contrast, stress and tone (cf. Lee) are all addressed. Issues about processing also extend to acquisition, multilingualism and language disorders. We address here concerns with processing phonological information by children (cf. Sereno), non-native speakers as well as speakers with language deficits (cf. Ryalls & Perkins). Phonological shapes of lexical items map on to the semantics and semantic categorisation has been an important research question in Professor Blumstein's work. Finally, the research presented here covers a wide range of methodology – acoustic analyses, eliciting speech production, behavioural as well as neurolinguistics experiments – all of which have been employed by her.

As this volume is going to press, Professor Blumstein announced that she will be retiring, 46 years after her start in academics at Brown. This news surprised all of us. Because she is so enthusiastic and passionate to advance science, it is easy to forget that Professor Blumstein has been at it for a long time. Our field would not be what it is today without Sheila's many seminal contributions spanning five decades. We all owe Sheila Blumstein a huge debt of gratitude and are fortunate to have worked with her. We proudly dedicate this book to her.

Acknowledgements: This volume stems from a workshop held at The Lords of the Manor (Cotswolds, UK) which was funded by the European Research Council (Grant FP7-IST-269670; PI A. Lahiri).

Sheila E. Blumstein
Phonetic categories and phonological features: Evidence from the cognitive neuroscience of language

Abstract: Despite the central role that phonetic features and segments play in linguistic theory, there is debate about their status in language processing as well as the nature of their representations. In this chapter, we consider recent research examining evidence from the cognitive neuroscience of language that may not only inform but also help resolve this debate. Specifically, we investigate the neural systems underlying phonetic category and phonetic feature invariance, and the role of segments and features in lexical access. Results from a series of functional neuroimaging studies provide evidence that there is an invariant representation for phonetic categories as well as an invariant representation for more abstract phonetic features. The neural areas activated suggest that the source of phonetic category invariance reflects computations over phonetic category membership, and phonetic feature representations are acoustic in nature but are based on more abstract properties of speech rather than directly sensory processes. Additionally, lexical representations in both auditory word recognition and spoken word production include both segments and the features that underlie them.

1 Introduction

Segments and the distinctive features that comprise them are critical theoretical constructs in linguistic theory. Indeed, historical language change, synchronic processes, and the broad principles that underlie the phonetic/phonological inventories of language could not be explained without them. That both segments and features influence and shape language systems suggest that they underlie the functional architecture of language for the speaker-hearer. Indeed, most language processing models include both segments and features as representational units (McClelland & Elman, 1986; Marslen-Wilson, 1987). Nonetheless, there still

---

Sheila E. Blumstein, Department of Cognitive, Linguistic & Psychological Sciences, Brown University

remains debate about the status of these theoretical constructs in language processing as well as the nature of the representations that underlie them. In this chapter, we will consider recent research in our lab that has attempted to speak to these issues, specifically, examining evidence from the cognitive neuroscience of language.

2 Segments and Features in Language

With regard to historical language change, one can find examples of both segmental as well as feature changes that alter the sound system inventory of particular languages. For example, in the Great English Vowel Shift, a change which occurred over several centuries (1350–1700), affected the segmental vowel inventory of English: the high vowels [i] and [u] became diphthongs [ai] and [aw] respectively, and each of the remaining vowels were raised in height, e. g. [a:] → [e:], [e:] → [i:], [o:] → [u:]. Grimm's law, on the other hand, is an example of a feature change which affected a class of sounds. In this case, Proto-Indo-European stop consonants underwent a series of changes in the development of German: voiceless stops became voiceless fricatives – a change in the feature [obstruent]; voiced stops became voiceless stops and voiced aspirated stops became voiced stops or fricatives – both changes reflecting a change in laryngeal features.

Synchronically, morphophonological processes in which the sound realization of two morphemes changes as they combine in word formation often involve the assimilation of one distinctive feature to another. Thus, in English, the past tense of a verb (i. e. "ed") undergoes voicing assimilation; it is either voiced, [d], or voiceless, [t], depending on the voicing of the preceding verb stem. This alternation occurs irrespective of the manner of articulation of the final consonant of the verb stem, e. g. walk[t], beg[d], kiss[t], raze[d]. New words added to the language also obey these general processes, e. g. 'he xerox[t] / google[d] the manuscript.'

Finally, distinctive features play a role not only in distinguishing between and among the segments or phonetic categories of a language, but they also shape the sound inventories of languages. Indeed, phonetic/phonological systems of language are not comprised of a 'random' selection of sounds. Rather, the sounds of a language typically group themselves in terms of 'natural classes' defined in terms of a set of shared distinctive features (Greenberg, 1963; Halle, 1964). Consonants are organized across such dimensions as manner of articulation, place of articulation, and voicing, and vowels across such dimensions as tongue height, frontback, and rounding. These natural classes provide the organizational framework for the sound inventories of language resulting in phonological inventories that tend to be symmetrical. Thus, it is common to have a language with a class of labial, alveolar, and velar voiced and voiceless stop consonants, and unusual to have a language with a voiced labial stop consonant, a voiced velar stop consonant, and a voiceless alveolar consonant (see Figure 1).

	Bilabial	**Alveolar**	**Velar**
Stop			
voiceless	p	t	k
voiced	b	d	g
Nasal	m	n	ŋ
Fricative			
voiceless	f	s	
voiced	v	z	

	Bilabial	**Alveolar**	**Velar**
Stop			
voiceless		t	
voiced	b		g
Nasal			ŋ
Fricative			
voiceless	f		
voiced		z	

Figure 1: An example of a typical (top grid) and an atypical (bottom grid) stop, nasal, and fricative phonetic inventory

3 The Invariance Problem

The invariance problem is one that cuts across a number of cognitive domains. Simply defined, it is the ability to perceive the same object or category across a number of sources of variability. For example, we recognize the same face or object across a number of different visual transformations including rotation, size, illumination and distance. And we recognize an object such as a specific instance of a 'cup' as belonging to the class of objects *cup* despite differences in any number of visual attributes or features. In both cases, the viewer must be able to distinguish and process those visual changes that are 'distinctive' and change the identity of the face or the object in question from those visual changes that do not change the identity of the object or the face.

The invariance problem extends to language, and in particular, to the processing of speech. Dating from the seminal work of Haskins Laboratories (Liberman et al., 1967), much research in the field has focused on solving the invariance problem – namely, determining how the listener maintains perceptual stability for the phonetic categories of speech in the face of variability. And there are many sources of variability: speech naturally occurs in a noisy environment, and speakers have different vocal tract sizes, speak different dialects, and produce speech with imprecision, all resulting in a variable acoustic input.

There is also variability intrinsic to the properties of speech. Listeners perceive the same phonetic category despite changes in the acoustic properties signaling that category, e. g. they perceive a voiceless stop as voiceless whether it is cued by different 'weightings' of voice-onset time and degree of aspiration (Repp, 1982), and listeners perceive the same phonetic category across differences in vowel context, e. g. they perceive the initial consonant as [d] in the three syllables [da], di], [du]. In all cases, at some level of processing, the listener must be able to extract those properties which are 'distinctive', i. e. distinguish one phonetic category or segment from another, and those which are not. For example, the listener must be able to distinguish a 'pear' from a 'bear' or a 'pear' from a 'peer', whether spoken by the same or different speaker and whether the speech occurs in a noisy or quiet environment.

A number of different hypotheses have been proposed to account for the invariance problem in speech. One class of theories assumes that the mapping process from acoustic input to sound structure representation normalizes the input to a common invariant representation, with the variability in the input filtered out as 'noise' (see Goldinger, 1998 for review). In one proposal, the form of the invariance is acoustic; namely, the acoustic input is transformed into more generalized spectral-temporal patterns which correspond to phonetic features (Stevens & Blumstein, 1978; Blumstein & Stevens, 1980; Kurowski & Blumstein, 1987). For example, higher order acoustic patterns relating to the shape of the onset spectrum as rising, falling, or compact have been proposed to correspond to labial, alveolar, and velar places of articulation in stop consonants respectively, with the shape of the spectrum remaining invariant across vowel context, speaker, and manner of articulation. Another approach proposes that there may be multiple acoustic properties associated with a particular feature. These properties may be weighted differently and vary as a function of context, but nonetheless they give rise to an invariant acoustic pattern (McMurray & Jongman, 2011).

An alternative view is that the form of the invariance is motor or gestural; namely, the acoustic input is mapped on to the motor or gestural patterns used in producing or articulating speech (for review see Galantucci, Fowler & Turvey, 2006; Liberman et al., 1967; Fowler, 1986; Fowler, Shankweiler & Studdert-Kennedy, 2015). For example, although the starting frequencies and directions of the formant transitions differ for [di] and [du], the articulatory gestures for the production of alveolar stop consonants are purportedly the same. Thus, it has been hypothesized that object constancy in speech perception is derived from vocal tract gestures.

In both the theory of acoustic invariance and the motor/gestural theory of speech perception, a single invariant representation underlies each lexical entry. This view is distinguished from the second class of theories that assumes that variability in the speech signal is not 'noise' to be filtered out, but rather it provides critical information that is both used and retained by the listener in processing speech (Johnson & Mullenix, 1997). In this view, variability not only provides critical information for perceiving speech as the speech input is unfolding, but it is also retained and ultimately encoded, forming part of the neural representation of speech (Pisoni, 1997). These episodic memory traces are proposed to not only extend to the processing of the sounds of speech but also to the representations of words in the lexicon. In this view, the lexical representation of a word is not invariant but rather there are multiple episodic representations for a particular word with the representations retaining details of the acoustic input (Goldinger, 1996; Mullenix, Pisoni & Martin, 1989; but cf. Pufhal & Samuel, 2014).

Despite the richness of the literature and of the theories proposed, none have actually 'solved' the invariance problem. That is, none have succeeded in providing an explicit characterization of the computations necessary to map from variable input to stable percept. And at this stage, it is not clear how behavioral evidence and acoustic or physiological measures will provide the answer. One possibility is to examine whether evidence from cognitive neuroscience can provide a window into how the neural processing system 'solves' the invariance problem. In particular, it would be informative to know whether particular neural regions show 'invariant' neural responses to phonetic categories in the face of different sources of variability. Identifying those areas may provide evidence for the nature of the representations underlying invariance. For example, if those neural areas are sensory, it would be consistent with the notion that phonetic category representations are acoustic; if they are motor, it would suggest that phonetic category representations are articulatory or gestural; and if they are represented in the speech/lexical processing stream in posterior temporal and parietal areas, it would be consistent with the notion that phonetic category representations maintain 'traces' of the variable input. Indeed, invariant neural responses to phonetic categories in different regions of the phonetic processing stream could provide critical constraints on extant theories of phonetic invariance.

Consideration of the invariance problem raises the issue of the nature of the representational units used in processing speech. As discussed earlier, evidence from phonological processes in language suggests that phonetic features are basic representation units. And there is strong evidence that at least at some level of processing the segment and phonetic feature are basic processing units.

In particular, slips of the tongue in normal individuals (Fromkin, 1971; 1973) and speech output errors of aphasic patients (Blumstein, 2000) are typically based on segmental or phonetic feature changes. They rarely, if ever, involve whole syllables. Similarly, patterns of speech perception errors in both normals (Miller & Nicely, 1955) and aphasic patients (Blumstein, Baker & Goodglass, 1977) are based on the misperception of segments and the number of phonetic feature properties that they share.

Segments and phonetic features also appear to play a role in lexical access. As we will discuss below, lexical access is influenced by the phonological similarity between and among words in the lexicon. This phonological similarity is based on the extent to which phonetic segments and phonetic features are shared (Luce & Pisoni, 1998; Milberg, Blumstein & Dworetzky, 1988). The question then is whether invariant neural patterns emerge not only for phonetic categories, e. g. [d] across sources of variability, e. g. [di] or [du], but also for shared phonetic features that constitute natural classes, e. g. voiceless in [p], [t], or [k].

3.1 Phonetic Category Invariance

The seminal work of Haskins Laboratories demonstrated that speech perception is categorical (Liberman et al., 1967). Namely, the perception of an acoustic continuum that systematically ranges in acoustic steps from one phonetic category, e. g. [d], to another [t], is perceived by the listener categorically. Listeners identify a range of stimuli at one end of the continuum as belonging to a particular category, and at the other end of the continuum a different category. There are typically one or two stimuli along the continuum for which their responses are at chance (considered the boundary between the two phonetic categories). Critically, discrimination of stimulus pairs across the continuum is good for those stimulus that are between phonetic categories, i. e. identified by the listener as belonging to different phonetic categories (e. g. [d] vs. [t]), and is poor for those stimuli within phonetic categories, i. e. identified by the listener as belonging to the same phonetic category (d_1 vs. d_2).

Further behavioral research has shown that there is a structure to phonetic categories (Miller, 1994). In particular, perception of within phonetic category stimuli is not all-or-none; rather, it is graded. As the stimuli along the continuum approach the phonetic boundary, phonetic categorization latencies are slower (Andruski, Blumstein & Burton, 1994), and goodness ratings are worse (Miller & Volaitis, 1989). Moreover, discrimination judgements are slower for within phonetic category stimulus pairs compared to acoustically identical pairs (Pisoni & Tash, 1974).

An fMRI study conducted in our lab (Blumstein, Myers & Rissman, 2009) showed, not surprisingly, that the neural system is sensitive to both within and between phonetic category differences. In particular, we examined the perception of voice-onset time (VOT), a temporal cue that distinguishes initial voiced and voiceless stop consonants. Stimuli included 5 [da]-[ta] stimuli that ranged in 10 ms steps from 0–40 ms. Thus, there were 2 exemplar endpoint [d] and [t] stimuli, 2 within category stimuli, and one boundary stimulus. During scanning, subjects' task was to categorize the stimuli as either [d] or [t]; both performance and reaction-time measures were taken. Results showed sensitivity to phonetic category structure throughout the phonetic processing stream. Of most importance, graded activation for the endpoint, within category, and boundary stimuli emerged in the inferior frontal gyrus (IFG) and cingulate with increased activation as the stimuli approached the phonetic category boundary (endpoint < within-category < boundary stimuli). Additionally, the posterior middle temporal gyrus (MTG) and angular gyrus (AG) showed increased activity to the 'best fit', i.e. endpoint stimuli compared to either the within or boundary value stimuli. Joanisse, Zevin & McCandliss (2007) also showed sensitivity in temporo-parietal areas to between compared to within phonetic category stimuli varying in place of articulation {da]-[ga]. Taken together, these results indicate that the neural system is sensitive to acoustic fine structure and that differences emerge across the phonetic processing stream.

The findings that that there are perceptual sensitivities to both within and between phonetic category stimuli provide a means for determining whether there are neural areas that respond to acoustic differences between phonetic categories while showing a similar neural response to within phonetic category differences. Such results would indicate that there is a neural area that treats within and between phonetic category stimuli differently but treats within category stimuli the same, despite the fact that the acoustic difference between the stimuli along the continuum is the same.

To examine this question, we utilized an adaptation paradigm (Myers et al., 2009; cf. Grill-Spector & Malach, 2001; Grill-Spector, Hension & Martin, 2006). Here subjects received a string of [da]-[ta] stimuli varying in VOT: one stimulus (either an endpoint [da] or [ta]) was repeated 4 times followed by a stimulus which was either acoustically the same as the preceding stimuli or it differed in VOT. The acoustically different stimuli varied from the standard stimulus by 25 ms VOT, but one was either a within phonetic category change or was a between phonetic category change. An increase in neural activation when there was an acoustic change indicates sensitivity to the acoustic dimension (in this case VOT).

Results showed sensitivity to both within and between category changes in the posterior superior temporal gyrus (STG) consistent with the view that this area is involved in early sensory processing of speech. Critically, a pattern consistent with phonetic category invariance emerged in the left inferior frontal sulcus. This area showed sensitivity to between phonetic category changes but failed to show sensitivity to within phonetic category changes. This invariant neural response to phonetic variability (i. e. similar patterns of activation to within category stimuli) suggests that the IFG treats the stimulus input as perceptually equivalent.

These findings provide evidence that the basis for phonetic category invariance is neither acoustic nor motor. Had that been the case invariant neural responses should have emerged either in temporal areas including the superior temporal gyrus and/or superior temporal sulcus reflecting acoustic invariance or they should have emerged in frontal areas that have shown activation under certain conditions during speech perception tasks including the pars opercularis (BA44 of the inferior frontal gyrus (IFG)), the supplementary motor area (SMA), ventral premotor areas (BA6), and possibly primary motor cortex (BA4) reflecting motor/gestural invariance (Fadiga et al., 2002; Watkins Strefella & Paus, 2003; Wilson et al., 2004; Pulvermuller et al., 2006; Wilson & Iacoboni, 2006).

Interestingly, the invariant phonetic category response that emerged in the inferior frontal sulcus is in an area that has been implicated in research with non-human primates in visual categorization (Freedman et al., 2002). In this study, Freedman et al. trained monkeys to categorize a continuum of 'cats' and 'dogs' that were visually morphed in equal steps. The lateral prefrontal cortex showed an invariant response to members within a category but showed sensitivity to between the 'cat' and 'dog' category.

Thus, it appears that phonetic category invariance reflects computations reflecting decision processes on phonetic category membership. Such computations are likely necessary given that phonetic category boundaries are not fixed, but rather are probabilistic; the phonetic category boundary changes as a function of any number of variables including speaker, context, the presence or absence of other acoustic cues, and speaking rate. In this sense, phonetic category invariance is a higher order computation that takes into account these and potentially other variables that influence the perceptual boundary between phonetic categories.

As indicated earlier, there are many sources of variability. Another form of variability that represents a challenge for phonetic category invariance is speaker. Variations across speakers is particularly interesting because for the listener recognizing speaker differences is critical; it is essential to know which person or persons said 'Help!' and at the same time it is essential to know that the variable acoustic output of the speakers maps on to the same phonetic category or word. Thus, the neural system of the listener must be able to respond in an invariant way to phonetic identity across speakers and also to differentiate between and among speakers.

To further explore phonetic category invariance, we examined whether there was a specific neural area that showed phonetic category invariance across speakers (Salvata, Blumstein & Myers, 2012). As described earlier, this question is of particular interest given the behavioral findings suggesting that listeners maintain a 'trace' of a speaker in the underlying representation of a word. Although there have been studies examining speaker changes in producing phonetic information (Belin & Zatorre, 2003; Wong, Nusbaum & Small, 2004; Formisano et al., 2008), they did not explicitly explore whether there is a neural area that shows phonetic category invariance across speakers. To investigate this question, we utilized an adaptation paradigm comparing conditions that changed phonetic category only, (e. g., $[ta]_{S1} [ta]_{S1} [ta]_{S1} [ta]_{S1} [ga]_{S1}$), speaker only (e. g. $[ta]_{S1} [ta]_{S1} [ta]_{S1} [ta]_{S1} [ta]_{S2}$), both phonetic category and speaker (e. g. $[ta]_{S1} [ta]_{S1} [ta]_{S1} [ta]_{S1} [ga]_{S2}$) or no change (e. g., $[ta]_{S1} [ta]_{S1} [ta]_{S1} [ta]_{S1} [ta]_{S1}$). Results showed an invariant speaker response in the superior temporal gyrus. These findings suggest that extraction of phonetic category information independent of speaker occurs relatively early in the phonetic processing stream (in the anterior portion of the STG), rather than in temporo-parietal areas (pSTG, angular gyrus, supramarginal gyrus) which are involved in those processes involved in lexical access (i. e. mapping sound structure to lexical form and lexical access).

It may not be surprising that phonetic category invariance emerges in different neural areas depending on the source of the variability in the acoustic signal; phonetic category invariance emerged in the inferior frontal sulcus when the acoustic properties for the phonetic category were varied and it emerged in the superior temporal gyrus when the speaker varied. Acoustic properties are an inherent part of the speech signal ultimately providing cues to the phonetic dimensions of speech. In contrast, speaker information provides acoustic information that is extrinsic to phonetic dimensions. Indeed, Pufhal and Samuel (2014) showed that listeners retained the 'trace' of an environmental sound that accompanied the presentation of a lexical item, even though the environmental sound ('dog barking') had no semantic or phonological relation to the target word ('termite'). On their own merits, such findings present a challenge to the view that speaker information is an intrinsic part of the lexical representation of a word. The neural results also suggest that at some level of processing lexical representations may be independent of speaker information.

3.2 Phonological Feature Invariance

A series of recent studies has provided evidence that the auditory cortex extracts what appears to be generalized properties of speech sounds that correspond to phonetic/phonological features. Using a variety of neural methods including fMRI (Arsenault & Buchsbaum, 2015), MEG (Obleser, Scott & Eulitz, 2006), and electrocorticography (ECoG) (Chang et al., 2010; Mesgarani et al., 2014), researchers have shown selective responses in the superior temporal cortex to consonant parameters including the class of stop consonants, fricative consonants, nasal consonants, place of articulation, voicing, and also to vowel parameters (front-back, low-high) (Mesgarani et al., 2014; Obleser et al., 2006). These findings provide strong evidence that the acoustic fine structure of speech maps on to more generalized spectro-temporal parameters associated with phonological features. Moreover, they suggest that the basis of this mapping is acoustic not motor, consistent with theories of acoustic invariance in speech (Stevens & Blumstein, 1978; Blumstein & Stevens, 1981).

Our lab has extended this research by specifically examining the extent to which the neural system shows an invariant response to voicing across manner of articulation [s] and [t] vs. [z] and [d], on the one hand, and distinguishes voicing between these different manners of articulation, [s] vs. [z] and [t] vs. [d], on the other (Guediche et al., 2015). Voicing is a particularly relevant dimension because although its acoustic manifestation involves glottal excitation, the details of the acoustic properties giving rise to voicing in stops and fricatives are different. The critical acoustic parameter distinguishing voicing in stop consonants is voice-onset time, the temporal relation between the release of the stop closure and the onset of glottal excitation. Typically, voiceless stop consonants in English have a VOT ranging from 30–150 ms and voiced stop consonants have a VOT range from 0–25 ms. In contrast, voicing in fricative consonants is characterized by the presence or absence of glottal excitation at the acoustic boundaries of the frication noise (Pirello, Blumstein & Kurowski, 1997; Stevens et al., 1992). The average duration of alveolar fricatives is on the order of 170 ms and voiceless fricative consonants are characterized by zero voicing within this interval, whereas voiced consonants are characterized by 20–30 ms of voicing within this interval.

These difference between the acoustic cues for voicing in stop and fricative consonants indicate that duration of glottal excitation cannot be used as a cue to group voiceless stop consonants (with a VOT of 30+ms) and voiceless fricative consonants (absence of voicing in the frication noise) or to group voiced stop consonants (VOT of 0–25) and voiced fricative consonants (20–30 ms of voicing) (see Figure 2). Moreover, simply the presence of voicing cannot be used as a classification measure for grouping voiced stops and fricatives and voiceless stops and fricatives since voicing occurs in nasals, liquids, and glides, as well as in vowels. That the fine details of the acoustic realization of voicing across stops and fricatives are different means that the phonological feature of voicing is a relatively abstract property. The question we asked is whether, despite these acoustic differences, the neural system treats voicing across stops and fricatives as the same (Guediche et al., 2015).

As in the previously discussed studies investigating phonetic category invariance, an adaptation paradigm was utilized. Four naturally produced syllables, [ta], [da], [sa], [za] were used in creating four experimental conditions: Voicing Change, Manner Change, Both Voicing and Manner Change, or No Change. Results showed different patterns of activation in the STG and the IFG. As expected, the STG was sensitive to voicing across manner of articulation. That is, it showed differences in the neural activation patterns between voicing in stop consonants and voicing in fricative consonants. In contrast, an invariant response to voicing across manner of articulation emerged in the IFG. Here, the magnitude of the BOLD response did not differ between voicing changes in stop consonants, i. e. [t] vs. [d], and voicing changes in fricative consonants, i. e. [s] vs. [z].

	Fricatives		Stops	
	Voiced	Voiceless	Voiced	Voiceless
Location of Voicing Cue	within fricative noise interval		between release of stop closure and onset of voicing	
Voicing Duration	20–30ms	0 ms	0–25	30–150

Figure 2: Acoustic cues to voicing for fricatives and stop consonants

The emergence of feature invariance is consistent with the view that there is a feature-based organization of the phonemic inventory of language. That a pattern of invariance emerged in the IFG suggests that phonological features are based on more abstract properties of speech rather than directly sensory processes. As described earlier, the cues to voicing in stops and fricatives are not the same; despite the fact that glottal excitation is characteristic of voicing in both manners of articulation, the actual parameters defining the contrast between voiced and voiceless stops and voiced and voiceless fricatives are different. Indeed, low-level sensory processes would treat voicing across manner of articulation as different, and such differences in activity emerged, not surprisingly, in the STG.

4 Segments, Features, and the Lexicon

To this point, we have focused on the neural systems underlying phonetic categories and features by examining neural responses to syllables. However, what is critical for language processing is whether phonetic categories, i. e. segments, and the features comprising them are the representational units for words. As discussed earlier, behavioral evidence suggests that indeed both segments and features underlie lexical representations.

We now turn to neural evidence showing that the organizational properties of the lexicon reflect segments and features as well. To this end, we examine a series of studies that have investigated lexical access by assessing potential differences in neural activity as a function of the similarity of a target word to other words in the lexicon. These studies are based on behavioral research showing that word recognition is influenced by neighborhood density, defined as the number of words that can be identified by substituting, deleting, or adding a segment in any position to a given target word. Critically, density reflects the number of words that share *segmental properties* with the target word. Listeners show slower reaction-time latencies in word recognition tasks such as lexical decision to words that have many neighbors and are thus in high density neighborhoods compared to words that have few neighbors and are thus in low density neighborhoods (Luce & Pisoni, 1998). It has been proposed that these results reflect the network-like architecture of the lexicon in which not only a given target word is activated upon presentation but words that share phonological properties with the target word are also partially activated. Thus, the greater the lexical density of a neighborhood, the greater the competition in accessing or selecting the target word leading to increased errors as well as slowed latencies.

In a series of studies, we examined whether there were neural areas that were specifically sensitive to neighborhood density. In the first study (Prabhakaran et al., 2006), participants performed an auditory lexical decision task in which both word and nonword stimuli varied in neighborhood density. (A density neighborhood can be created for nonwords by determining the number of words that are created when substituting, adding, or deleting a segment to a nonword stimulus). FMRI results showed increased activation for high density compared to low density words in the supramarginal gyrus (SMG). In a similar study, Okada and Hickok (2006) showed activation in the posterior STG as a function of lexical density. The increased activity shown in both studies presumably reflects increased demands and hence neural processing resources required to access a word that has a lot of neighbors that compete for access. Importantly, these areas have been implicated in phonological processing and mapping sound structure to the lexicon (Celsis et al., 1999; Gold & Buckner, 2002; Caplan, Gow & Makris, 1995).

Neither the Prabhakaran et al. (2006) nor the Okada & Hickok studies (2006) showed a density effect for nonwords. These findings suggest that the locus of the neighborhood density effect was lexical, reflecting access to the lexicon, rather than prelexical, reflecting the phonotactic probabilities of possible words in the language. Had the effect been prelexical, nonwords should have induced a neighborhood density effect, which they did not.

Further research has shown that the neural system shows lexical density effects not only in auditory word recognition but also in spoken word production. This work was based on prior behavioral research showing that the production of voicing in stop consonants is influenced by the presence of a voiced lexical competitor (Base-Berk & Goldrick, 2009). Namely, VOT was longer for words that had a voiced minimal pair (e. g. tart-dart) compared to ones that did not (e. g. tar; *dar is not a word). Further behavioral work in our lab showed that this lexically-conditioned variation was actually driven by overall lexical density, not by the presence or absence of a voiced minimal pair (Fox, Reilly & Blumstein, 2015). In this study, participants read words either in isolation or in biased or neutral contexts. They produced longer VOTs for words beginning with voiceless stop consonants that were from a high neighborhood density, irrespective of whether that word had a voiced minimal pair or not and independent of whether the word was produced in isolation or in a biased or neutral context.

We examined the neural substrates of the effect of lexical density in spoken word production (Peramunage et al., 2011). Here, VOT was used as a proxy for lexical density (see Fox, Reilly & Blumstein, 2015 for discussion). That is, words beginning with voiceless stop consonants that had voiced minimal pair competitors were from high density neighborhoods and voiceless stop consonants that did not have voiced minimal pairs were from low density neighborhoods. Participants read aloud a set of words while in the scanner. Their productions were recorded and subsequently analyzed for VOT. Similar to Prabhakaran et al.'s (2006) study investigating auditory word recognition, Peramunage et al.'s (2011) results examining spoken word production showed modulation of activity as a function of lexical density in the supramarginal and left superior temporal gryi. A similar density effect emerged in the inferior frontal and precentral gyri as well. Taken together, these findings suggest that both segments and the features that represent them are a part of the lexical representations of words, and that neighborhood density not only influences lexical access and word selection (as shown by activation in temporo-parietal areas) but also the articulatory processes involved in planning and ultimately implementing the word (as shown by activation in frontal areas).

5 Summary

In his seminal work, Noam Chomsky (1965) made a distinction between language competence (what a speaker-hearer 'knows') and language performance (what a speaker actually 'does'). This distinction helped drive a dichotomy between the theory of language and its use. Both segments and features are critically important constructs in linguistic theory, and, although most language processing models also include segments and features as representational units, there has been debate in the psycholinguistic literature about their status. Here, we showed that a cognitive neuroscience approach not only informs this debate but also may help resolve it. Neuroimaging findings provide evidence for phonetic category invariance such that there is a common representation for a phonetic category across sources of variability including both acoustic-phonetic and speaker variation, and this representation is acoustic in nature. There is also evidence for phonological feature invariance such that there is a common representation for more abstract properties of phonology reflecting natural classes. Finally, fMRI results show that lexical representations include both segments and the features that represent them, and are reflected not only in auditory word recognition but also in spoken word production.

Taken together, these findings emphasize the critical importance of converging evidence from linguistic theory, psycholinguistics, and cognitive neuroscience. Each approach provides unique insights. None alone are sufficient to provide an explanatory model of the nature of human language and the processes and mechanism that underlie it. However, together they afford a means of integrating these insights into a unitary theory/model of language.

Acknowledgements: This research was supported in part by NIH Grant R01 DC006220 from the National Institute on Deafness and Other Communication Disorders. The content is solely the responsibility of the authors and does not necessarily represent the official views of the National Institute on Deafness and Other Communication Disorders or the National Institutes of Health.

References

Andruski, J. E., Blumstein, S. E. & Burton, M. (1994). The effect of subphonetic differences on lexical access. *Cognition 52*(3). 163–187.

Arsenault, J. S. & Buchsbaum, B. R. (2015). Distributed neural representations of phonological features during speech perception. *The Journal of Neuroscience 35*(2). 634–642.

Baese-Berk, M. & Goldrick, M. (2009). Mechanisms of interaction in speech production. *Language and Cognitive Processes 24*. 527–554.

Belin, P. & Zatorre, R. J. (2003). Adaptation to speaker's voice in right anterior temporal lobe. *Neuroreport 14*(16). 2105–2109.

Blumstein, S. E. (2000). Deficits of speech production and speech perception in aphasia. In R. Berndt Ed. *Handbook of Neuropsychology*, 2nd edition, Vol.2. The Netherlands: Elsevier Science.

Blumstein, S. E., Baker, E. & Goodglass, H. (1977). Phonological factors in auditory comprehension in aphasia. *Neuropsychologia 15*, 19–30.

Blumstein, S. E. & Stevens, K. N. (1980). Perceptual invariance and onset spectra for stop consonants in different vowel environments. *Journal of the Acoustical Society of America 67*. 648–662.

Blumstein, S. E. & Stevens, K. N. (1981). Phonetic features and acoustic invariance in speech. *Cognition 10*(1). 25–32.

Blumstein, S. E., Myers, E. B. & Rissman, J. (2005). The perception of voice onset time: an fMRI investigation of phonetic category structure. *Journal of Cognitive Neuroscience 17*(9). 1353–1366.

Caplan, D., Gow, D. & Makris, N. (1995). Analysis of lesions by MRI in stroke patients with acoustic-phonetic processing deficits. *Neurology 452*. 293–298.

Celsis, P., Boulanouar, K., Doyon, B., Ranjeva, J. P., Berry, I., Nespoulous, J. L. & Chollet, F. (1999). Differential fMRI responses in left superior temporal gyrus and left supramarginal gyrus to habituation and change detection in syllables and tones. *NeuroImage 9*. 133–144.

Chang, E. F., Rieger, J. W., Johnson, K., Berger, M. S., Barbaro, N. M. & Knight, R. T. (2010). Categorical speech representation in human superior temporal gyrus. *Nature Neuroscience 13*(11). 1428–1432.

Chomsky, N. (1965). *Aspects of the theory of syntax*. Cambridge, MA: MIT Press.

Formisano, E., De Martino, F., Bonte, M. & Goebel, R. (2008). "Who" is saying "what"? Brain-based decoding of human voice and speech. *Science New York, N.Y. 322*. 970–973.

Fowler, C. A. (1986). An event approach to the study of speech perception from a direct-realist perspective. *Journal of Phonetics 14*(1). 3–28.

Fox, N., Reilly, M. & Blumstein, S. E. (2015). Phonological neighborhood competition affects spoken word production irrespective of sentential context. *Journal of Memory and Language 83*. 97–117.

Fowler, C. A., Shankweiler, D. & Studdert-Kennedy, M. (2015). Perception of the speech code revisited: Speech is alphabetic after all. *Psychological Review 123*(2). 125–150.

Freedman, D. J., Riesenhuber, M., Poggio, T. & Miller, E. K. (2002). Visual categorization and the primate prefrontal cortex: neurophysiology and behavior. *Journal of Neurophysiology 882*. 929–941.

Fadiga, L., Craighero, L., Buccino, G. & Rizzolatti, G. (2002). Speech listening modulates the excitability of tongue muscles: A TMS study. *European Journal of Neuroscience 15*(2). 399–402.

Fromkin, V. A. (1971). The non-anomalous nature of anomalous utterances. *Language 47*(1). 27–52.

Galantucci, B., Fowler, C. A. & Turvey, M. T. (2006). The motor theory of speech perception reviewed. *Psychonomic Bulletin & Review 13*. 361–377.

Gold, B. T. & Buckner, R. L. (2002). Common prefrontal regions coactivate with dissociable posterior regions during controlled semantic and phonological tasks. *Neuron 35*(4). 803–812.

Goldinger, S. D. (1996). Words and voices: episodic traces in spoken word identification and recognition memory. *Journal of Experimental Psychology: Learning, Memory, and Cognition 22*(5). 1166–1183.

Goldinger, S. D. (1998). Echoes of echoes? An episodic theory of lexical access. *Psychological Review 105*(2). 251–279.

Greenberg, J. H. (ed.) (1963). *Universals of language*. Cambridge: MIT Press.

Grill-Spector, K., Hension, R. & Martin, A. (2006). Repetition and the brain: neural models of stimulus-specific effects. *Trends in Cognitive Science 10*. 14–23.

Grill-Spector, K. & Malach, R. (2001). fMRI-adaptation: a tool for studying the functional properties of human cortical neurons. *Acta Psychologica 107*. 293–321.

Guediche, S., Minicucci, D., Shih, P. & Blumstein, S. E. (2015). Sensitivity of the neural system to phonetic features and phonological patterns: An fMRI investigation. Manuscript.

Halle, M. (1964). On the bases of phonology. In Fodor, J. A. & Katz, J. J. Eds. *The Structure of Language*. New Jersey: Prentice-Hall.

Joanisse, M. F., Zevin, J. D. & McCandliss, B. D. (2007). Brain mechanisms implication in the preattentive categorization of speech sounds revealed using fMRI and a short-interval habituation trial paradigm. *Cerebral Cortex 17*(9). 2084–2093.

Johnson, K. & Mullenix, J. W. (eds.). (1997). Complex representations used in speech processing: overview of the book. *Talker variability in speech processing*. 1–8.

Kurowski, K. & Blumstein, S. E. (1987). Acoustic properties for place of articulation in nasal consonants. *The Journal of the Acoustical Society of America 81*(6). 1917–1927.

Liberman, A. M., Cooper, F. S., Shankweiler, D. P. & Studdert-Kennedy, M. (1967). Perception of the speech code. *Psychological Review 74*(6). 431–461.

Luce, P. A. & Pisoni, D. B. (1998). Recognizing spoken words: The neighborhood activation model. *Ear and Hearing 19*(1). 1–36.

Marslen-Wilson, W. (1987). Functional parallelism in spoken word-recognition. *Cognition 25*. 71–102.

Miller, J. L. (1994). On the internal structure of phonetic categories: a progress report. *Cognition 50*(1–3). 271–285.

Mullennix, J. W., Pisoni, D. & Martin, C. S. (1989). Some effects of talker variability on spoken word recognition. *Journal of the Acoustical Society of America 85*. 365–378.

McClelland, J. L. & Elman, J. (1986). The TRACE model of speech perception. *Cognitive Psychology 18*. 1–86.

McMurray, B. & Jongman, A. (2011). What information is necessary for speech categorization? Harnessing variability in the speech signal by integrating cues computed relative to expectations. *Psychological Review 118*(2). 219–246.

Mesgarani, N., Cheung, C., Johnson, K. & Chang, E. F. (2014). Phonetic feature encoding in human superior temporal gyrus. *Science 343*(6174). 1006–1010.

Milberg, W., Blumstein, S. & Dworetzky, B. (1988). Phonological processing and lexical access in aphasia. *Brain and Language 34*(2). 279–293.

Miller, G. A. & Nicely, P. E. (1955). An analysis of perceptual confusions among some English consonants. *The Journal of the Acoustical Society of America 27*(2). 338–352.

Miller, J. L. & Volaitis, L. E. (1989). Effect of speaking rate on the perceptual structure of a phonetic category. *Perception & Psychophysics 46*(6). 505–512.

Myers, E. B., Blumstein, S. E., Walsh, E. & Eliassen, J. (2009). Inferior frontal regions underlie the perception of phonetic category invariance. *Psychological Science 20*. 895–903.

Obleser, J., Boecker, H., Drzezga, A., Haslinger, B., Hennenlotter, A., Roettinger, M., Eulitz, C. & Rauschecker, J. P. (2006). Vowel sound extraction in anterior superior temporal cortex. *Human Brain Mapping 27*. 562–571.

Obleser, J., Scott, S. K. & Eulitz, C. (2006). Now you hear it, now you don't: transient traces of consonants and their nonspeech analogues in the human brain. *Cerebral Cortex 16*(8). 1069–1076.

Okada, K. & Hickok, G. (2006). Identification of lexical–phonological networks in the superior temporal sulcus using functional magnetic resonance imaging. *Neuroreport 17*(12), 1293–1296.

Peramunage, D., Blumstein, S. E., Myers, E. B., Goldrick, M. & Baese-Berk, M. (2011). Phonological neighborhood effects in spoken word production: An fMRI study. *Journal of Cognitive Neuroscience 23*(3). 593–603.

Pirello, K., Blumstein, S. E. & Kurowski, K. (1997). The characteristics of voicing in syllable-initial fricatives in American English. *Journal of the Acoustical Society of America 101.* 3754–3765.

Pisoni, D. B. (1997). Some thoughts on 'normalization' in speech. In Johnson, K. & Mullinex, J. W. Eds. *Talker Variability in Speech Processing.* New York: Academic Press.

Pisoni, D. B. & Tash, J. (1974). Reaction times to comparisons within and across phonetic categories. *Attention, Perception & Psychophysics 15*(2). 285–290.

Prabhakaran, R., Blumstein, S. E., Myers, E. B., Hutchison, E. & Britton, B. (2006). An event-related fMRI investigation of phonological-lexical competition. *Neuropsychologia 44.* 2209–2221.

Pufahl, A. & Samuel, A. G. (2014). How lexical is the lexicon? Evidence for integrated auditory memory representations. *Cognitive Psychology 70.* 1–30.

Pulvermüller, F., Huss, M., Kherif, F., Moscoso del Prado Martin, F., Hauk, O. & Shtyrov, Y. (2006). Motor cortex maps articulatory features of speech sounds. *Proceedings of the National Academy of Sciences 103.* 7865–7870.

Raizada, R. D. S. & Poldrack, R. A. (2007). Selective amplification of stimulus differences during categorical processing of speech. *Neuron 56.* 726–740.

Rapp, B. & Goldrick, M. (2000). Discreteness and interactivity in spoken word production. *Psychological Review 107.* 460–99.

Salvata, C., Blumstein, S. E. & Myers, E. B. (2012). Speaker invariance for phonetic information: an fMRI investigation. *Language and Cognitive Processes 27*(2). 210–230.

Stevens, K. N. & Blumstein, S. E. (1978). Invariant cues for place of articulation in stop consonants. *Journal of the Acoustical Society of America 64.* 1358–1368.

Stevens, K. N., Blumstein, S. E., Glicksman, L., Burton, M. & Kurowski, K. (1992). Acoustic and perceptual characteristics of voicing in fricatives and fricative clusters. *Journal of the Acoustical Society of America 91.* 2979–3000.

Watkins, K. E., Strafella, A. P. & Paus, T. (2003). Seeing and hearing speech excites the motor system involved in speech perception. *Neuropsychologia 41.* 989–994.

Wilson, S. M., Saygin, A. P., Sereno, M. I. & Iacoboni, M. (2004). Listening to speech activates motor areas involved in speech production. *Nature Neuroscience 7.* 701–702.

Wilson, S. M. & Iacoboni, M. (2006). Neural responses to non-native phonemes varying in producibility: Evidence for the sensorimotor nature of speech perception. *NeuroImage 33.* 316–325.

Wong, P. C. M., Nusbaum, H. C. & Small, S. L. (2004). Neural bases of talker normalization. *Journal of Cognitive Neuroscience 16*(7). 1173–1184.

Allard Jongman and Bob McMurray
On invariance: Acoustic input meets listener expectations

Abstract: Speech perception has been classically framed in terms of the widespread variability in speech acoustics. Factors like speaking rate, coarticulation, and speaker affect virtually all phonetic measurements or "cues". However, our understanding of this problem has been built on the basis of small-scale phonetic work, one cue and context at a time. We present findings based on a large corpus of fricatives that suggest that the massive variability in speech may not be insurmountable, but rather can be described as the simple additive product of multiple known factors. At any given moment, listeners have expectations about the anticipated value of cues like formant frequency or fricative spectrum as a function of contextual factors like talker and vowel. Perception is then based on the difference between the actual cue values heard and these expectations. We briefly describe two additional experiments that demonstrate that manipulation of listeners' expectations can change the accuracy of fricative identification, and improve listeners' ability to predict the subsequent vowel. Finally, we present new data on the relative contributions of place and voicing cues which suggest that there are several acoustic cues that can be considered invariant. However, this information alone is not sufficient to account for listeners' identification of fricatives. To approximate the performance of human listeners requires many cues, and these cues need to be interpreted relative to expectations derived from context.

1 Introduction

One of the principal goals of research on speech perception is to characterize the defining properties of speech sounds that occur in natural language, and to establish how the listener extracts these properties and uses them to identify linguistic units like phonemes or words. Sixty years of phonetic research have demonstrated that determining the acoustic cue or cues that uniquely characterize particular (classes of) speech sounds is a serious, if not insurmountable,

---

Allard Jongman, Department of Linguistics, University of Kansas
Bob McMurray, Department of Psychology, Department of Linguistics, University of Iowa

challenge. Not unexpectedly, the major obstacle in this endeavor is the variability typically found in the speech signal. This lack of invariance derives from a variety of sources, including variation in vocal tract size (across talkers), phonetic context, and speech tempo. Such variability often results in an imperfect one-to-one correspondence between acoustic cue and phonetic percept (e. g., Liberman et al., 1967) in which any given cue can reflect the influence of multiple factors (talker, multiple segments, and pure noise), The basic problem, then, is how perceptual constancy or invariance is achieved in the presence of such varying information.

We are by no means the first or the last to confront this question. This long-running debate has centered on the question of whether or not there are invariant acoustic markers for various phonological distinctions. This question goes beyond the nature of the speech signal, as it has often served as a crucible for larger theoretical debates about the nature of speech as an auditory or gestural process (Fowler, 1986; Diehl & Kluender, 1989; Sussman et al., 1998), or debates about the types of cognitive operations needed to understand speech (Mermelstein, 1978; Nearey, 1990; Smits, 2001b), and it is fundamental to the notion of what a phonological feature is (e. g., Blumstein & Stevens, 1981; Lahiri & Reetz, 2010; McMurray, Cole & Munson, 2011). Thus, understanding whether there is invariance in the speech signal, and the form it takes is central to our understanding of speech perception, phonology, and psycholinguistics.

The purpose of this chapter is three-fold. First, we review this long-standing debate on invariance both to highlight the seminal contributions of Sheila Blumstein's work, and to frame the issue more broadly. Second, we present a review of our own recent work on this issue. While our model stresses the lack of invariance in the signal, it also argues that some measure of invariance can be achieved via fairly simple domain-general processes. We end with a new phonetic analysis of fricatives that highlights the complex constellation of invariant and non-invariant cues when we consider the range of factors that simultaneously influence the production of a fricative.

The Search for Invariance

Much research has attempted to derive distinct spectral patterns that correspond to phonetic dimensions, such as place and manner of articulation, from the acoustic waveform. While there is no widely agreed upon definition of invariance, for the present purposes we suggest that invariance is achieved if some identified property of the speech signal reliably reflects a phonological distinction, and is not affected by contextual factors like talker, speaking rate and so forth.

If such invariant properties can be found, this would support a relatively straightforward bottom-up model of perception as a form of template matching. Consequently, the issue of invariance has been seen as central to debates about the nature of the speech perception system. The extent to which invariant cues for various phonological distinctions can be found offers a proof of concept that domain-general auditory processes might be successful in speech perception. In contrast, if invariance cannot be found, more complex perceptual processes (analysis by synthesis, relative cue encoding, and so forth) may offer a more compelling account.

This search for acoustic invariance was initially driven by engineering advances. While physical descriptions of speech in terms such as frequency and intensity date back at least as far as 1830 (Willis, 1830), the invention of the sound spectrograph in 1945 was the major technological discovery that made the analysis and visualization of the speech signal possible (see Jongman 2013, for a brief historical review). As the sound spectrograph became commercially available after WWII, researchers began to document the acoustic properties of speech sounds. Haskins Laboratories was at the forefront of this movement. A group at Haskins had been contracted to design a reading machine for the blind, a high priority as disabled veterans returned from the front. In theory, designing such a machine should be fairly straightforward: an optical sensor would scan each printed letter, each of the 26 letters would be associated with a distinct or arbitrary sound, and all the users would have to do is learn the association between each sound and letter. However, even after extensive training, the 'reading' rates of the trainees remained painfully slow, well below the rate at which speech is perceived. This prompted the research group, most notably Alvin Liberman, to study the speech signal in an attempt to determine how speech conveyed information so much more efficiently than the reading machine (see Liberman, 1996; Shankweiler & Fowler, 2015).

In this endeavor, he was helped by two technological advances: the aforementioned spectrograph and the Pattern Playback. Developed at Haskins (Cooper et al., 1952), the Pattern Playback machine produced sound from a graphic representation of the acoustic signal. These two technological advances enabled the Haskins group to contribute significantly to our understanding of the relation between acoustic properties and their perception. This work was fundamental to identifying the range of cues that listeners use to identify speech. It became clear that a stop-vowel syllable has a release burst, formant transitions from the burst into the vowel, and that the vowel has a number of distinct formant frequencies. The Pattern Playback in turn allowed us to determine which of these acoustic properties was necessary for a specific percept. For example, could a clear /k/ still be perceived if either the burst or the formant transitions were removed?

Early studies did not find any consistent mapping between acoustic properties and phonetic features (e. g., Cooper et al., 1952; Schatz, 1954; Delattre, Liberman & Cooper, 1955). For example, it was found that a given burst frequency or formant transition did not always elicit the same percept; a stimulus with a burst located at 1500 Hz was perceived as /p/ when followed by the vowel /i/ but as /k/ when followed by /ɑ/. Indeed, this now well-understood property of coarticulation is one of the critical features of speech that enables it to convey information more efficiently than the reading machine. But at the same time, it represents a form of context dependency of acoustic cues that is a serious challenge to the identification of invariant acoustic properties. The lack of this one-to-one mapping between acoustic property and perceived phoneme eventually led Liberman and colleagues to settle on articulation rather than acoustics as the source of the invariance, as laid out in the Motor Theory of Speech Perception (Liberman et al., 1967; Liberman & Mattingly, 1985; Galantucci, Fowler & Turvey, 2006).

Subsequent research, aided by yet another technological breakthrough, challenged Liberman's claim that acoustic invariance was not to be found. A new spectral analysis technique, Linear Predictive Coding (LPC), became available in the late 1960s and provided a different view of the speech signal. Specifically, instead of the spectrogram's visualization of release bursts, formant transitions, and steady-state formants as separate events, LPC analysis integrates spectral information over a brief time window (typically 20–40 ms) and produces a global spectral shape abstracting over these individual articulatory/acoustic events. This integrated spectral representation may be more similar to what our auditory system computes.

Research using LPC suggested that reliable acoustic properties could indeed be found in the speech signal and led Sheila Blumstein and Ken Stevens to their theory of Acoustic Invariance. (e. g., Stevens & Blumstein, 1981; Kewley-Port, 1983; Lahiri, Gewirth & Blumstein, 1984, Forrest et al., 1988; Sussman, McCaffrey & Matthews, 1991). For example, Blumstein & Stevens (1981) showed that the overall shape of the spectrum computed over the first 25 ms of the stop release burst provided invariant information about the stop's place of articulation. Each place was represented by a unique spectral shape that was retained across changes in the talker or vowel context. Subsequent work on acoustic invariance replaced these static onset spectra with a more dynamic approach that focused on relative changes in the distribution of energy between the spectrum computed at burst onset and that computed at vowel onset (Lahiri et al., 1984; see also Kewley-Port & Luce, 1984). This metric was shown to be a highly accurate and stable cue to place of articulation across a number of languages. In addition, follow-up perception experiments confirmed that listeners do indeed identify place of articulation based on the relationship between burst and vowel onset properties (Lahiri et al., 1984). In sum, Blumstein, Stevens, and colleagues showed that invariant cues to features such as place of articulation, manner of articulation, and voicing are indeed present in the acoustic signal and that listeners use these cues in their perception.

This work offered a powerful proof of concept that there may be invariant information for phonological contrasts, information that is statistically reliable across many tokens of the same sound. Further, it led to a flurry of ideas about what the form of these invariant properties might be, and consequently, the form of the representations that listeners must use to store them. Blumstein and Stevens initially envisioned this invariance as a complex spectro-temporal pattern or template that is associated with a given phonological feature. However, motivated in part by the presence of such invariance, a number of other research groups began to identify even simpler forms of invariance by looking at combinations of small numbers of acoustic cues (e. g., measurable values). For example, Port & Dalby (1982) proposed the ratio of the duration of the consonant to the vowel as a rate-invariant cue; and Sussman and colleagues proposed locus equations as a simple invariant cue to place of articulation (Sussman et al., 1998; see McMurray, Rhone & Hannaway, 2016, for a review). While the nature of these invariant cues was quite different than the complex representations suggested by Blumstein and Stevens, both lines of work offered support for relatively simple bottom-up approaches to perception based on matching templates, or simply computing thresholds for these compound cues.

These approaches were not without their own limitations, however. It was difficult to find cues for many phonemic contrasts. More importantly, in their focus on the information in the signal, these approaches lacked clear models of categorization to describe how listeners used this invariant information to extract linguistic units. However, in the late 1970s, inspired by advances in mathematical psychology, and in computational modeling, Gregg Oden and Dominic Massaro developed the Fuzzy Logical Model of Perception (FLMP; Oden & Massaro, 1978). FLMP and a number of related models (e. g., Normal A Posteriori Probability (NAPP), Nearey 1990, 1997; Weighted Gaussian Mixture Models, Toscano & McMurray, 2010) offered a precise mathematical formulation of the categorization problem as one of linearly weighting and combining multiple continuous cues. It also offered a new view of how to describe *what* is invariant. Critically, motivated by the extensive work on trading relations (e. g., Repp, 1982), FLMP argued that invariance may not be found in any single cue (indeed, listeners had been shown to use many cues for most speech sounds), but rather it may be defined as a region in high-dimensional (multiple-cue) space.

These ideas reframed the nature of the invariant information that listeners may retain and use. However, they also fundamentally built on Blumstein and

Stevens' insight – that lurking across all the variability in the acoustic signal, there are reliable acoustic markers of speech contrasts. Moreover, the ability to link these insights to listener behavior offered two key advances. First, the richer listener models offered a way to account for perceptual effects of things like visual speech that were long thought to be a marker of motor or gestural accounts. Second, and more importantly, the ability to link perceptual performance to acoustic cues (either in a corpus of measurements or stimulus set) offered a platform for testing the sufficiency of a hypothesized set of cues to account for behavior, something which we have built on in our own work (McMurray & Jongman, 2011) including the research reported here. These kinds of demonstrations offered powerful support to the idea that given the invariance in the signal listeners may be able to engage relatively simple, domain-general and bottom-up processes to identify phonemes.

All told, this line of work offered important support for the idea that some invariance could be found in the signal, and that listeners therefore may be able to classify speech using domain-general sorts of mechanisms. However, the case was by no means complete: invariant cues had not been found for all types of phonemes, and there was some sense that they may not be (e. g., Ohala, 1996; Lindblom, 1996). More importantly, there were few demonstrations that one could convert these invariant properties of the signal into categories with an accuracy that approached listeners. This latter point was crucial as one must not just establish that there *is* invariant information, but also that it is *sufficient* to account for listener-like levels of accuracy.

However, other theoretical developments in speech changed the nature of the argument over invariance in more significant ways. Much of the prior work on invariant acoustic cues suggested that the invariance in the signal is used by listeners to form a sort of template which can be applied to the noisy signal to extract categories. However, the 1980s also saw a paradigm shift with respect to the status of variability in the speech signal. Since Liberman's pioneering work, acoustic variability had always been considered a nuisance ('noise') which had to somehow be removed to reveal the underlying structure of the speech signal. The removal of this noise is a process referred to as 'compensation' or 'normalization'.

In contrast, researchers like Elman & McClelland (1986) pointed out that variability need not be a problem since it is "lawful"; that is, variability in the acoustic (or articulatory) realization of speech categories is predictable from context and may in fact be helpful rather than harmful to speech comprehension. The 1990s produced a wealth of studies that suggested that fine-grained acoustic information is not removed during speech processing but in fact retained to aid lexical access. In part due to Blumstein's seminal work we now know that word recognition is sensitive to within-category variation in phonetic cues like voice onset time (Andruski, Blumstein & Burton, 1994; Utman, Blumstein & Burton, 2000; McMurray, Tanenhaus & Aslin, 2002; McMurray et al., 2008). That is, listeners are not just storing that a speech sound was /b/ or /p/, but they seem to also be preserving how far or close that token was to their /b/ prototype (see also Miller, 1997).

Work since then has further shown that listeners can harness a wide range of fine-grained information including indexical detail (Creel, Aslin & Tanenhaus, 2008; Goldinger, 1998), word-level prosody (Salverda, Dahan & McQueen, 2003), coarticulation (Marslen-Wilson & Warren, 1994; Dahan et al., 2001), and alternations like reduction (Connine, 2004; Connine, Ronbom & Patterson, 2008) and assimilation (Gow, 2003). In many of these cases, such detail aids processing by allowing listeners to anticipate upcoming material (Martin & Bunnel, 1981, 1982; Gow, 2001, 2003), resolve prior ambiguity (Gow, 2003; McMurray, Tanenhaus & Aslin, 2009) and disambiguate words faster (Salverda, Dahan & McQueen, 2003). Consequently, the idea of simply identifying phonemes based on whatever invariant information can be found seemed to undersell the richness of the perceptual process.

Such evidence has led some to reject normalization altogether in favor of exemplar approaches (e. g. Pisoni, 1997; Port, 2007) which preserve continuous detail. Exemplar models (e. g., Goldinger, 1998) offer a somewhat different take on invariance. These models argue that rather than storing a single abstract form of a given phonological category (or word), listeners retain multiple exemplars of each word in a relatively unanalyzed form that includes substantial fine phonetic detail. This detail necessarily includes both phonologically relevant information (e. g., VOT, formant frequencies) as well as contextual factors (indexical properties of the talker, speaking rate and so forth). This ability to match incoming speech at a more holistic level allows the system to implicitly accommodate for contextual factors without explicit normalization procedures.

Deep inside an exemplar model, however, acoustic invariance may play an important role. The prior phonetic work on invariance derived invariance across many recordings of many talkers. As such, the invariant information that was found phonetically fundamentally reflects stable statistical properties (in a high-dimensional space) across all of the tokens containing a given speech sound. This is exactly the kind of information that will also be observed distributed across the exemplar space. Thus, at a deep level exemplar models are likely to take advantage of similar invariant properties, even if they don't explicitly represent it. It is not clear that such models *require* there to be invariance, but to the extent that the exemplar "cloud" is based on a similar sample of speech to prior phonetic studies, it is likely that such invariance will be there. Where exemplar models differ (functionally) is that they can also take advantage of second-order lawful relationships between phonetic cues and factors like talker to improve on the basis offered by acoustic invariance.

As a whole, then, this body of work has established that there may be a substantial amount of more or less invariant information to be found in the speech signal. Yet it has not determined if this is sufficient to account for listener behavior. Similarly, there are several promising models explaining how perception can harness this information, but with few exceptions (Nearey, 1997), it is not clear these have been tested on phonetic corpora with substantial variability. Addressing these issues is crucial for realizing the promise of the invariance approach started by Stevens and Blumstein. We have recently developed a computational framework in which assumptions about the specific content of acoustic cues and the category structure can be directly evaluated. We will start by summarizing this approach here (for more detail, see McMurray & Jongman, 2011; Apfelbaum et al., 2014; Apfelbaum & McMurray, 2015); we will also present new results from additional modeling and behavioral experiments.

2 Comparing models of speech categorization

Our investigation started with this goal of linking variability in a corpus of phonetic measurements to listener perception. We had a large set of recordings of the fricatives of English including many different talkers and coarticulatory contexts. We measured a very large number of cues for each token. And we had listeners' perception of a subset of these tokens. With this as a base, our goal was to develop a framework for comparing models of how listeners use information in the speech signal.

We set out to compare three influential approaches to speech perception. First, we sought to evaluate our version of the early theories of **Acoustic Invariance**, the idea that a small number of highly invariant cues would be sufficient for perception. The listener extracts these invariants and maps them onto linguistic dimensions such as place and manner of articulation. As these cues are invariant, there is no need for listeners to perform any compensation or normalization for contextual factors.

Second, in cue-integration models like FLMP and NAPP listeners rely on a multitude of acoustic cues; while individual cues may vary in how well they specify a certain speech sound, the integration of many cues should yield robust phonetic categorization in a high-dimensional space. This assumption is shared with exemplar models (though as we'll describe below, our initial modeling framework did not implement an exemplar model; but see Apfelbaum &

McMurray, 2015). Cue-integration models do not take a principled stance with respect to the need for compensation. In some, cues are used in a relatively raw manner (FLMP, NAPP); in others, context (e. g., talker or neighboring phoneme) can be used for compensation. Here we focused on models that use raw cues so as to address the question of whether adding additional cues over and above the most invariant ones is helpful.

Finally, we examined what we call *relative cue* models. These models (which we describe in more depth later) implement a form of compensation in which cues are recoded relative to listeners' expectations (Cole et al., 2010). F0, for example, is coded as high for a man, or low for a voiceless stop. This recoding need not discard fine-grained detail (in fact, it may help listeners access it: Cole et al., 2010). This compensation is likely functionally similar to many other versions of compensation such as HICAT (Smits, 2001a, b) and perhaps even accounts like gestural parsing (Fowler, 1986).

Our goal was to develop simple models of listener behavior and then to pit these models against a large corpus of natural measurements of speech. We selected the English fricatives as the target of our investigation since they represent a large number (8) of categories and since some of the acoustic cues to fricatives are thought to be invariant while others are determined by context. In addition, previous research had identified a large number of potential cues. This work suggests that place of articulation can be distinguished by the four spectral moments (mean, variance, skewness and kurtosis of the frequency spectrum of the frication) (Forrest et al., 1988; Jongman, Wayland & Wong, 2000; Maniwa, Jongman & Wade, 2009), and by spectral changes in the onset of the subsequent vowel, particularly the second formant (Jongman, Wayland & Wong, 2000; Fowler, 1994; Maniwa, Jongman & Wade, 2009). Duration and amplitude of the frication are also related to place of articulation, primarily distinguishing sibilants from non-sibilants (Behrens & Blumstein, 1988; Baum & Blumstein, 1987; Crystal & House, 1988; Jongman, Wayland & Wong, 2000; Maniwa, Jongman & Wade, 2009; Strevens, 1960). Voicing is cued by changes in duration (Behrens & Blumstein, 1988; Baum & Blumstein, 1987; Jongman, Wayland & Wong, 2000; Maniwa, Jongman & Wade, 2009) and spectral properties (Stevens et al., 1992; Jongman, Wayland & Wong, 2000; Maniwa, Jongman & Wade, 2009).

Our corpus consisted of the 8 fricatives of English (/f, v, θ, ð, s, z, ʃ, ʒ/) followed by each of the 6 vowels /i, e, æ, ɑ, o, u/. Twenty talkers (10 females) produced three repetitions of each stimulus embedded in a carrier sentence for a total of 2880 tokens. Jongman et al. (2000) provide a detailed acoustic analysis of 14 acoustic cues including spectral moments (measured at multiple locations in the signal), spectral peak frequency, fricative duration and amplitude, relative amplitude, and F2 at vowel onset. McMurray & Jongman (2011) added 10 more cues including F1, F3, F4, and F5 at vowel onset, low frequency energy in the fricative, and the amplitude in the F3 and F5 frequency region in both the fricative and the vowel. We felt that these 24 cues (see Table 1) provided a very comprehensive representation of the acoustic/phonetic properties of these fricatives.

Table 1: Cues Measured in McMurray & Jongman (2011)

Cue	Description
MaxPF	Frequency with highest amplitude in the frication.
DUR_F	Duration of frication
DUR_V	Duration of vocalic portion
RMS_F	Amplitude of frication
RMS_V	Amplitude of vocalic portion
$F3AMP_F$	Narrow band amplitude of frication at F3
$F3AMP_V$	Narrow band amplitude of vowel at F3
$F5AMP_F$	Narrow band amplitude of frication at F5
$F5AMP_V$	Narrow band amplitude of vowel at F5
LF	Low Frequency: Mean RMS <500 Hz in frication
F_0	Pitch at vowel onset
F1	1st formant frequency of vowel
F2	2nd formant frequency of vowel
F3	3rd formant frequency of vowel
F4	4th formant frequency of vowel
F5	5th formant frequency of vowel
M1	Spectral mean in first half of frication
M2	Spectral variance in first half of frication
M3	Spectral skewness in first half of frication
M4	Spectral kurtosis at three windows in frication noise
$M1_{trans}$	Spectral mean at fricative/vowel juncture
$M2_{trans}$	Spectral variance at fricative/vowel juncture
$M3_{trans}$	Spectral skewness at fricative/vowel juncture
$M4_{trans}$	Spectral kurtosis at fricative/vowel juncture

Our first question was whether our fricative corpus contained any invariant cues that were not affected by contextual variables such as speaker and vowel quality. Here, prior approaches focused largely on statistical comparisons of a given cue as a function of a phonological feature or of contextual factors (e. g., does a cue differ significantly with respect to place of articulation). We took it one step farther, by using a hierarchical regression approach which allows us to estimate the amount of variance in each cue that was accounted for by contextual factors (talker, coarticulation) and by the relevant phonological factors. Thus, we used separate regression analyses to compare the amount of variance in each cue due to dimensions such as voicing and place of articulation as well as context factors like talker. Given this sort of model, we can define invariance in statistical terms, using Cohen and Cohen's (1983) definition of effect size: a cue is invariant if it showed a large effect ($R^2 > .15$) of a single feature (e. g., place of articulation, voicing) and, at most, small effects ($R^2 < .05$) of context. Using these criteria, none of the 24 cues could be considered invariant. Relaxing our criteria somewhat, we designated 9 cues as nearly invariant (large effect of a single feature ($R^2 > .30$), small to moderate effects of context ($R^2 < .17$). These 9 cues are shown in Table 2.

Table 2: Results from regression analyses examining effects of Speaker and Vowel on phonetic features including voicing, place of articulation, and sibilance. R^2_{change} values are shown. These 9 cues are relatively unaffected by speaker and vowel context.

Cue	Cue for	Context Effects	
		Talker	Vowel
RMS_F	Sibilance ($R^2 = .419$)	Moderate ($R^2 = .081$)	n.s.
$F5AMP_F$	Sibilance ($R^2 = .39$)	Moderate ($R^2 = .07$)	Small ($R^2 = .012$)
$F3AMP_F$	Sibilance ($R^2 = .24$)	Moderate ($R^2 = .07$)	Small ($R^2 = .028$)
	Place/sibilants ($R^2 = .44$)		
M2	Sibilance ($R^2 = .44$)	Small ($R^2 = .036$)	n.s.
	Place/sibilants ($R^2 = .34$)		
MaxPF	Place/sibilants ($R^2 = .50$)	Moderate ($R^2 = .084$)	n.s.
M1	Place/sibilants ($R^2 = .55$)	Moderate ($R^2 = .122$)	n.s.
M3	Place/sibilants ($R^2 = .37$)	Moderate ($R^2 = .064$)	n.s.
DUR_F	Voicing ($R^2 = .40$)	Large ($R^2 = .16$)	Small ($R^2 = .021$)
LF	Voicing ($R^2 = .48$)	Moderate ($R^2 = .11$)	Small ($R^2 = .004$)

These results show that few cues come close to an invariant or primary cue. In fact, even with this relaxed criterion there were no cues that invariantly distinguished place of articulation in non-sibilants. Instead, vowel quality, talker, and fricative identity affect virtually every cue studied. All of the cues we measured are multiply determined by largely the same information (vowel, talker, fricative) and this may present problems for models that simply conflate these sources of information.

3 Relating acoustics to perception

We next set out to compare three claims about how listeners categorize speech sounds (fricatives in our case): a) a small number of invariant cues can distinguish the 8 fricatives; b) a large number of cues is sufficient without compensation; and c) compensation is required. To achieve this, we used the fricative cues to train a generic categorization model. Model performance was then compared to listener performance. To gauge listener performance, we collected perceptual identification data for a subset of the fricatives. To keep the perception experiment manageable, we selected tokens produced by 10 (5 female) of our 20 speakers. In addition, we included only three vowels (/i, ɑ, u/) and a single token. Thus, listeners identified 240 tokens (8 fricatives x 3 vowels x 10 speakers). We will discuss the perception data when we assess model performance below. By manipulating the cues available to the model and whether or not compensation was applied, we assessed the information required to yield listener-like performance.

The categorization model was trained on all of the tokens in the corpus minus those that were used in the perception experiment. It was given a much more powerful sort of training than listeners are likely to have had, as it was given both the acoustic measurements and the intended productions, and had to acquire the mapping between them. Thus, it represents something akin to an ideal observer model, asking how much information is present in that cue set under the best of circumstances. The categorization model was built on logistic regression, which was selected because it was a) general purpose, b) had few assumptions, and c) mapped closely onto cue integration models like FLMP and NAPP. Briefly, logistic regression first weights and combines multiple cues linearly. This is then transformed into a probability (e. g., the probability of an /f/ given the cues). Weights are determined during training to optimally separate the categories. For each fricative in the training set, the model generates a set of probabilities of choosing each of the 8 fricatives.

Acoustic Invariance

Among the 9 nearly invariant cues shown in Table 1, none were even modestly invariant for place of articulation in the non-sibilants (/f, v, θ, ð/). We therefore added four additional cues, two of which were strongly associated with both place of articulation and context, and two of which were moderately correlated with place and context. We then trained the categorization model with only these 13 nearly invariant cues, without any form of compensation. Mean categorization accuracy was 79 % and fell well below human listeners' performance (91 %). Moreover, the model did not approximate the patterns of errors observed in our listeners. For example, the model did substantially worse on the non-sibilant fricatives and failed to capture the fact that human fricative perception was worst in the context of the vowel /i/.

Cue Integration

We next trained the categorization model with all 24 cues, without any form of compensation. Mean categorization accuracy increased to 82%, still well below human listeners' performance (91%). While this model resembled the pattern of listeners' confusions more closely, it still failed to predict worse performance in the context of /i/.

The fact that the addition of 11 cues (from 13 to 24) only slightly improved the categorization model's performance suggests that simply adding more cues will not result in human-like accuracy. This was unexpected, but it makes sense in retrospect since all of these cues are the product of a much smaller number of underlying physical events: speech gestures. If the spectral mean of an /ʃ/ is a bit higher than it should be (closer to an /s/), that probably derives from the fact that the tongue is positioned a bit more to the front than it should be. Since many of the secondary cues to fricative place (e. g., F2 at onset) are also products of tongue position, they too will reflect this slightly deviant tongue position – they won't help cope with this ambiguity. This redundancy also extends to context. Our phonetic analyses illustrate that most cues are the simultaneous product of multiple factors including talker and coarticulation. Consequently, if spectral mean (for example) is affected by talker and by the neighboring vowel, adding another cue that is also affected by these factors, won't necessarily improve perception. We therefore subjected these cues to a form of compensation to determine if compensation would boost model performance.

Compensation

Finally, we trained the categorization model with all 24 cues, this time with compensation. Our approach to compensation is inspired by previous research on overlap in articulatory gestures. For example, Fowler & Brown (2000) observed that a partially nasalized vowel is perceived as more oral when it is followed by a nasal as compared to an oral stop. They offered a 'parsing' account: Since English does not use nasalized vowels contrastively, the lowering gesture of the velum to open the nasal cavity is assigned to the stop (a result of anticipatory coarticulation). Thus, listeners actively parse the components of the variability into their underlying sources in order to reach a more invariant representation (see also Fowler, 1986). Gow (2003) presents a version of this process that is built on auditory, rather than gestural features. And Cole et al. (2010; McMurray, Cole & Munson, 2011) extended this to show that parsing can be successfully applied to phonetic cue measurements as well to dramatically clean up the signal.

Building on this earlier work (Cole et al., 2010; McMurray, Cole & Munson, 2011), we implemented a very simple form of this type of parsing. Rather than treating absolute F0 as meaningful, F0 can be recoded relative to the expected F0 of that talker or gender (e. g., it is 20 Hz lower than would be expected for a man). This accounts for these sources of variance, and what's left over (the residual, or the variance in a cue value that cannot be attributed to talker or other factors) can then be used as information for the next stage of perception. In the earliest work applying this to vowel formants (long the poster-child for lack of invariance), we demonstrated that this simple scheme (implemented with linear regression) can account for 95 % of the variance in F2 and 90 % of the variance in F1 across a set of recordings that contained multiple coarticulatory influences and 10 different talkers. This suggests that acoustic variability is more lawful and decomposable than perhaps acknowledged (though see Elman & McClelland, 1986).

Up until that point, however, such a scheme had not been tested in a way that links the variability in the signal to listeners' behavior. Fricatives seemed to provide an ideal situation, since almost half of the cues were observed to be highly context-sensitive: For 10 of the 24 cues, context variables (speaker and vowel) accounted for over 25 % of the variance. Our implementation of this form of compensation was simple: we used linear regression to partial the effects of vowel and speaker from the cue values for each token before entering them into the categorization model. Briefly, each acoustic measure is first entered as the dependent variable of a linear regression in which the cue value is predicted from explicit information about talker and vowel. This regression predicts cue values for any cue as produced by a particular speaker in a particular vowel context. We then compute the difference between actual and predicted value (residual). Next, these residuals are used as the training set for the logistic regression which identifies the fricative categories.

This process represents a form of rescaling. The "prediction" from the regression can be seen as the model's expectation for what that cue value should be (e. g., this F0 came from a man, so it should be low). The residual then is how different from these predictions the actual value is. Since residualization is done with subtraction, no information is really lost (from an individual cue value for an individual token), so this is not an example of "normalization" that eliminates fine-grained detail in the signal. Rather, as Cole et al show, this process actually enhances the fine-grained detail in the signal (in their case vowel-to-vowel coarticulatory information), making it more available.

When we trained the model on all 24 cues with compensation as described above, categorization accuracy rose to 90 %, nearly identical to human performance (91 %). As shown in Figure 1, the compensation model not only approximates listener performance for each fricative and each speaker, it is also the only model that captures the vowel context effect (Figure 1B). Further, when we next tested listeners on the frication alone (substantially reducing their ability to identify the talker/vowel, and thus to perform this compensation), we found that the raw cue model offered a better fit to the data. These results show that human performance can be matched with a simple categorization model as long as many cues are included (no single cue is crucial) and these cues are encoded veridically and continuously. In addition, cues are encoded relative to expected values derived from context (e. g. speaker and vowel). Finally, these results do not appear to derive from our use of logistic regression as a categorization model (which implements something like a prototype model). We have now used the same cues to train connectionist networks and exemplar models, which are much more sophisticated and powerful categorization engines. In both cases, relative cues offered better performance and a closer match to listeners (Apfelbaum & McMurray, in press).

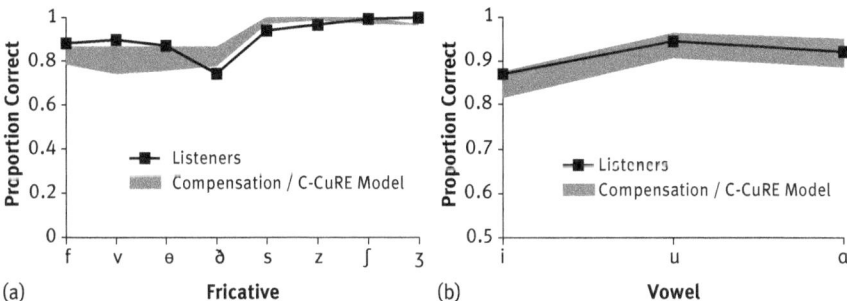

Figure 1: Performance of the compensation model and human listeners on the complete-syllable condition. Listener performance is indicated in black. Model performance is represented by the gray range that is bounded by the performance of the model using the probabilistic rule (on the bottom) and the discrete-choice rule (on the top). A) As a function of fricative. B) As a function of vowel context. (From McMurray & Jongman, 2011).

We named this approach C-CuRE (Computing Cues Relative to Expectations; McMurray & Jongman, 2011). Crucially, the implication of C-CuRE is that the information enabling speech perception is not the raw acoustic signal per se but the difference between the acoustic signal and what was expected. This encoding relative to expectations is similar to what is known as predictive coding in other cognitive domains such as vision and motor control (see Clark 2013 for a review). For example, event perception appears to rely on predictions about upcoming information; violation of these expectations signals event boundaries (Zacks et al., 2007).

Further Tests

C-CuRE is based on a computational model. It not only predicts human performance with a high degree of accuracy, it also makes concrete predictions that can be tested behaviorally. One such prediction is that high-level expectations can improve perceptual analysis and lead to greater accuracy. In our previous work, we compared both human and model performance in situations in which they heard the complete syllable and those from which the vowels had been removed. With these more reduced stimuli, we observed that the raw cue-integration model's performance (74 %) matched human performance (76 %); however, when adding the cues in the vowel, model performance (82 %) significantly undershot human performance (91 %). Thus, when adding vocalic cues to the fricatives, human performance drastically improved (from 76 % to 91 %) but model performance showed only a moderate gain (from 74 % to 82 %). Adding the secondary cues in the vocalic portion was not enough to match listeners' performance. This suggests that without the vowel, listeners could not identify the talker or context to categorize the cues in the frication, and were thus forced to rely on raw cues. The vowel contributes toward contingent categorization: listeners identify vowel and talker and use this information to better interpret the fricative cues.

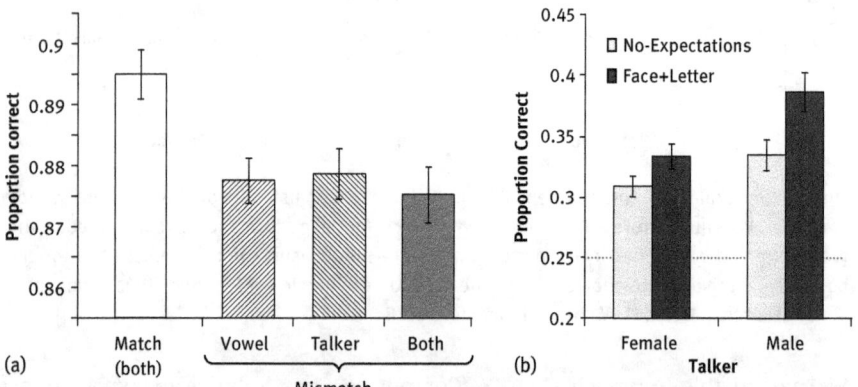

Figure 2: Results of follow-up tests of C-CuRE. A) Results from Apfelbaum et al., 2014. Shown is accuracy of fricative identification as a function of whether the vocoid and frication matched on talker, vowel, both, or neither. B) Results from McMurray & Jongman (2016). Shown is accuracy at anticipating the final vowel after hearing the fricative alone, or after hearing the fricative alone while viewing the face of the talker and the letter corresponding to the fricative.

We recently tested this prediction in a perception experiment with cross-spliced fricative-vowel syllables (Apfelbaum et al., 2014). Fricatives do not contain sufficient information to unambiguously identify vowel or talker; rather, listeners must obtain that information from the vocoid which holds strong cues for speaker and vowel, but only weak cues for the fricative. We thus manipulated the vocalic portion of a fricative-vowel pair to mislead the listener about which speaker may have generated the cues in the frication, or which vowel may have conditioned them. Specifically, we created various combinations of the fricatives /f, θ, s, ʃ/ and the vowels /i, ae, ɑ, u/ as produced by two female and two male speakers. The resulting syllables could match in terms of both talker and vowel, mismatch in terms of either or both (e. g., /s/ before /i/ spoken by a man paired with /u/ spoken by a female). Crucially, the vowel was always spliced from a token of the same fricative so that the bottom-up cues in both portions matched the correct fricative. Thus, the bottom-up cues to the fricative were always matching and correct. We presented these syllables to listeners who had to indicate which fricative they heard. Results showed that performance was impaired (as measured in terms of both accuracy and reaction time) when fricatives were heard in the context of mismatching vowels or speakers (Figure 2A). This finding is consistent with C-CuRE in that mismatching vowel and speaker information changed the way bottom-up information was used by listeners such that they misinterpreted the cues to frication.

Most recently, we tested C-CuRE's prediction that giving listeners more information about the source of a fricative should enable them to better use fine-grained detail to make predictions (McMurray & Jongman, 2016). In this case, we presented listeners with the 8 English fricatives (the vowels following the fricative had been digitally removed) and asked them to identify the missing vowel as one of /i, ae, ɑ, u/. The crucial manipulation here was that in addition to this standard speech perception task (the 'no expectations' condition), we included a second condition in which participants executed the same task but in which each trial was preceded by a picture of the face of the speaker as well as the letter(s) representing the fricative (e. g., 'f', 'sh') (the 'expectations' condition).

Our results (Figure 2B) show that even without expectations provided by context, listeners were consistently above chance at predicting the upcoming vowel. This is consistent with a long history of work showing that listeners can use anticipatory coarticulation in fricatives (Yeni-Komshian & Soli, 1981) and in other speech sounds (Martin & Bunnel, 1981; Gow, 2001; Salverda, Kleinschmidt & Tanenhaus, 2014). More importantly, however, listeners' vowel identification was significantly better in the expectations condition than in the no expectations condition. Traditional accounts of speech perception have difficulty explaining this advantage as the context provides no direct evidence for what vowel is coming up. However, C-CuRE specifically predicts this benefit because contextual knowledge (in this case, about the fricative and speaker) allows listeners to better interpret the acoustic signal. For example, if the listener knows that the sound was an /s/ spoken by a female, slight deviations from that expectation due to coarticulation will be more detectable and lead to a more accurate identification of the vowel.

These results go beyond previous findings that listeners can use fine-grained coarticulatory information to predict adjacent phonemes (Gow, 2001; Martin & Bunnell, 1981; Salverda, Kleinschmidt & Tanenhaus, 2014; Yeni-Komshian & Soli, 1981). In most of these cases, the information being used for prediction is direct, bottom-up support for the next phoneme (e. g., coarticulation), and it is not clear that these predictions are used as the basis of comparison. However, in our experiments, predictions must be based on contextual, rather than phonetic information. Here, *contextual information* refers to factors that affect the speech signal systematically but do not serve as information about a particular segment (Repp, 1982). For example, knowing the talker does not tell the listener if an upcoming sound is bilabial or alveolar – it helps the listener interpret the cues for place of articulation. This suggests a more complex form of prediction that has not been investigated either empirically or theoretically.

So what does this approach say about invariance? On the one hand, it seems to argue, by a classical definition, that it's not there and it is not sufficient for perception. No truly invariant cues were found in this corpus and a model trained on our best cues performed far below listener levels. On the other hand, at a deeper level, the fact that we were able to extract the right information using linear regression suggests that the various factors that drive the lack of invariance are in fact linearly separable in the signal. In fact, Cole et al. show that for F1 and F2 of two vowels the combination of talker, vowel identity, and neighboring consonant and vowel can predict up to 90 % of the variance. Thus, the information is not hopelessly lost, it just needs to be actively discovered by processes like parsing and expectation-relative coding. As a result, even as this model clearly challenges the simple bottom-up model of perception that was assumed as part of acoustic invariance theory, at the highest level it supports the notion that there is clear information in the signal to support perception using fairly simple mechanisms.

4 New Results: The role of bottom-up information in C-CuRE

Our prior work leading up to the C-CuRE model (Apfelbaum & McMurray, 2015; McMurray & Jongman, 2011) showed conclusively that even when we combine a massive number of cues (24) there was not sufficient information in the signal to unambiguously identify fricatives at listener-like levels of accuracy. This may seem counterintuitive as one might expect that while any individual cue may be highly variable, the addition of more redundant cues should help overcome that. Indeed, when students are presented with data showing how variable individual cues are the almost immediate response is "why not add more cues?". However, as we described, the redundancy of the additional cues may also be their downfall. If a primary cue is ambiguous or context-dependent, the secondary, tertiary cues are likely to be so as well. Instead, we demonstrated that a model which uses a more top-down or interactive approach offers a much better account – if perception is based on the difference between top-down expectations and the bottom-up signal, we can not only get more accurate classification, but we see classification performance that looks more like listeners.

This theoretical approach to speech perception suggests that perception may not be best described purely as a process of bottom-up template-matching or categorization. Rather, it is more akin to a process of accounting for or explaining the data (the perceptual input). That is listeners are identifying the talker, forming expectations about what the speech signal should sound like for that talker, and then comparing the incoming speech to those talkers. Under this description, what they are really doing, then, is accounting for one set of properties as the consequence of talker-related variation, and then using what is left over to do useful work.

At the broadest level, this has some similarities to ideas like analysis by synthesis (Liberman & Mattingly, 1985), gestural parsing (Fowler & Smith, 1986), and more recent Bayesian accounts (Feldman, Griffiths & Morgan, 2009) of speech in that the goal of speech perception is to account for all the variance in the signal as the product of some set of overlapping "causes" (talker, place of articulation, and other factors). However, at the same time, data explanation can also work quite nicely in purely auditory frameworks – we have shown it can be implemented with linear regression (as a product of statistical learning, McMurray & Farris-Trimble, 2012), and it is not very different from the way that interactive activation models (Elman & McClelland, 1986; McClelland & Elman, 1986) carve up the speech stream into words.

While this seems to put all the onus on top-down or expectation-driven processing, one should not ignore the important role of bottom-up categorization in such systems. That is, in order to engage in such processing, listeners must identify factors like the first phoneme or the talker (presumably using bottom-up mechanisms in part) before they can account for their effects on later factors. In this light, the kind of basic templates that Blumstein and Stevens introduced us to can play a crucial role in expectation-relative coding schemes like C-CuRE.

More importantly, it is not clear that expectation-relative processing is needed for every possible combination of factors affecting speech acoustics. It is probably not the case that listeners have a homunculus that turns on or off expectation generation and comparison for some contrasts but not others. Rather, given the particular structure of the variance associated with two factors (e. g., talker and nasality), there may be little additional benefit to accounting for variance in one thing before processing another. In these situations, we may find that, superficially at least, perception looks like a largely bottom-up process.

Phonemes and features: On the independence of Place and Voicing in fricatives

The studies described above focused on the influence of factors external to the target fricative, the talker and the neighboring vowel. However, a history of both theoretical and empirical work has also examined factors internal to the target sound such as the interaction of place and voicing features for a single consonant (Oden, 1978; Sawusch & Pisoni, 1974). This is important because it can speak to the question of what the fundamental representations of phonemes are. Can phonemes be decomposed simply into features, or do they have a more unary status. Crucially, in the context of this chapter, such an investigation speaks to a more refined understanding of what (if anything) is invariant in the speech signal.

This has not been examined in the context of fricative perception. More importantly, given our understanding of this corpus of measurements, we can simultaneously examine how this plays out given overlapping variance from both talker and vowel.

Acoustic Analysis

We started with an examination of the acoustic cues. Our goal here was to document whether place and voicing had unique effects on each cue, and importantly, to examine the distribution of this across the 24 cues to fricatives analyzed by McMurray & Jongman (2011). These cues are summarized in Table 1. As in our prior work, we used linear regressions conducted on each cue to determine how much variance in that cue was predicted by various factors including talker, neighboring vowel, and many others. In these regressions, sets of dummy codes were constructed for each factor (e. g., 19 dummy codes for the 20 talkers, plus 5 dummy codes for the 6 vowels and so forth). These were the independent variables in the regression and always added to the model as a set (all the talker variables were added together). Regressions were conducted hierarchically, allowing us to quantify the unique variance accounted for by each factor. For example, to quantify the amount of variance accounted for by place of articulation over and above the effect of talker, we added the talker dummy codes on the first step of the model and computed the R^2. Next, we added the place of articulation dummy codes, and computed the increase in R^2 (R^2_Δ) as the unique variance in that cue that was accounted for by place of articulation over and above talker. Due to the strong (and variable) effect of context (talker and vowel) across the different cues, all of the regressions added talker and vowel first, and then looked at the contribution of place and/or voicing over and above that.

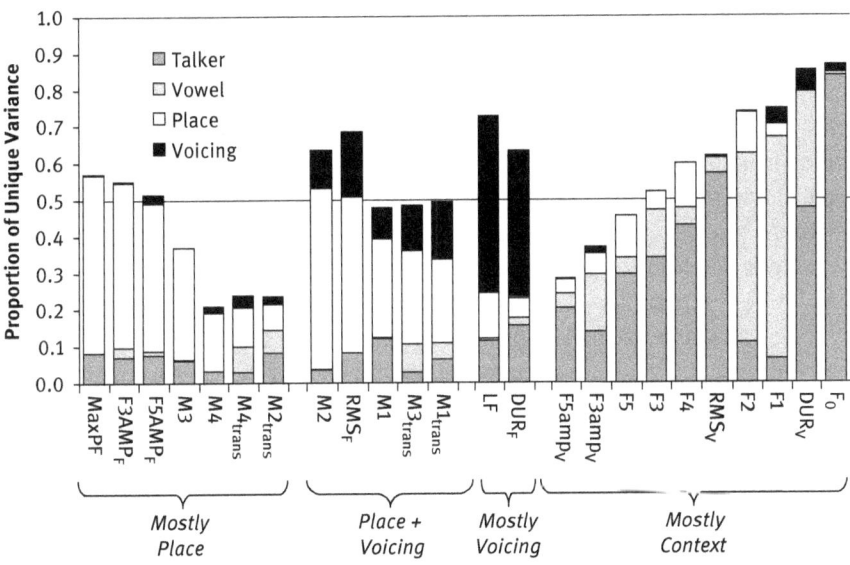

Figure 3: Proportion of unique variance contributed by Talker, Vowel, Place of articulation, and Voicing for each acoustic cue.

We first examined the relative contribution of the effect of context (talker and vowel) vs. place and voicing cues. Figure 3 shows the results for each of the 24 cues. The total height of each bar indicates the total proportion of variance accounted for by all four factors; the different shaded regions represent the proportion of variance associated with just one factor. The cues are sorted (horizontally) into roughly four groups: cues that seemed most strongly associated with place, voicing or both, and those most strongly associated with contextual factors (talker + vowel).

A couple of broad generalizations can be drawn from this. There are clearly about four cues (MaxPF through M3) for which the majority of the variance is due to place of articulation, two (LF and DUR_F) for which the majority is due to voicing, and another 5 which show only moderate or small influences of context and large effects of both place and voicing.

By these standards, there do appear to be a fair number of cues one might want to call "invariant", cues for which a purely bottom-up template matching (e. g., Blumstein & Stevens, 1979; Blumstein & Stevens, 1980) might be sufficient for categorization. Indeed, this is not surprising – it is just a finer-grained analysis of what was presented before (Table 2). If these cues are available, then why were the models based on raw cues in McMurray & Jongman (2011) unable to achieve high levels of performance? We suspect the answer is that while all of these cues are not strongly related to context factors, they are also not perfectly related to place and voicing. For most of them, context, place, *and* voicing accounted for a total of around 50 % of the variance – that means that 50 % of the variance in these cues may not be lawfully related to the obvious factors (we hesitate to call it truly random or noise). Consequently, even as place of articulation may be the strongest predictor of MAXPF (for example), MAXPF may not be that great of a predictor of place. As a result, the contribution provided by the other cues ($F5AMP_V$ through F_0) may be important as additional sources of information, and these may strongly benefit from expectation-relative coding or other forms of context compensation.

We next wanted to look at the relative influence of place and voicing on each cue (our primary goal). Here, since a large number of the cues were quite context-dependent, we wanted to be able to look at the contributions of place and voicing over and above the large effect of context. Thus, the unique contributions of these two factors were recomputed as the proportion of the remaining variance (e. g., if talker and voicing accounted for 40 % of the variance, and place accounted for an additional 20 %, it was recoded as 20 / (100 – 40) = 33 % of the additional variance. These proportions are plotted in Figure 4. The order of the cues is not the same as in Figure 3 to highlight a number of new relationships.

Viewed in this way, many of the cues that looked quite insignificant in Figure 3 are suddenly quite useful. For example, with respect to F0, place and voicing together accounted for less than 2.2 % of the variance in absolute terms, but after accounting for the large amount of context variability, this was actually 14.3 % of the remaining variance. Given this, we see a very clear distribution of cues, with 14 cues responding almost entirely to place of articulation (after talker and vowel are removed), 4 cues with very large effects of voicing (but not place) and 6 cues with some effects of both.

Given this, there does appear to be some evidence that after accounting for the variance in talker and neighboring vowel, fricative place and voicing have at least some independent instantiation in the set of cues that distinguish fricatives. However, it is unclear what role (if any) the six cues that respond to both might play.

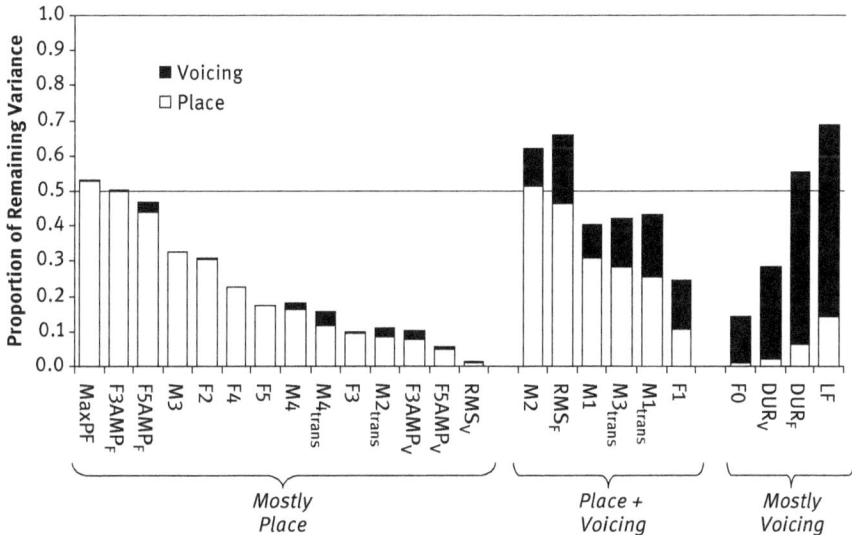

Figure 4: Proportion of remaining variance contributed by Voicing and Place of articulation for each acoustic cue, after effects of context (Talker and Vowel) have been removed.

Classification Analysis

Our next analysis sought to examine the information distributed across all of these cues. In particular, we wanted to assess the independence of voicing and place decisions, given the variance structure across cues. We did this by using multinomial logistic regression to predict the intended fricative using a near-optimal weighting of all 24 cues. Here, accuracy serves as a measure of how well the cues distinguish the 8 fricatives.

For these analyses, we started with one of two baseline models – either a model trained on raw cues, or one trained on cues which were computed relative to talker and vowel expectations. We trained the model to identify place (4AFC) from these cues and recorded the accuracy. We next residualized these cues for voicing and retrained the model. This simulates a situation in which the model knows the voicing of the token, and may now be able to use that to improve classification of place of articulation. To the extent that voicing and place decisions may be contingent (in fricatives) we should see gains in accuracy. This was then repeated for models trained to identify voicing (this time partialing out place).

Models were trained and tested with a K-fold procedure in which 1/20th of the data (144 tokens) was randomly selected and held out from training to use for test; we then repeated the procedure 20 times until all of the trials had served as test trials. This whole procedure was then repeated 10 times to get a stable estimate of accuracy across different random foldings. As in McMurray & Jongman (2011), model accuracy was evaluated in two ways: using the raw probabilities output by the model (the probabilistic rule) and making a discrete choice for each token (the outcome with the highest probability). These are presented as a range of accuracy in the figures below.

Figure 5 shows the results for place of articulation. Models performed well overall, averaging in the low to mid 80 % range. As in our prior work, models trained on raw cues performed worse than models trained on cues relative to talker and vowel (Figure 5A). However, in both cases, there was no benefit for the model knowing voicing (the difference between the gray and black ranges) – those models performed identically to ones with cues that were not relative to voicing. We broke these results down in a number of ways (e. g., by voicing, sibilance, etc.) and found no cases where residualizing by voicing was helpful. For example, Figure 5B shows the results using context-relative cues as a baseline for each of the four places of articulation. While clearly the non-sibilants (labiodental and interdental) were much harder, knowing the voicing did not improve performance; and for the sibilants, it may have offered slightly worse performance.

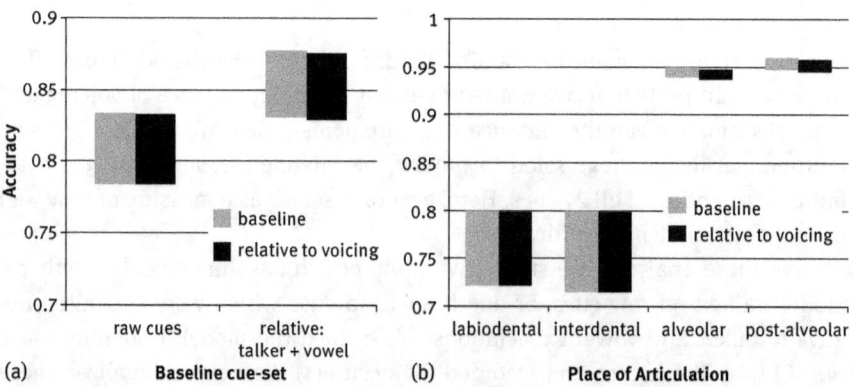

Figure 5: Classification accuracy (panel A: fricatives; panel B: place of articulation) of a model trained on 24 raw acoustic cues and a model trained on cues which were computed relative to talker and vowel expectations. 'Relative to voicing' represents accuracy when the voicing of each token is explicitly provided to the model.

Figure 6 shows similar findings for models trained to identify voicing. Performance is quite a bit higher, both because the cues are likely more distinct and because the model is being asked to perform an easier (2AFC) task. Again, we see that context-relative cues (talker and vowel) show better performance than raw cues. However, again, partialing out place of articulation appears to offer no better performance over the baseline models. As before, we broke this down by voicing, place of articulation, sibilance, talker gender, etc. Figure 6B, which shows performance as a function of place of articulation, is quite representative – in no case did we observe that cues computed relative to place of articulation were better for distinguishing voicing than cues that were not relative to place.

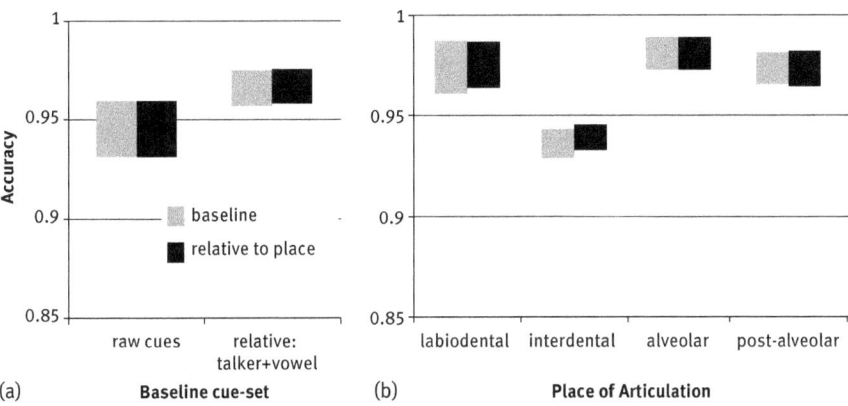

Figure 6: Classification accuracy (panel A: fricatives; panel B: place of articulation) of a model trained on 24 raw acoustic cues and a model trained on cues which were computed relative to talker and vowel expectations. 'Relative to place' represents accuracy when the place of articulation of each token is explicitly provided to the model.

5 Conclusions

C-CuRE provides a novel way to conceptualize and investigate the relation between the acoustic properties of speech and the perception of phonetic categories. Building on previous research into the nature of invariance and variability in the acoustic or articulatory signal, we suggest that the exact nature of any individual cue is not that important. Rather, we must consider a large number of cues. And more importantly, rather than thinking of how these cues are used in a simple, bottom-up framework, we must consider perception as part of a data explanation process in which listeners are actively parsing the variance in a set of cues into various components. We argue that this can be accomplished by relative cue encoding – encoding these cues relative to expected values derived from context (e. g. speaker and vowel), is crucial to match listeners' accuracy. Listeners use any and all cues available and use their experience and expectations. In addition to auditory or lexical properties, these expectations can derive from relatively abstract sources such as social expectations about what a male or female speaker should sound like.

However, expectation-driven processing does not mean there is no role for bottom-up acoustic information. While compensation occurs as the signal is interpreted relative to expectations driven by categories, listeners must categorize the first sound before they can account for its effects on the second sound. Our modeling of the relative contributions of place and voicing cues suggests that there are several acoustic cues that can be considered invariant. However, while it is the case that these invariant cues were more strongly correlated with place or voicing than with talker or vowel, they did not provide strong, unambiguous information about these dimensions; and their information can be amplified if context factors like talker and vowel are taken into account. In sum, then, there is some degree of invariant acoustic information in the speech signal that maps onto linguistic dimensions such as place of articulation and voicing. At a linguistic level, this supports the notion of fairly independent featural specifications for fricatives. However, this information alone is not sufficient to account for listeners' identification of fricatives. To approximate the performance of human listeners requires many cues, and these cues need to be interpreted relative to expectations derived from context.

More importantly, these analyses, suggest that the simple form of invariance that speech perception researchers have been seeking for so long may not be found universally, and certainly not for fricatives. However, at the same time, the fact that this information can be decomposed and used as a simple linear process suggests that the deep insight offered by the acoustic invariance approach may be true – there is lawful information in the signal that can be recovered by listeners with a minimum of fuss using domain-general mechanisms.

Acknowledgements: The authors would like to thank Keith Apfelbaum, Natasha Bullock-Rest, Ariane Rhone & Joan Sereno for helpful discussions on fricative perception and relative cue encoding during the development of these various projects. We also thank Sheila Blumstein for her trailblazing contributions to the phonetics, psycholinguistics, and cognitive neuroscience of speech perception. This research was supported by DC 008089 awarded to BM.

References

Andruski, J. E., Blumstein, S. E. & Burton, M. W. (1994). The effect of subphonetic differences on lexical access. *Cognition*, *52*, 163–187.

Apfelbaum, K. S., Bullock-Rest, N., Rhone, A., Jongman, A. & McMurray, B. (2014). Contingent categorization in speech perception. *Language, Cognition and Neuroscience*, *29*, 1070–1082.

Apfelbaum, K. S. & McMurray, B. (2015). Relative cue encoding in the context of sophisticated models of categorization: Separating information from categorization. *Psychonomic Bulletin & Review*, *22*, 916–943.

Baum, S. R. & Blumstein, S. E. (1987). Preliminary observations on the use of duration as a cue to syllable-initial fricative consonant voicing in English. *Journal of the Acoustical Society of America*, *82*, 1073–1077.

Behrens, S. J. & Blumstein, S. E. (1988). Acoustic characteristics of English voiceless fricatives: A descriptive analysis. *Journal of Phonetics*, *16*, 295–298.

Blumstein, S. E. & Stevens, K. N. (1979). Acoustic invariance in speech production: Evidence from measurements of the spectral characteristics of stop consonants. *Journal of the Acoustical Society of America*, *66*, 1001–1017.

Blumstein, S. E. & Stevens, K. N. (1980) Perceptual invariance and onset spectra for stop consonants in different vowel environments. *Journal of the Acoustical Society of America*, *67*, 648–662.

Blumstein, S. E. & Stevens, K. N. (1981). Phonetic features and acoustic invariance in speech. *Cognition*, *10*, 25–32.

Clark, A. (2013). Whatever next? Predictive brains, situated agents, and the future of cognitive science. *Behavioral and Brain Sciences*, *36*, 181–204.

Cohen, J. & Cohen, P. (1983). *Applied multiple regression/correlation analysis for the behavioral sciences* (2nd edition). Hillsdale, NJ: Erlbaum.

Cole, J. S., Linebaugh, G., Munson, C. & McMurray, B. (2010). Unmasking the acoustic effects of vowel-to-vowel coarticulation: A statistical modeling approach. *Journal of Phonetics*, *38*, 167–184.

Connine, C. (2004). It's not what you hear but how often you hear it: On the neglected role of phonological variant frequency in auditory word recognition. *Psychonomic Bulletin & Review*. *11*, 1084–1089.

Connine, C., Ranbom, L. & Patterson, D. (2008) Processing variant forms in spoken word recognition: The role of variant frequency. *Perception & Psychophysics*, *70*, 403–411.

Cooper, F. S., Delattre, P. C., Liberman, A. M., Borst, J. M. & Gerstman, L. J. (1952). Some experiments on the perception of synthetic speech sounds. *Journal of the Acoustical Society of America*, *24*, 597–606.

Creel, S. C., Aslin, R. N. & Tanenhaus, M. K. (2008). Heeding the voice of experience: The role of talker variation in lexical access. *Cognition*, *106*, 633–664.

Crystal, T. & House, A. (1988). Segmental durations in connected-speech signals: Current results. *Journal of the Acoustical Society of America*, *83*, 1553–1573.

Dahan, D., Magnuson, J. S., Tanenhaus, M. K. & Hogan, E. M. (2001). Subcategorical mismatches and the time course of lexical access: Evidence for lexical competition. *Language and Cognitive Processes*, *16*, 507–534.

Delattre, P., Liberman, A. M. & Cooper, F. S. (1955) Acoustic loci and transitional cues for consonants. *Journal of the Acoustical Society of America*, *27*, 769–773.

Diehl, R. L. & Kluender, K. R. (1989). On the objects of speech perception. *Ecological Psychology*, *1*, 121–144.

Elman, J. & McClelland, J. (1986). Exploiting Lawful Variability in the Speech Wave. In J. S. Perkell & D. Klatt (Eds.) *Invariance and Variability in Speech Processes*, 360–380. Hillsdale, NJ: Erlbaum

Feldman, N. H., Griffiths, T. L. & Morgan, J. L. (2009). The influence of categories on perception: Explaining the perceptual magnet effect as optimal statistical inference. *Psychological Review*, *116*, 752–782.

Forrest, K., Weismer, G., Milenkovic, P. & Dougall, R. N. (1988). Statistical analysis of word-initial voiceless obstruents: Preliminary data. *Journal of the Acoustical Society of America*, *84*, 115–124.

Fowler, C. A. (1986). An event approach to a theory of speech perception from a direct-realist perspective. *Journal of Phonetics*, *14*, 3–28.

Fowler, C. A. (1994) Invariants, specifiers, cues: An investigation of locus equations as information for place of articulation. *Perception & Psychophysics*, *55*, 597–611.

Fowler, C. & Brown, J. (2000). Perceptual parsing of acoustic consequences of velum lowering from information for vowels. *Perception & Psychophysics*, *62*, 21–32.

Fowler, C. & Smith, M. (1986). Speech perception as "vector analysis": An approach to the problems of segmentation and invariance. In J. Perkell & D. Klatt (eds.) *Invariance and variability in speech processes*,123–136. Hillsdale, NJ: Erlbaum.

Galantucci, B. Fowler, C. A. & Turvey, M. T. (2006). The motor theory of speech perception reviewed. *Psychonomic Bulletin and Review 13*, 361–377.

Goldinger, S. D. (1998) Echoes of Echoes? An episodic theory of lexical access. *Psychological Review*, *105*, 251–279.

Gow, D. (2001) Assimilation and anticipation in continuous spoken word recognition. *Journal of Memory and Language*, *45*, 133–139.

Gow, D. W. (2003). Feature parsing: Feature cue mapping in spoken word recognition. *Perception & Psychophysics*, *65*, 575–590

Jongman, A., Wayland, R. & Wong, S. (2000). Acoustic characteristics of English fricatives. *Journal of the Acoustical Society of America*, *106*, 1252–1263.

Jongman, A. (2013). Acoustic Phonetics. *Oxford Bibliographies in Linguistics*. Edited by M. Aronoff. New York: Oxford University Press, 2013-03-19. URL: http://www.oxfordbibliographies.com/view/document/obo-9780199772810/obo-9780199772810-0047.xml?rskey-=8kNg37&result=42&q=

Kewley-Port, D. (1983). Time-varying features as correlates of place of articulation in stop consonants. *Journal of the Acoustical Society of America*, *73*, 322–335.

Kewley-Port, D. & Luce, P. A. (1984). Time-varying features of initial stop consonants in auditory running spectra: A first report. *Perception & Psychophysics*, *35*, 353–360.

Lahiri, A., Gewirth, L. & Blumstein, S. E. (1984). A reconsideration of acoustic invariance for place of articulation in diffuse stop consonants: evidence from a cross-language study. *Journal of the Acoustical Society of America*, *76*, 391–404.

Lahiri, A. & Reetz, H. (2010). Distinctive features: Phonological underspecification in representation and processing. *Journal of Phonetics*, *38*, 44–59.

Liberman, A. M. (1996). *Speech: A special code*. Cambridge, MA: MIT Press.

Liberman, A. M., Cooper, F. S., Shankweiler, D. P. & Studdert-Kennedy, M. (1967). Perception of the speech code. *Psychological Review*, *74*, 431–461.

Liberman, A. M. & I. G. Mattingly. (1985). The motor theory of speech perception revised. *Cognition*, *21*, 1–36.

Lindblom, B. (1996). Role of articulation in speech perception: Clues from production. *Journal of the Acoustical Society of America*, *99*, 1683–1692.

Maniwa, K., Jongman, A. & Wade, T. (2009) Acoustic characteristics of clearly produced fricatives. *Journal of the Acoustical Society of America*, *125*, 3962–3973.

Marslen-Wilson, W. & Warren, P. (1994). Levels of perceptual representation and process in lexical access: Words, phonemes, and features. *Psychological Review*, *101*, 653–675.

Martin, J. G. & Bunnell, H. T. (1981). Perception of anticipatory coarticulation effects. *Journal of the Acoustical Society of America*, *69*, 559–567.

Martin, J. G. & Bunnell, H. T. (1982). Perception of anticipatory coarticulation effects in vowel-stop consonant-vowel sequences. *Journal of Experimental Psychology: Human Perception and Performance*, *8*, 473–488.

McClelland, J. L. & Elman, J. L. (1986). The TRACE model of speech perception. *Cognitive Psychology*, *18*, 1–86.

McMurray, B., Aslin, R., Tanenhaus, M., Spivey, M. & Subik, D. (2008). Gradient sensitivity to within-category variation in speech: Implications for categorical perception. *Journal of Experimental Psychology, Human Perception and Performance*, *34*, 1609–1631.

McMurray, B., Cole, J. S. & Munson, C. (2011). Features as an emergent product of computing perceptual cues relative to expectations. In Ridouane, R. & Clement, N. (eds.), *Where do Features Come From?*, 197–236. Amsterdam: John Benjamins Publishing.

McMurray, B. & Farris-Trimble, A. (2012) Emergent information-level coupling between perception and production. In A. Cohn, C. Fougeron & M. Huffman (eds.), *The Oxford Handbook of Laboratory Phonology*, 369–395. Oxford, UK: Oxford University Press.

McMurray, B., Rhone, A. & Hannaway, K. (2016) Relativity in speech perception: From locus equations to predictive coding. In A. Agwuele and A. Lotto (eds.) *Essays in Speech Processes: Language Production and Perception*, 30–67. Sheffield, UK: Equinox Publishing

McMurray, B. & Jongman, A. (2011). What information is necessary for speech categorization? Harnessing variability in the speech signal by integrating cues computed relative to expectations. *Psychological Review*, *118*, 219–246.

McMurray, B. & Jongman, A. (2016). What comes after [f]? Prediction in speech is a product of expectation and signal. *Psychological Science*, *27*, 43–52.

McMurray, B., Tanenhaus, M. & Aslin, R. (2002). Gradient effects of within-category phonetic variation on lexical access, *Cognition*, *86*, B33-B42.

McMurray, B., Tanenhaus, M. K. & Aslin, R. N. (2009) Within-category VOT affects recovery from "lexical" garden paths: Evidence against phoneme-level inhibition. *Journal of Memory and Language*, *60*, 65–91.

Mermelstein, P. (1978). On the relationship between vowel and consonant identification when cued by the same acoustic information. *Perception & Psychophysics*, *23*, 331–336.

Miller, J. L. (1997). Internal structure of phonetic categories. *Language and Cognitive Processes*, *12*, 865–869.

Nearey, T. M. (1990). The segment as a unit of speech perception. *Journal of Phonetics*, *18*, 347–373.

Nearey, T. M. (1997). Speech perception as pattern recognition. *Journal of the Acoustical Society of America*, *101*, 3241–3254.

Oden, G. (1978). Integration of place and voicing information in the identification of synthetic stop consonants. *Journal of Phonetics*, *6*, 83–93.

Oden, G. & Massaro, D. W. (1978). Integration of featural information in speech perception. *Psychological Review*, *85*, 172–191.

Ohala, J. (1996). Speech perception is hearing sounds, not tongues. *Journal of the Acoustical Society of America*, *99*, 1718–1725.

Pisoni, D. B. (1997). Some thoughts on "normalization" in speech perception. In K. Johnson and J.W. Mullennix (eds.), *Talker Variability in Speech Processing*, 9–32. San Diego: Academic Press.

Pisoni, D. B. & Sawusch, J. R. (1974). On the identification of place and voicing features in synthetic stop consonants. *Journal of Phonetics*, *2*, 181–194.

Port, R. F. (2007). How are words stored in memory? Beyond phones and phonemes. *New Ideas in Psychology*, *25*, 143–170.

Port, R. F. & Dalby, J. (1982). Consonant/vowel ratio as a cue for voicing in English. *Perception & Psychophysics*, *32*, 141–152.

Repp, B. H. (1982). Phonetic trading relations and context effects: New evidence for a phonetic mode of perception. *Psychological Bulletin*, *92*, 81–110.

Salverda, A. P., Dahan, D. & McQueen, J. (2003). The role of prosodic boundaries in the resolution of lexical embedding in speech comprehension. *Cognition*, *90*, 51–89.

Salverda, A. P., Kleinschmidt, D. & Tanenhaus, M. K. (2014). Immediate effects of anticipatory coarticulation in spoken-word recognition. *Journal of Memory and Language*, *71*, 145–163.

Sawusch, J. R. & Pisoni, D. B. (1974). On the identification of place and voicing features in synthetic stop consonants. *Journal of Phonetics*, *2*, 181–194.

Schatz, C. D. (1954). The role of context in the perception of stops. *Language*, *30*, 47–56.

Shankweiler, D. & Fowler, C. A. (2015). Seeking a reading machine for the blind and discovering the speech code. *History of Psychology*, *18*, 78–99.

Smits, R. (2001a). Evidence for hierarchical categorization of coarticulated phonemes. *Journal of Experimental Psychology: Human Perception and Performance*, *27*, 1145–1162.

Smits, R. (2001b). Hierarchical categorization of coarticulated phonemes: A theoretical analysis. *Perception & Psychophysics*, *63*, 1109–1139.

Stevens, K. N. & Blumstein, S. E. (1981). The search for invariant acoustic correlates of phonetic features. In P. D. Eimas & J. L. Miller (eds.), *Perspectives on the Study of Speech*, 1–39. New Jersey: Erlbaum.

Stevens, K. N., Blumstein, S. E., Glicksman, L., Burton, M. & Kurowski, K. (1992). Acoustic and perceptual characteristics of voicing in fricatives and fricative clusters. *Journal of the Acoustical Society of America*, *91*, 2979–3000.

Strevens, P. (1960). Spectra of fricative noise in human speech. *Language and Speech*, *3*, 32–49.

Sussman, H. M., McCaffrey, H. A. & Matthews, S. A. (1991). An investigation of locus equations as a source of relational invariance for stop place categorization. *Journal of the Acoustical Society of America*, *90*, 1309–1325.

Sussman, H. M., Fruchter, D., Hilbert, J. & Sirosh, J. (1998). Linear correlates in the speech signal: The orderly output constraint. *Behavioral and Brain Sciences*, *21*, 241–259.

Toscano, J. C. & McMurray, B. (2010). Cue integration with categories: Weighting acoustic cues in speech using unsupervised learning and distributional statistics. *Cognitive Science*, *34*, 434–464.

Utman, J. A., Blumstein, S. E. & Burton, M. W. (2000). Effects of unsystematic and rule-governed acoustic variation on word recognition. *Perception and Psychophysics*, *62*, 1297–1311.

Willis, R. (1830). On the vowel sounds, and on reed organ pipes. *Transactions of the Cambridge Philosophical Society*, *3*, 231–269.

Yeni-Komshian, G. H. & Soli, S. D. (1981). Recognition of vowels from information in fricatives: Perceptual evidence of fricative-vowel coarticulation. *Journal of the Acoustical Society of America*, *70*, 966–975.

Zacks, J. M., Speer, N. K., Swallow, K. M., Braver, T. S. & Reynolds, J. R. (2007). Event perception: A mind/brain perspective. *Psychological Bulletin*, *133*, 273–293.

Emily Myers, Alexis R. Johns, F. Sayako Earle and Xin Xie
The invariance problem in the acquisition of non-native phonetic contrasts: From instances to categories

Abstract: The invariance problem refers to the challenge that listeners face when confronted with acoustic variability in speech sounds as they attempt to map these sounds to few phonological categories. This problem is compounded in the adult non-native language learner, in that the listener must overcome processing biases that prevent the perception of key differences among tokens within the native language category. Evidence from behavioral and neural data suggests that phonetic category learning can be described as a two-stage process, in which categorical sensitivity first emerges in frontal brain structures, and subsequently "tunes" perceptual areas in the temporal lobes. Moreover, sleep appears to modulate non-native category learning. Taken together, these findings provide new insight regarding the overall trajectory of phonetic learning that results in heightened sensitivity to non-native sounds.

1 Introduction

For any language user, the object of language comprehension is to take the acoustic signal and map it to the lexical, syntactic, and semantic structures that enable the listener to extract meaning. A fundamental obstacle to this goal occurs very early in the processing stream when the speech signal is mapped onto the sounds of one's language. It has long been observed that the acoustics that characterize the sounds of speech are variable (Liberman, Cooper, Shankweiler & Studdert-Kennedy, 1967; Lisker & Abramson, 1964; Peterson & Barney, 1952). The acoustic tokens that a listener ultimately maps to a given

---

Emily Myers, Department of Speech, Language and Hearing Sciences, University of Connecticut
Alexis R. Johns, Brandeis University Memory & Cognition Lab
F. Sayako Earle, College of Health Sciences, University of Delaware
Xin Xie, Department of Brain and Cognitive Sciences, University of Rochester

phoneme (such as /t/) may vary within different instances of a given speaker's production, across speakers, according to the surrounding phonological context due to coarticulation, and can vary given different speech rates, dialects, and speaking registers. As such, the challenge for the listener seems substantial: one must sort through this multidimensional acoustic variability in order to extract the relevant parameters to access phonemic identity. This problem, termed the 'invariance problem for speech' has occupied speech perception researchers for the past sixty years.

How then, do listeners map such acoustic variability to the limited inventory of speech sounds? One approach to the invariance problem is to posit that there is a dimension or combination of dimensions of the signal which is constant irrespective of the talker, the phonological context, and other sources of variability. Two dominant types of theories have attempted to find these invariant dimensions. One perspective is that higher-order acoustic properties of speech sounds provide invariant cues to phoneme identity, even when surface-level acoustic properties are variable. Work from Stevens and Blumstein (Blumstein & Stevens, 1979, 1980; Stevens & Blumstein, 1978) showed that for some phonemic contrasts, higher-order acoustic properties such as spectral shape following a stop burst can serve to reliably categorize that stop even as phonological context changes. A competing perspective from a class of theories known as motor or gestural theories of speech perception posits that perceptual constancy instead arises through access to shared gestural or motor codes for producing each phoneme that are proposed to be a source of constancy amidst potential variability (Galantucci, Fowler & Turvey, 2006; Liberman & Mattingly, 1985).

An alternative approach suggests that no such inherent invariances need be present in the input. Instead the listener constructs on-the-fly perceptual schemes to process acoustic variability in speech. This kind of system requires that listeners adjust their perceptual criteria dynamically for each talker, phonological context, speech rate, accent, etc. Depending on the context, acoustic and/or articulatory cues may be re-weighted in order to accommodate the particular demands of that listening environment (Francis & Nusbaum, 2002; Holt & Lotto, 2006). In this view, listeners may still take advantage of perceptual constancies in the input, but also reweight the relative contribution of different cues as the listening context changes.

Even if listeners are able to use acoustic or motor invariances in the input, they must learn how these properties map to phonemes within a language. For example, speakers of various languages might rely on different acoustic properties to signal the same phonetic contrast (McAllister, Flege & Piske, 2002). Similarly, if motor invariances serve as anchors for perception, it is logical to posit that the link between the acoustic signal and the motor representation must be learned through an individuals' monitoring of his/her own productions. Alternatively, if phonetic perception is constructed through context-guided dynamic weighting of different acoustic cues, a listener would have to be exposed to a large range of variability (e. g., different phonological environments, different talkers, different speech rates, etc.) in order to support generalization to novel environments (Bradlow, Pisoni, Akahane-Yamada & Tohkura, 1997; Lively, Logan & Pisoni, 1993). The types of input that facilitate speech sound learning, the mechanisms that underlie learning and generalization, and the neural systems that support learning are the subject of the current chapter.

1.1 Non-native speech sound learning in adulthood

Most individuals learning a second language after puberty show evidence of incomplete acquisition of the speech sound system. This is most observable in speech production: a substantial majority of late L2 learners have a perceptible non-native accent (Flege, MacKay & Meador, 1999). Incomplete acquisition is also apparent in perception: differences among non-native speech sounds can be very difficult, if not impossible for adults to perceive, even with substantial real-world experience (Flege, 1991; Flege et al., 1999) as well as directed training (Golestani & Zatorre, 2009). An unanswered question is precisely why adults show comparatively poor perception of non-native speech contrasts, especially when some aspects of language processing such as lexical semantics and simple properties of grammar, can successfully reach native-like expertise (Clahsen & Felser, 2006; Sanders & Neville, 2003; Weber-Fox & Neville, 1996).

1.2 Perceptual narrowing and the loss of neural plasticity for speech sound learning

Infants show sensitivity to most (if not entirely all) phonological contrasts in the world's languages (Eimas, Siqueland, Jusczyk & Vigorito, 1971; Polka & Werker, 1994; Sundara, Polka & Genesee, 2006; Werker & Tees, 1999), an ability which is gradually lost over the first two years of life. This phenomenon has been termed 'perceptual narrowing', the end result of which is an adult system that is highly proficient at native sound processing, but consequently struggles to distinguish novel speech sounds. This maturational process has prompted the hypothesis that early neural tuning to the sounds of one's native language interferes with subsequent L2 learning, (the Native Language Neural Commitment hypothesis,

Kuhl et al., 2008; Kuhl, Conboy, Padden, Nelson & Pruitt, 2005). A logical extension of the Native Language Neural Commitment hypothesis is that a loss of neural plasticity is at the root of failures in adult non-native speech sound acquisition (Kuhl, 2010). Rigidity in the neural system, specifically a lack of neural plasticity in the perceptual system handling speech sounds, is assumed be a barrier to learning speech sounds after the critical period.

It has been surprisingly difficult to show exactly how neural plasticity for speech sound perception changes as children mature. Current literature on the neural bases of infant speech sound learning suggests that changes in either theta or gamma band activity between 6 and 12 months of age are related to increasing sensitivity to native-language contrasts compared to non-native contrasts, which parallels infants' behavioral sensitivities to the same contrasts (Bosseler et al., 2013). Yet these results only hint at a mechanism for this shift in neural activity. Kuhl and colleagues propose that perceptual narrowing may be a result of an attentional process in which attention shifts from more frequent instances in their input (statistical learning) to category-level information in the input (Bosseler et al., 2013). In short we know that perceptual narrowing occurs because infants develop specific expertise in the sounds of their own language to the exclusion of sounds in other languages, and we have an emerging picture of the neural systems that change alongside perceptual narrowing, yet there is no agreed-upon explanation for why the adult system should show such inflexibility.

Loss of sensitivity to non-native contrasts might not simply be the *normal* developmental trajectory, it may also be *beneficial* for the language-learning child. Infants who retain an ability to perceive difficult non-native contrasts at 7 months show paradoxically *lower* vocabulary development at 30 months than infants who lose this sensitivity early (Kuhl et al., 2005). One interpretation of this finding is that the ability to focus on only those sound contrasts that cue differences in meaning allows the infant learner to ignore extraneous (and computationally demanding) acoustic information that might distract them from word learning. The end result, however, is that as individuals mature, obstacles to speech sound learning grow.

1.3 The categorical cliff and climbing out of local minima: hazards of native language perceptual topography

The adult language learner differs from the infant language learner not only in the qualities of the adult learning system (i. e., potential losses in plasticity) but also differs in the initial conditions of the perceptual space. Adult L2 language learners by definition have a fully-acquired L1 perceptual system which has become specialized for sounds of their native language. One consequence of this specialization is that at least some speech sounds become perceived categorically (Liberman, Harris, Hoffman & Griffith, 1957). That is, while adult listeners readily perceive differences between two speech sounds drawn from different sound categories (e. g., /d/ vs. /t/), they are less able to perceive differences between sounds that fall within the same category. Categorical perception is especially evident for short-duration speech sounds such as stops, but is observed to a lesser extent for vowels and fricatives as well (Fry, Abramson, Eimas & Liberman, 1962; Healy & Repp, 1982; Liberman et al., 1967).

Categorical perception may be facilitatory for native language speech processing but it can be detrimental to adults learning non-native speech contrasts. If two non-native speech sounds fall within the boundaries of one native language sound, the adult listener will often be unable to differentiate these sounds. Best's Perceptual Assimilation Model (Best & McRoberts, 2003; Best, McRoberts & Goodell, 2001) predicts that non-native contrasts will be more difficult to perceive (and presumably, also more difficult to acquire) when the sound is heard as an exemplar of a native-language category, but slightly easier to acquire if listeners can perceive the non-native sound as a 'not-as-good' exemplar of their native language sound, and rather easy when the sound is unlike any sound in the listener's inventory (Best, McRoberts & Sithole, 1988). A paradigmatic case is the Hindi dental vs. retroflex voiced stop contrast. For English-speaking listeners, both sounds are perceived as variants of an alveolar /d/ sound. As such, distinguishing the dental from the retroflex sound is difficult for native-English listeners (Golestani & Zatorre, 2004; Pruitt, Jenkins & Strange, 2006; Swan & Myers, 2013).

The similarity of non-native sounds to existing native-language categories may be characterized in terms of the acoustic similarity (or gestural similarity) between sounds (Best & Hallé, 2010; Best & Tyler, 2007). Speech perception can be described as a process of mapping the acoustic token into a perceptually-warped acoustic space, with the center of the phonetic category occupying a local minimum in this space (Guenther & Gjaja, 1996; Guenther, Husain, Cohen & Shinn-Cunningham, 1999; Kuhl, 1991). A non-native speech sound which is close in acoustic space to an existing, native-language category will be drawn towards the center of this probability distribution, whereas sounds which are further away will be subject to less pull from the native language sound. This view generates the prediction that (a) the closer a non-native speech sound is to a native-language sound, the more difficult it will be to learn and (b) native-language speech sounds with denser probability distributions will exert a stronger pull on the to-be-learned non-native sounds.

1.4 Paying attention to attention

An alternative approach attributes non-native speech learning difficulties not to the topography of the native language perceptual map, but rather to differences in the way attention is directed to acoustic parameters in the input (Holt & Lotto, 2006; Francis & Nusbaum, 2002). Certain aspects of any given speech sound will be diagnostic of its identity (e. g., formants for vowels) but other parameters will be irrelevant or redundant (e. g., pitch for vowels). Importantly, these parameters may vary significantly by language, by position in the word, and even by talker. For instance, English combines duration and spectral cues to distinguish the /i/ vs. /I/ contrast. However, English speakers appear to preferentially weight spectral cues in identifying these sounds, whereas native speakers of Finnish, a language that uses duration phonemically in vowel contrasts, will tend to weight duration cues more strongly than spectral cues (Ylinen et al., 2010).

Similarly, a shared acoustic dimension may distinguish between sounds across two languages, but the location of the boundary along that dimension may differ. For instance, English voiced and voiceless stops in stressed, syllable-initial position differ primarily in voice onset time (VOT), which is the time between the release of the constriction in the oral cavity and the onset of the vocal fold vibration signaling the start of the vowel (Lisker & Abramson, 1964). While the VOT value that marks the boundary between voiced and voiceless stops can vary based on speaking rate, place of articulation, and talker (Allen, Miller & DeSteno, 2003; Miller, 1994; Volaitis & Miller, 1992), in general stops with VOTs less than about 20 msec VOT will be perceived by native English speakers as voiced, whereas those with VOTs greater than 30 msec will be perceived as voiceless. Other languages (e. g., Spanish) also use a VOT distinction to signal differences in voicing, but the boundary will fall close to 0 msec VOT, with stops with negative VOTs (prevoiced) being perceived as voiced and those with positive VOTs perceived as voiceless (Lisker & Abramson, 1964).

Taken together, a listener's task when confronted with a novel speech sound contrast is to determine (a) which acoustic dimensions are diagnostic for that contrast and (b) the location in acoustic space of the boundary between sounds. Attention to Dimension (A2D) models posit that the task of the listener is to shift auditory attention appropriately towards the correct acoustic dimension (Francis & Nusbaum, 2002). This may involve directing attention to a previously unattended dimension, as in the case of Finnish speakers learning to weight spectral cues over durational cues for vowel perception in English. Alternatively, this process may involve perceptual re-warping along a dimension that was previously attended (Francis, Baldwin & Nusbaum, 2000; Francis & Nusbaum, 2002; Guenther et al., 1999) such that a portion of acoustic space that was perceptually collapsed is now expanded, as in the case of an English speaker learning to perceive the new boundary location for stop contrasts in Spanish. These models take as a given the idea that attention can be dynamically adjusted based on the language context (e. g., "am I hearing Finnish or English vowels?").

A strength of A2D models is that they capture the dynamic nature of the speech perception system in a bilingual listener, in which different criteria may be used as the listener switches between languages. Moreover, A2D models can be adapted to describe the flexibility in processing as listeners adjust to other relevant features even within the native language environment. For instance, this kind of mechanism might assist a listener in recognizing an idiosyncratic version of a sound linked to a given talker – for instance, in listening to a talker with a lisped /s/ sound (see Section 3 for a discussion of flexibility in native language speech sound perception).

2 Optimal and limiting conditions for non-native speech sound learning

Learning a non-native speech sound category requires two steps. First, the learner must discover the properties of acoustic space which are relevant for the to-be-learned contrast. Second, the learner must be able to generalize from the learning context to new exemplars. These processes likely rely on different mechanisms, have distinct timelines, and tap distinct neural resources. In particular, as we argue below, sleep and memory processes play a crucial role in both retention of learned information and generalization to new contexts.

2.1 Perceptual learning of non-native speech contrasts

We take as given that successful learning of a non-native phonological contrast will result in accurate identification of sounds that map to the learned sound categories, this being the minimum prerequisite for mapping these sounds ultimately onto words in L2. However the extent to which L2 contrasts are processed like native-language contrasts is less clear. One hallmark of native-language speech contrasts is, as stated previously, that sounds tend to be categorically perceived. Recall that the key metric of categorical perception is that two phonetic tokens which fall into separate learned categories will be easy to discriminate, whereas those two tokens that fall within the same category will be more difficult (or even impossible) to tell apart. We propose that the success of non-native speech acquisition can be measured not only by the accuracy of a listener in *identifying* a non-native sound, but by the degree to which non-native contrasts are perceived categorically.

Phonetic learning can benefit from several sources of information. On the one hand, listeners may be able to track the statistical distribution of auditory tokens in the input in order to discover the perceptual space that new speech sounds occupy. Since this process is proposed to be independent of the recognition of acoustic tokens as members of any particular phonetic category, the use of this kind of information is referred to as 'bottom-up' because it proceeds from lower-level details of the input (Hayes-Harb, 2007; Maye, Werker & Gerken, 2002). However, the use of statistical cues to learn non-native speech sound categories has been less attested in the literature. In addition to distributional information, listeners may also be able to exploit information in the input regarding the presence of perceptual categories. This kind of information is referred to as 'top-down' information because it originates at a higher level of processing.

2.2 Top-down induction of categorical sensitivities

In laboratory studies, top-down information is provided to participants via explicit feedback or the association of the auditory input with a visual object. In the real world, top-down information about phonetic category status can come from learning minimal pairs and explicit classroom instruction. Notably, with sufficient repetition, provision of top-down information is enough to increase listener sensitivity to contrasts that fall into two learned categories (Golestani & Zatorre, 2009; McCandliss, Fiez, Protopapas, Conway & McClelland, 2002; Swan & Myers, 2013), and will transfer to discrimination tasks.

For instance, in a study from our lab, native English-speaking listeners were trained on a synthesized acoustic continuum which ranged from a dental to retroflex to velar CV syllable, that is, from /d̪a/ to /ḍa/ to /ga/ (Swan & Myers, 2013). Participants were trained to categorize tokens from this three-way continuum into two distinct categories, with one group trained to place the boundary between the dental and retroflex sounds, and the other group trained to place the boundary between the retroflex and velar sounds (see Figure 1). While participants in both groups achieved success in learning the category boundary, of interest was whether categorization training transferred to an untrained skill: that is, the ability to discriminate tokens that either fell within a learned category or fell between the two learned categories. For the dental/retroflex contrast, participants who had been trained to categorize dental and retroflex sounds into different categories showed enhanced discrimination after training, whereas participants who had been trained such that dental and retroflex sounds both fell within the same category showed no change in discrimination (Figure 2). Notably, passive exposure to the same type of input produced no changes in discrimination. Taken together, this suggests that explicit feedback to the participant was necessary to induce shifts in between-category sensitivity (McCandliss et al., 2002; McClelland, Fiez & McCandliss, 2002).

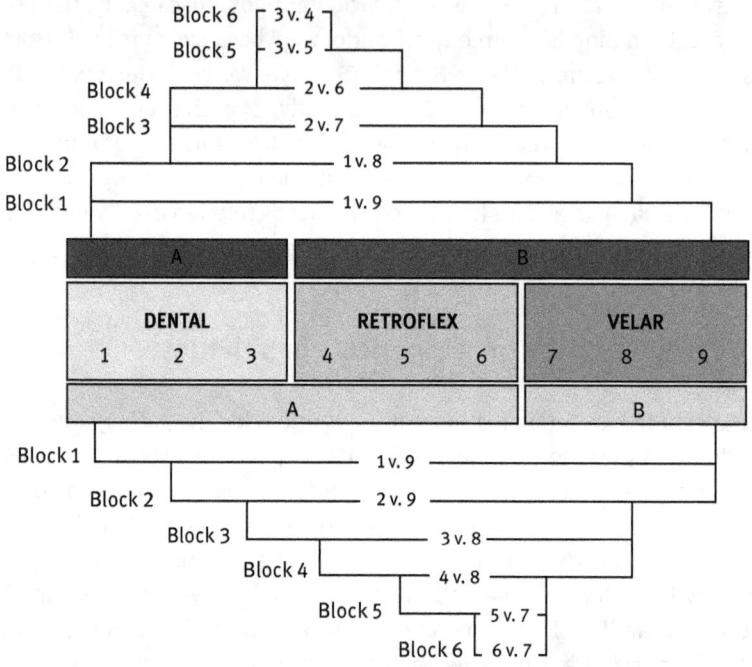

Figure 1: From (Swan & Myers, 2013). Schematic of perceptual fading training schedule. Nine-point continuum shown in center, appropriate category labels denoted with 'A' and 'B'. Dental/Retroflex group shown with upper pattern and Retroflex/Velar group with lower pattern. Category labels induce boundary-dependent perceptual warping in learned speech categories. Second Language research, 29(4), 391–411.

In their seminal study of categorical perception, Liberman and colleagues propose that the relative ease of discriminating between-category compared to within-category contrasts might result from one (or both) of two mechanisms: *acquired similarity* (also known as *acquired equivalence*) or *acquired distinctiveness* (Liberman et al., 1957). The acquired similarity account states that over the course of learning, sensitivity to within-category contrasts declines while sensitivity to between-category contrasts is maintained. In contrast, acquired distinctiveness reflects increased sensitivity to between-category contrasts in the face of maintained sensitivity to within-category contrasts. Evidence for acquired similarity in certainly seen in the developmental literature, in which there is substantial evidence for loss of sensitivity to non-native contrasts as infants mature (Eimas et al., 1971; Werker & Tees, 1984), but fewer observed instances of increases in sensitivity to native language contrasts (Polka, Colantonio & Sundara, 2001).

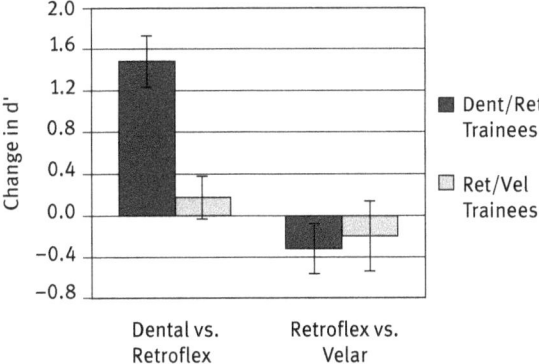

Figure 2: Changes in discrimination accuracy, as assessed by d', after training on one of two different boundary locations along a dental-retroflex-velar continuum. Black bars show data from a group that was trained to place the boundary between dental and retroflex items, the grey bars show the group that was trained to place the category boundary between the retroflex and velar stimuli. Error bars indicate standard error of the mean. Modified from Swan & Myers 2013. Category labels induce boundary-dependent perceptual warping in learned speech categories. Second Language research, 29(4), 391–411.

In general, limited evidence exists for acquired similarity related to novel sound contrasts learned in *adulthood*. A possible exception comes from a study by Guenther and colleagues (Guenther et al., 1999) which demonstrated that training listeners to identify items from a novel sound continuum produced poorer discrimination of tokens taken from within the learned category. However, studies have primarily shown that identification training tends to result in enhanced perception of between-category differences. The fact that re-warping of perceptual space is mainly revealed by increases in performance for between-category contrasts as compared to decreases in performance for within-category contrasts may be due to a fairly trivial reason. Given that adults already show relatively poor discrimination of non-native contrasts, there may be no direction to go but up: acquired distinctiveness is more probable. This notion was corroborated in a study from our lab investigating the effects of intense, multi-day categorization training on the acquisition of a non-native contrast (Myers, Mesite & Del Tufo, in prep). After ten days of identification training, with pre- and post-training assessments of discrimination every day, large increases in discrimination sensitivity were seen for stimulus pairs that fell between categories, whereas no significant change (either decrease or increase) was observed for pairs that fell within categories (Figure 3), controlling for the size of the acoustic interval between pairs. Interpreting this result from the stance of Attention-to-Dimension models of phonetic learning suggests that attention is allocated specifically to those portions of acoustic space (e. g., the boundary region of the continuum), which are useful for allowing listeners to distinguish among the trained categories, but not to the entire length of the continuum (Francis & Nusbaum, 2002). Taken together, these results show that even non-ecological, laboratory-based training can induce perceptual patterns that begin to resemble those of native language speech sounds, namely good discrimination of between-category sounds in the face of poor discrimination of within-category sounds.

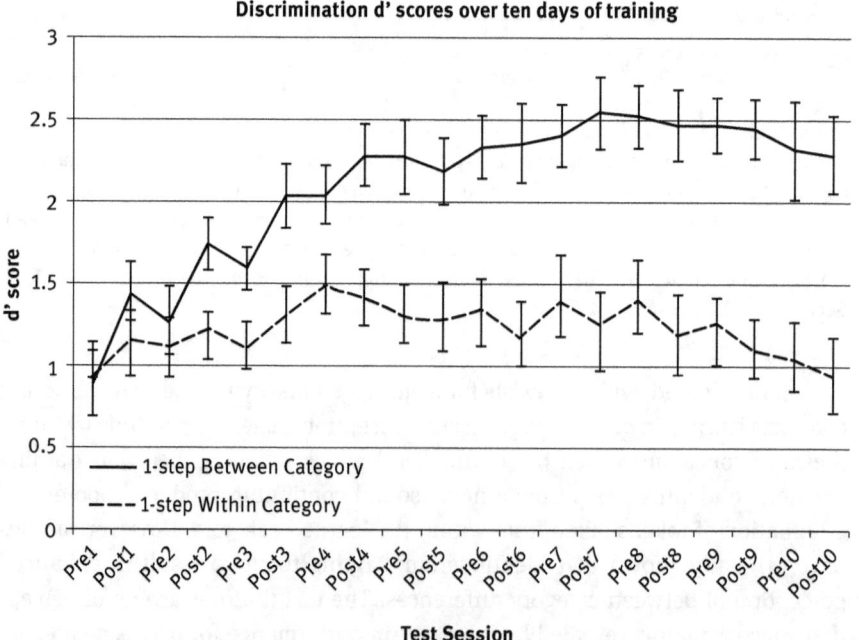

Figure 3: Myers, Mesite & Del Tufo, in prep. Participants were trained over ten sessions to categorize dental and retroflex tokens. Before (pre) and after (post) each training session, listeners performed an AX discrimination task on stimulus pairs that either fell within the trained category (1-step Within Category) or between trained categories (1-step Between Category). Error bars indicate standard error of the mean.

2.3 Neural pathways for non-native speech sound learning

Learning non-native contrasts induces changes in behavioral sensitivity which are accompanied by changes in neural pathways for speech sound processing, and an examination of the engagement of these regions over the course of training helps us understand which underlying cognitive mechanisms are recruited for speech sound learning. Before describing changes in this network, it is important to first understand the neural systems that underlie native speech sound processing.

In adults, mapping a native language speech sound from acoustics to meaning involves a network of brain areas with specific roles for processing aspects of the speech signal (see Blumstein & Myers, 2014 for review). While many brain areas are involved at some level in the perception of speech sounds, a temporal-to-frontal lobe pathway is crucial for phonetic perception. At the cortical level, speech sounds are processed by the bilateral temporal lobes, which show specialization for human speech sounds in general, and for native language speech sounds specifically (Chang et al., 2010; Hickok & Poeppel, 2004; Myers, 2014; Scott & Johnsrude, 2003). From the temporal lobes, additional processing may proceed to the left inferior frontal gyrus in regions within or adjacent to Broca's area (D'Ausilio, Craighero & Fadiga, 2012; Myers, Blumstein, Walsh & Eliassen, 2009).

Notably, the temporal lobes appear to show exquisite sensitivity to the structure of native language categories. Because speech sounds exist on a continuum, some sounds are better (or more representative) exemplars of their phonetic category (Miller, 1994). In the VOT domain, for instance, exemplars of /t/ with a VOT of about 70 msec are more typical than those with a VOT of 35 msec or 120 msec, although all of these tokens will be mapped by English speakers to the /t/ category. The bilateral temporal lobes show sensitivity to this internal structure of the phonetic category, showing activation in proportion to the 'goodness of fit' of a token to its phonetic category (Myers, 2007; Myers et al., 2009). This, together with evidence that the temporal lobes generally respond to fine-grained aspects of the speech signal, suggests that bilateral temporal lobes are a center for processing the structure of the phonetic category.

More controversial is the role of frontal regions in processing the sounds of speech (Hickok, Costanzo, Capasso & Miceli, 2011). Frontal brain regions are often seen to be engaged during speech tasks which require an overt response such as a phonetic categorization judgment, but less often in passive listening tasks. This leads to the assertion that these regions are only engaged when explicit decisions must be made (Hickok & Poeppel, 2007). Engagement of frontal regions is also seen when listeners are confronted with greater difficulty in processing, particularly when listening to speech in noise or when the signal itself is ambiguous

(D'Ausilio, Bufalari, Salmas & Fadiga, 2012; Myers, 2007). Therefore a critical question is whether the involvement of the frontal lobe for speech sound processing represents core and essential processes for language comprehension, or whether the frontal lobe performs a more auxiliary or supplemental role.

Other evidence from imaging studies suggests a larger role for the left frontal lobe in speech sound processing. In particular, the left IFG may play a significant role in phonetic category processing even in the absence of an explicit task (Myers et al., 2009). For instance in an fMRI study employing a passive listening task, neural sensitivity was measured in response to two different types of stimulus changes: changes in phonetic category (e. g., from /ta/ to /da/) as compared to changes in acoustics within a category (e. g., /ta/ with a VOT of 35 msec compared to /ta/ with a VOT of 60 msec). Only a left frontal region (but not temporal areas) showed an 'invariant' pattern of response, with sensitivity to changes in phonetic category but no sensitivity to within-category changes of an identical acoustic magnitude. Corroborating evidence comes from studies by Corroborating evidence comes from studies by Chevillet et al. (2013) and Lee et al. (2012), which both show evidence of categorical responses to phonetic stimuli along a continuum in the frontal lobe.

In sum, the literature on native language speech processing suggests that frontal (IFG) and posterior (superior temporal) brain regions subserve very different roles in the perception of the speech signal. While temporal regions may be responsible for processing the fine-grained, language-specific structure of the acoustic input, frontal structures appear to play a role in computing the phonetic category of the incoming stimulus.

How, then, does the brain process non-native speech sounds? In general, non-native or unfamiliar speech sounds elicit a smaller response in the temporal lobe (Callan, Callan, Tajima & Akahane-Yamada, 2006; Callan, Jones, Callan & Akahane-Yamada, 2004; Golestani & Zatorre, 2004). Non-native speech sounds have been shown to elicit a more bilateral (or right-lateralized) neural response, which is consistent with the view that initially, these sounds may not be automatically processed via the same neural networks that subserve native language processing. The question, of course, is whether non-native speech sound training can result in recruitment of the same neural pathways as are used for native language speech perception.

In brief, the answer is yes: several studies of non-native speech sound training have shown increases in post-training activation in the same network of areas associated with effective native-language speech processing, in particular in the superior temporal gyrus (Leech, Holt, Devlin & Dick, 2009; Wang, Sereno, Jongman & Hirsch, 2003), but also in inferior frontal regions and inferior parietal regions (Golestani & Zatorre, 2004; Ventura-Campos et al., 2013).

A complicating factor in any imaging study investigating non-native speech sounds is that the processing of these sounds is by definition more effortful than processing native-language sounds. If one compares activation for a difficult non-native speech categorization task with an easy native language speech categorization task, the regions revealed may reflect the greater *non-linguistic* resources engaged in effortful processing (e. g., working memory, attention, cognitive control) than they do differences in non-native speech processing per se. Moreover, not all non-native sounds are equally difficult to perceive – for instance, some non-native contrasts are easily distinguishable on the basis of acoustics alone (e. g., Best, McRoberts & Sithole, 1988).

A solution to these challenges is to probe neural sensitivity to the same acoustic tokens by comparing groups of individuals who have either been trained to categorize both sounds as members of the same category, or as members of different categories (Myers & Swan, 2012). As in Swan & Myers (2013, described above), participants were trained to identify tokens taken from a three-way dental-retroflex-velar continuum. After a brief categorization training session, neural sensitivity to these same speech sounds was assessed using fMRI. Critically, this study employed a habituation design, in which participants did not have to actively engage in metalinguistic categorization or discrimination tasks, but rather they monitored the speech stream for rare, anomalous high-pitched targets (which were themselves not analyzed further). Activation was compared for pairs of tokens which participants in one group had been trained to place into the same category (within-category pairs) and participants in the other training group had learned belonged to distinct categories (between category pairs). Only a set of bilateral frontal areas showed sensitivity to the learned phonetic category structure, showing differential activation to between-category compared to within-category contrasts. Given that these inferior frontal areas also subserve other, domain-general cognitive functions, this leads to the suggestion that early phonetic learning may not require a reshaping of perceptual sensitivities, per se, but rather may reflect a shift in attention as listeners implicitly learn which acoustic dimensions define the contrast of interest. This evidence best aligns with theories of non-native perception which implicate a redirection of attentional/cognitive resources as the crucial first step in phonetic learning.

Evidence suggests that extensive training with non-native speech sounds may in fact eventually begin to reorganize neural sensitivities in the temporal lobes, and hence to resemble native-language speech sounds more closely. Several studies of novel or non-native speech sound training which have extended over multiple days have shown increasing activity in temporal areas (Leech et al., 2009; Liebenthal et al., 2010; Wong, Perrachione & Parrish, 2007; see Myers, 2014 for review).

Taken together, these findings suggest that non-native speech sound learning is supported by a two-stage process (see Figure 4). For a naïve learner, speech sounds are initially processed in the temporal lobes, where the provisional status of these sounds is assigned, likely as members of a native language category. Next, frontal areas calculate the match between the hypothesized sound and other top-down data (e. g., explicit feedback from the experimenter as to the category identity). Frontal areas then exert a control signal back to the temporal lobes to tweak the tuning of phonetically-sensitive temporal areas in line with the categorical status of the speech sound. Over time this process results in a heightened perceptual tuning in the temporal lobes for the learned category.

The hypothesis that temporal-lobe tuning to phonetic category structure would emerge only after extensive training was investigated by training participants continuously for two weeks on the same Hindi dental vs. retroflex contrast (Myers, Mesite & Del Tufo, in prep). Before training, neural sensitivity to the learned contrast was minimal, and distributed primarily in frontal lobes. After training, sensitivity to phonetic category structure of the contrast (as measured by differences in processing for between- vs. within-category contrasts) was evident not only in frontal lobes, but also in superior temporal lobes. Of interest, the magnitude of the response in the temporal lobes was positively correlated with individual variability in sensitivity to the learned contrast. This evidence corroborates the view that over time, non-native speech sounds come to be processed in temporal lobe regions which come to be specifically tuned to handle these sounds.

We have suggested that frontal areas reflect more domain-general, cognitive processes that are deployed to mediate between the incoming perceptual signal and the category status of the token, while the temporal areas reflect more automatic, sensory-based processing. This asymmetry could also be couched in terms of another distinction between declarative and procedural knowledge. On the one hand, listeners are likely to arrive at strategies for processing which may be explicit and within the participant's awareness and control. On the other hand, effective processing of speech is likely to be rather automatic and not require extensive effortful processing. In fact, Chandrasekaran and colleagues have proposed that successful learning of non-native speech sound contrasts is most evident in individuals who shift to implicit, procedural processing systems early in learning (Chandrasekaran, Yi & Maddox, 2014). In the next section, we will consider how declarative and procedural systems are affected by sleep – a factor which is known to affect learning in other domains, but is relatively unexplored in non-native speech sound learning.

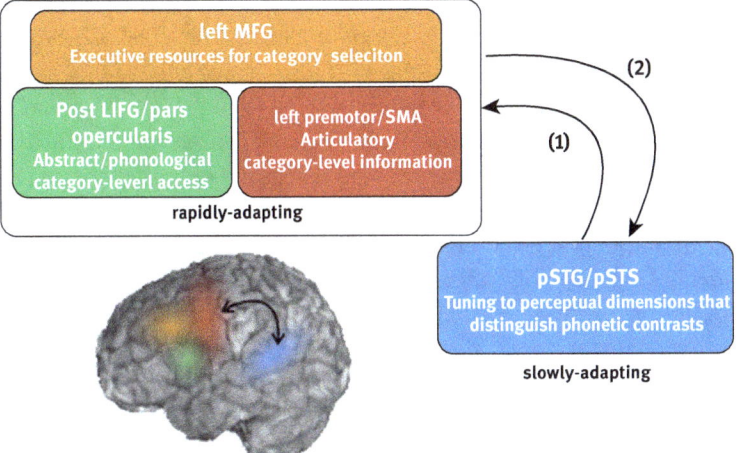

Figure 4: From Myers, 2014. Neural systems for the perception and learning of speech sound categories. Fine-grained sensitivity to acoustic dimensions that distinguish native speech sounds (e. g. VOT) is found in the posterior superior temporal gyrus (pSTG) and superior temporal sulcus (STS), which includes preferential sensitivity to speech categories, but to a lesser degree, also sensitivity to within-category variation. In perception, sounds which are not well-categorized by this tuning (e. g. ambiguous sounds) feed forward to categorical-level coding in the frontal lobe (1). For non-native category learning which relies on top-down feedback, category sensitivities may emerge first in the frontal lobe, then feed back to posterior temporal areas to guide long-term changes in perceptual sensitivity (2). Figure as originally published in Myers 2014. Emergence of category-level sensitivities in non-native speech sound learning. Frontiers in Neuroscience, 8, 238

2.4 Sleep and perceptual anchoring

While the process of non-native speech sound learning is often framed as a perceptual problem, it also challenges the memory systems. After discovering the appropriate acoustic dimensions to attend to, listeners must then maintain that information in memory over time as new instances are encountered. Simultaneously, the new speech sound information must be protected against interference from subsequent native tokens. Sleep is well known to play a significant role in stabilizing and enhancing procedural learning, including in the auditory domain (Atienza, Cantero & Stickgold, 2004; Brawn, Nusbaum & Margoliash, 2010; Fenn, Margoliash & Nusbaum, 2013; Fenn, Nusbaum & Margoliash, 2003). Of interest is whether sleep plays a similar role in stabilizing non-native phonetic learning and enabling listeners to generalize to new tokens.

Evidence from our lab suggests that sleep and post-training linguistic experience plays a dynamic role in acquiring distinctiveness in non-native phonetic contrasts (Earle & Myers, 2015b). In particular, sleep appears to enhance the transfer of categorization learning to discrimination tasks. The effect of sleep on training success was investigated in a series of studies in our lab. We first investigated whether the timing of training relative to sleep would affect the ultimate retention of the trained contrast. Monolingual English speakers were trained to identify a closed set of dental and retroflex stop tokens either in the morning or evening (Earle & Myers, 2015b). Each participant returned twice over 24 hours such that discrimination performance was assessed immediately after training, and after roughly 12 and 24 hour intervals. Based on the sleep-mediated consolidation literature on auditory skill learning, we predicted latent performance gains to be observed immediately after sleep, whether participants were trained in the evening or morning. Instead, we found that participants who were trained in the evening demonstrated steady gains in performance at each posttest, while the morning group maintained their training-induced gain throughout the day, but then degraded in performance overnight (see Figure 5). Given that the two groups showed comparable gains immediately after training, suggesting that the training session was similarly successful in both groups, these differences appeared unlikely to be due to circadian influences on initial learning. This presented a puzzle – why should individuals trained in the morning show no sleep-related benefit in learning?

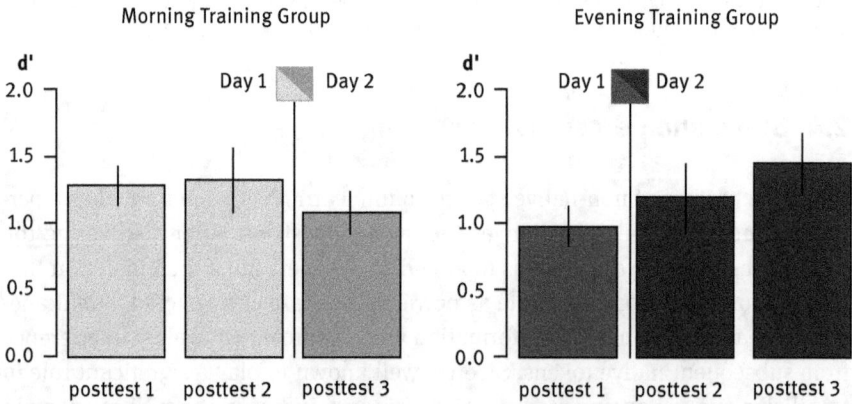

Figure 5: Discrimination performance on the dental-retroflex contrast in the 24 hours following training, by time of day of training (From Earle & Myers, 2015b).

In considering the divergent effects of sleep on the two groups, we speculated that the relevant difference may be in participants' experiences between training and sleep. Specifically, participants trained in the morning spent an entire school day speaking and hearing English before sleep, whereas those trained in the evening experienced less native-language experience between training and sleep. As dental and retroflex stops perceptually assimilate to alveolar /d/ for native speakers of English, we hypothesized that this post-training exposure to phonetically similar items eroded participants' memory for the learned contrast, and therefore interfered with the sleep-mediated enhancement of performance on the trained tokens. To test this hypothesis, participants were trained in the evening and exposed to one of two native language conditions immediately after training. One group was bombarded with a fifteen-minute train of /b/-initial syllables tokens, and the other was exposed to many /d/-initial syllables. Because the alveolar /d/ is perceptually similar to the trained contrast, we predicted that exposure to this segment would erode gains made during training, whereas exposure to the dissimilar /b/ sound would not. As expected, those who were exposed to /b/ tokens showed sleep-related enhancement of learning while the /d/ group showed decrements in performance and in fact a return to their baseline abilities (see Figure 6). We therefore suggest that post-training linguistic experience influences the extent to which subsequent sleep may either enhance or assimilate nonnative phonetic features.

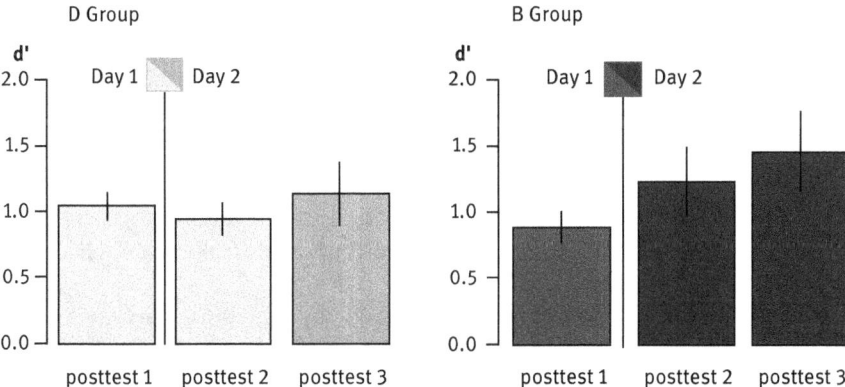

Figure 6: Discrimination performance on the dental-retroflex contrast in the 24 hours following training, by condition of exposure to interference (From Earle & Myers, 2015b).

Mechanistically, acquired distinctiveness implies a learning process by which attending selectively to a relevant set of acoustic-phonetic features becomes less effortful and more automatic over time. A model by Ashby, Ennis and Spierning (2007) assumes that there are two neural pathways between sensory association cortices and premotor areas that support perceptual category discrimination judgments. During initial learning, the model assumes dominant control by a slower cortical-striatal pathway in the procedural learning system, such that synapses active during responses eliciting 'correct' feedback are preferentially strengthened over those that are active during 'incorrect' trials or trials that elicit no feedback. Over time a more direct cortical-cortical pathway develops through Hebbian learning. The authors theorize that the mechanism underlying the development of categorization automaticity is the gradual transfer of control over task performance from the slower (cortical-striatal) pathway to the direct (cortical-cortical) pathway. Of particular relevance to this process, there is some evidence that rapid eye movement (REM) sleep facilitates localized cortical synaptic consolidation, and REM sleep has been found to enhance behavioral performance in procedural tasks (see Diekelmann & Born, 2010 for review). Taken together, the prediction for the role of REM sleep in category discrimination is to promote localized synaptic strengthening in cortical projections (e. g. Schwartz, Maquet & Frith, 2002) that facilitates the development of perceptual automaticity (Atienza et al., 2004; see Earle & Myers 2014 for review).

2.5 Generalization from instances to new talkers and phonological contexts

The invariance problem confronts learners head-on when they are asked to apply information learned about a non-native contrast from a given talker or phonological context to a new set of contexts. For instance, an adult talker with a relatively large vocal tract will have inherently different resonant frequencies than a child with a smaller vocal tract. Likewise, for reasons of idiolect or dialect, talkers often implement the same acoustic property in subtly different ways (see Drouin et al., this volume). Non-native phonetic perception must be robust enough to withstand talker changes.

In order for phonetic features to be applied to unfamiliar situations, a reasonable assumption is that acoustic-phonetic information must be extracted from acoustic instances and encoded in an abstract form. Previous literature suggests that sleep induces abstraction and integration of novel word forms with the pre-existing lexicon (Davis & Gaskell, 2009; Dumay & Gaskell, 2007; Gaskell & Dumay, 2003; Tamminen & Gaskell, 2008). By analogy, we predicted that the identification of dental and retroflex tokens by a category label becomes less reliant on the specific acoustic-phonetic experience of training, and therefore more generalizable after post-training sleep. This prediction was tested by training participants either in the morning or in the evening (Earle & Myers, 2015a) on a dental/retroflex contrast produced by a single talker. Each participant returned at roughly 12 and 24- hour intervals for reassessment. During each session, participants were asked to identify dental and retroflex tokens produced by a novel talker. While both morning-trained and evening-trained groups learned to identify the dental/retroflex sounds as spoken by the trained talker immediately after training, identification of the phonetic contrast in an untrained talker's voice was at chance until after a period of sleep (see Figure 7). This finding supports the assumption that sleep facilitates the abstraction of acoustic-phonetic features such that they can be applied to recognize category identity in tokens produced by unfamiliar talkers.

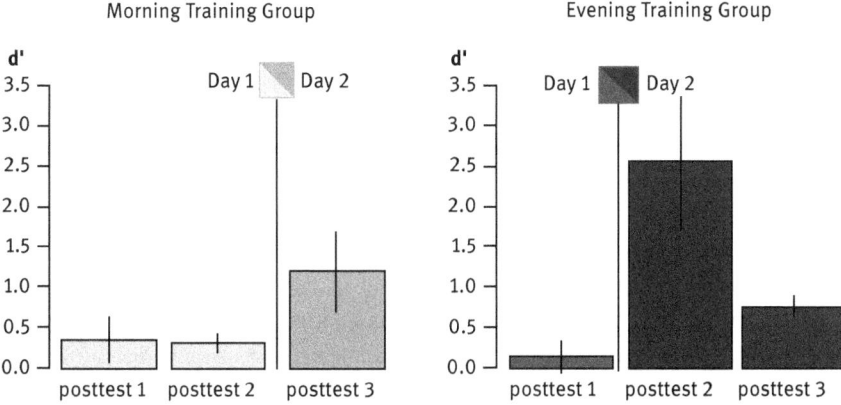

Figure 7: Identification performance on the dental-retroflex contrast produced by an unfamiliar talker in the 24 hours following training, by time of day of training. Reproduced with permission from Earle, F. S. & Myers, E. B. (2015a). Overnight consolidation promotes generalization across talkers in the identification of nonnative speech sounds. The Journal of the Acoustical Society of America, 137(1), EL91. Copyright 2015, Acoustical Society of America

In sum, adult non-native speech sound learning, while difficult, can result in perceptual sensitivity that begins to resemble that of native language categories. This is observable in behavior (acquired sensitivity) and in the recruitment of native-language neural structures for non-native perception as listeners become more proficient. At the same time, non-native speech learning is vulnerable to interference from one's native language phonology, and this interference can operate before and after training. One's native language phonology places constraints on the initial perception of non-native speech sounds in the sense that sounds that are similar to one's native language inventory are difficult to distinguish (Best et al., 2001). However, even after training, exposure to similar native language sounds may erode the newly learned information (Earle & Myers, 2015b). Recent evidence further shows that sleep plays a role in non-native speech sound acquisition, in strengthening the memory traces for the learned categories, as well as allowing listeners to generalize to new talkers.

3 Flexibility in the perception of native language speech sounds: idiolects and non-native accents

As argued above, acquisition of a non-native speech sound category involves a restructuring of existing sensitivities, and requires a fair degree of functional plasticity in the speech sound system. Listeners are similarly flexible to atypical phoneme utterances that occur within native language speech processing, whether these atypical pronunciations arise from foreign accents, regional dialects, or individual speech production patterns (idiolects). We argue that adaptation to nonstandard speech tokens in the context of one's native language involves processes that overlap with learning non-native phonetic contrasts. In particular, both situations require that listeners process acoustic input that does not precisely match existing language categories, in both situations listeners employ top-down information to solve perceptual ambiguity in the speech stream, and especially in the case of dialect or accent learning, listeners must learn to generalize from one speaker to another from that same language community. Of interest is how listeners accommodate non-standard speech tokens embedded in native language speech. For instance, it may be that listeners show a selective retuning of perceptual sensitivities in order to map the nonstandard speech token to the native language phonological category. Alternatively, listeners may employ a strategy whereby they loosen their criteria for what to include as a member of the phonetic category and thereby allow greater 'slip' in their perceptual mappings.

3.1 Perceptual adaptation to idiolect

Different speakers of a common dialect produce sounds in systematically unique ways, and listeners are sensitive to this talker-related variation in the phonetic content of speech (e. g. see Theodore et al., this volume). While systematic phonetic variability is a hallmark of one's idiolect, this kind of systematic variation can be simulated in the lab by presenting listeners with native-accented speech in which one phoneme is systematically altered. A set of studies using the 'perceptual learning for speech' paradigm has shown that listeners can use lexical-level information to adjust a phoneme category boundary to accommodate an ambiguous sound produced by a novel speaker even without explicit instruction to do so (Kraljic & Samuel, 2005; Norris, McQueen & Cutler, 2003). In this paradigm, listeners perform a lexical decision task on words in which sounds of a certain category (e. g.,/s/) are modified so as to be ambiguous between two categories (e. g.,

/s/ and /ʃ/), producing critical items such as 'dino[?]aur', where the? denotes the ambiguous token. This training set is analogous to a situation where a talker has a speech idiosyncrasy such as a lisp that affects only one segment. After the lexical decision task, listeners are asked to categorize a continuum of sounds from /s/ to /ʃ/ produced by the same talker, and show shifts in the category boundary which are consistent with the exposure they received in the lexical decision task. Of note, once listeners adapt to an ambiguous phoneme for one speaker, the adaptation usually does not generalize to new speakers (Eisner & McQueen, 2005). This suggests that once listeners learn that the talker produces certain sounds in an idiosyncratic way, they do not automatically apply this learning to other speakers, unless there is reason to infer that productions of the segment will be similar across speakers (as in the case for perceptual learning of stop consonants, Kraljic & Samuel, 2006, 2007). Such *a priori* assumption arises from long-term experience with different speakers of the native language. Without such experience available to L2 learners, non-native speech sound learning operates in a talker-specific manner – namely that generalization of non-native sound learning from one single talker to another talker is usually not possible unless the listener hears several talkers during training (Lively et al., 1993; Logan, Lively & Pisoni, 1991). This suggests that in order to take a talker-specific mapping scheme (e. g., "this talker produces voiceless stops with relatively shorter VOTs") and generalize it over a group of people within the same language community (e. g., "native speakers of Spanish have shorter VOTs for voiceless stops in their spoken English"), listeners must be clued in to how speakers of that language community sound, as well as understand when to apply the new phonetic mapping (e. g., recognize who is a speaker of Spanish).

The perception of a non-standard variant in native accented speech in general appears to emerge more rapidly, and persist longer that non-native phonetic learning, given similar amounts of exposure. In studies of adaptation to a talker idiolect, listeners rapidly map the characteristics of a novel speaker and only overwrite those initial mappings if a listener notices that the mispronunciation can be attributed to some external source, such as holding a pen in the mouth (Kraljic & Samuel, 2011; Kraljic, Samuel & Brennan, 2008). The shift in phonetic category boundary is stable over at least 24 hours (Eisner & McQueen, 2006), and will generalize to novel positions in a word (Jesse & McQueen, 2011). Taken together, this pattern suggests that adaptation to a single non-standard segment in the context of otherwise canonical forms presents a far easier and more automatic task than learning to distinguish similar-sounding non-native sounds.

Like non-native speech sound acquisition, the process of adapting to a non-standard token in the context of native accented speech may follow a similar frontal-to-temporal shift over the course of learning. In an fMRI study of perceptual learning for speech, neural sensitivity to the shift in category boundary conditioned by the perceptual learning for speech paradigm was observed in right frontal regions throughout the learning trajectory (Myers & Mesite, 2014). However, both anterior and posterior left temporal regions showed sensitivity to the category shift that only emerged after several blocks of exposure. Together with previous work on non-native speech sound learning, this study suggests that neural plasticity for re-categorizing the sounds of speech recruits a similar neural pathway whether those sounds are non-native speech sounds or are non-standard sounds embedded in native language speech.

3.2 Perceptual adaptation to non-native accents

In non-native speech sound acquisition, listeners must cope with a new phonological system. In accented speech, listeners are confronted with a similar acoustic challenge: non-native accented talkers transfer (completely or incompletely) acoustic properties of their native language phonological system to their L2 speech. Moreover, non-native speech may contain more acoustic variability in general than native-language speech, likely due to inconsistent application of the L1 rules in L2 speech (Wade, Jongman & Sereno, 2007). Both deviation from the native norms and within-talker variability in the realization of a phonetic category may lead to perceptual difficulty with foreign-accented speech, resulting in prolonged processing time and decreased accuracy in spoken word recognition (Munro & Derwing, 1995a, 1995b). Experience with a foreign accent can help native listeners adapt to accented speech and consequentially improve speech intelligibility of speakers of the accent (Weil, 2001; Clarke & Garrett, 2004). A key question is whether adaptation to accented speech resembles the process of non-native speech sound learning.

First of all, similar to acquisition of non-native phonetic categories, perceptual learning of accented speech is guided by top-down information. As listeners encounter foreign-accented speech, established lexical knowledge can inform them of a poor mapping from the acoustic signal to native phonetic categories and elicit adjustments in the sound-to-category mappings (Eisner, Melinger & Weber, 2013; Reinisch & Holt, 2014; Sumner, 2011). For instance, a French-accented /p/ sound is acoustically more similar to a /b/ than a /p/ when mapped onto distributions of native English. However, when French-accented /p/ tokens are heard in real English-words like '*paint*', listeners recalibrate the category boundary between /b/ and /p/; further, they generalize the adjusted mapping to novel tokens produced by the same speaker (Sumner, 2011). In addition, adaptation to high intelligible speech (which potentially provides clearer and more consistent top-down feedback) is faster than adaptation to low intelligible speech (Bradlow & Bent, 2008).

Second, listeners are quite sensitive to the bottom-up information along multiple acoustic dimensions. In addition to a recalibration of the between-category boundary location, listeners also discover the acoustic dimensions that are most relevant for phonemic distinctions in a particular accent. For example, vowel duration is diagnostic of a voicing contrast for word-final stops in native English, but not in Mandarin-accented English. Evidence from our lab (Xie, Theodore & Myers, under review) indicates that as native-English listeners adapt to a Mandarin-accented speaker, they shift their attention to burst length as an informative source to distinguish voiceless stops from voiced tokens at word-final positions (e. g., *seat* or *seed*). Such re-weighting in acoustic cues contributes to a reorganization of phonetic structure beyond the boundary region, producing changes in the tokens that listeners judged as 'good' members of a phonetic category.

Third, exposure to talker variability facilitates generalization across talkers, as in non-native category learning (Lively et al., 1993; Logan et al., 1991). While talker-specific adaptation seems robust, listeners generally do not transfer what they learn from one accented talker to another (Bradlow & Bent, 2008; Jongman, Wade & Sereno, 2003). In contrast, exposure to a group of talkers who share an accent may enhance subsequent word recognition for a novel talker with the same accent (Bradlow & Bent, 2008; Sidaras, Alexander & Nygaard, 2009; but see Wade et al., 2007; Clarke, 2000 for negative evidence). The question is what do listeners learn from the multiple-talker exposure that allows them to generalize across talkers? It is possible that the increased variability in the form of multiple talkers causes a general relaxation of the matching rule from nonstandard speech signals to category representations. Studies show that listener are more tolerant of acoustic mismatches in noncanonical forms of speech tokens (such as reduced speech, speech in noise, accented speech) than those in canonical forms (Brouwer, Mitterer & Huettig, 2012; McQueen & Huettig, 2012; Witteman, Weber & McQueen, 2013). A general relaxation may also account for the finding of Baese-Berk, Bradlow & Wright (2013) which shows that training with a group of foreign-accented speakers with various accents improved word recognition for an untrained accent. Alternatively, it is possible that the multiple-talker exposure benefits generalization by allowing listeners to selectively attend to particular aspects of the speech input (for instance, certain regions in the perceptual space or specific acoustic dimensions) that are stable across talkers but are relevant for making linguistic distinctions. Much less evidence is available to provide a rigorous test of this hypothesis. Of note, foreign speakers may demonstrate inconsistent variability in the realization of phoneme contrasts (Wade et al., 2007).

Our own work shows that cross-talker generalization of adaptation to foreign-accented phonemes is mediated by perceptual similarities among talkers, and in particular, by similarities along specific acoustic dimensions (Xie & Myers, under review). As such, when talkers did not show sufficient systematicity, listeners did not generalize to a novel talker.

Of note, even amidst multiple nonstandard cues in accented speech, listeners can still accurately track the specific variation tagged to a nonstandard phoneme, suggesting that listeners adjust to the specific qualities that make the phoneme nonstandard (e. g., Reinisch & Holt, 2014; Eisner et al., 2013). Variability in production, per se, does not seem to be an obstacle to adaptation. In addition, as listeners adapt to nonstandard phonemes spoken in a foreign accent, they may be more tolerant of variability in production than they are with native variants (compare Witteman et al., 2013 and Kraljic & Samuel, 2005) such that both canonical and noncanonical tokens (produced by the same speaker) are accepted as members of an intended category. Listeners will adapt to a nonstandard phoneme spoken in a foreign accent even if the speaker sometimes pronounces the phoneme in an unaccented way (Witteman et al., 2013). Lastly, although behavioral outcomes of accented speech training report successful learning of accents, eye tracking measurements nonetheless highlight the added difficulty and uncertainty listeners experience in the process of phoneme adaptation for accented speech (Trude, Tremblay & Brown-Schmidt, 2013). Thus, adaptation to foreign-accented speech may be more effortful than accommodating idiosyncratic native accents and in a way resembles non-native phoneme learning when the foreign-accented tokens deviate substantially from native norms.

4 Limits to flexibility in speech sound perception and unanswered questions

Obstacles to flexibility for speech sound perception are not insurmountable. While categorical perception does dominate the speech perception process, listeners show a large degree of adaptability in learning non-native speech tokens, and with sufficient input, timed appropriately, and with appropriate feedback, many listeners can show success in learning new speech sounds. We argue that this success is mediated by a neural pathway which engages first frontal systems, and then over time, temporal systems for perception. This pattern suggests a learning system which first engages category-level information, and only later re-tunes perceptual areas in order to facilitate perception of the learned sounds in the longer term. This learning process is facilitated by sleep. Sleep serves to both protect the learned information from interference from similar-sounding tokens in one's native language, but it also enables listeners to abstract away from the training tokens in order to generalize to a new talker of the same language.

Remarkably similar patterns emerge in perception of non-standard tokens in the context of idiolects or accents – however, learning in those situations appears to be quicker, requires fewer tokens, and is perhaps more robust than in speech sound learning. It may be that accents and dialects present less of an obstacle to learning precisely because listeners are mapping non-standard perceptual information to existing, stable phonological and lexical representations. This implies that what makes non-native speech sound learning hard whereas the perception of accented speech relatively easy is not the properties of the acoustic input (hearing non-standard input), but rather the challenge of creating new speech sound categories for functional use. Whereas perception of accented or non-standard native language speech engages an entire network of phonological, lexical, and semantic processing resources, training on non-native sounds is often impoverished (training on isolated sounds or meaningless syllables, or on a very few novel words). This raises the question of whether training listeners on non-native speech sounds embedded in native-accented speech could facilitate non-native speech sound learning over time through the engagement of the robust native language processing system.

In general, the speed with which listeners map non-standard tokens onto new categories suggests that fast-acting mechanisms are at play during learning, at least during early stages of learning. It seems unlikely that the perceptual sensitivities which take babies at least 12 months to acquire are the same mechanisms which allow adults to begin to perceive differences between similar speech sounds after only thirty minutes of training. As argued above, the speed of learning suggests that learning mechanisms must involve the dynamic, intelligent deployment of perceptual/attentional resources to the signal, and with very little input. However, these on-the-fly schemas are unlikely to be created fresh for each new speaker, new phonological context, etc. Over time, novel instances must accumulate in order to allow for this kind of generalization such that new tokens from the same talker and new talkers of the same accent or language can be easily recognized. We speculate that this process is facilitated by both sleep and a frontal-to-temporal transfer of neural sensitivity.

There is much that is still unknown about the limits of plasticity in speech sound perception. For instance, it is unknown whether the evening benefit for speech sound training transfers to real-world language learning situations. Moreover, while interference from one's native language seems to account for training declines over time, we do not know whether this interference is operating at the acoustic-phonetic level, an abstract phonological level, or an articulatory level (or all three). Finally, while advances have been made in strategies for speech sound training, it still remains the case that very few L2 learners fully acquire a new sound system in adulthood. There may be hard biological limits on the ability of the neural systems which handle speech to fully adapt to non-standard tokens, even given unlimited input and ideal learning conditions.

References

Allen, J. S., Miller, J. L. & DeSteno, D. (2003). Individual talker differences in voice-onset-time. *The Journal of the Acoustical Society of America*, *113*(1), 544–552.
Ashby, F. G., Ennis, J. M. & Spiering, B. J. (2007). A neurobiological theory of automaticity in perceptual categorization. *Psychological Review*, *114*(3), 632–656.
Atienza, M., Cantero, J. L. & Stickgold, R. (2004). Posttraining sleep enhances automaticity in perceptual discrimination. *Journal of Cognitive Neuroscience*, *16*(1), 53–64.
Baese-Berk, M. M., Bradlow, A. R. & Wright, B. A. (2013). Accent-independent adaptation to foreign accented speech. *The Journal of the Acoustical Society of America*, *133*(3), EL174–180.
Best, C. C. & McRoberts, G. W. (2003). Infant perception of non-native consonant contrasts that adults assimilate in different ways. *Language and Speech*, *46*(Pt 2–3), 183–216.
Best, C. T. & Hallé, P. A. (2010). Perception of initial obstruent voicing is influenced by gestural organization. *Journal of Phonetics*, Phonetic Bases of Distinctive Features, *38*(1), 109–126.
Best, C. T., McRoberts, G. W. & Goodell, E. (2001). Discrimination of non-native consonant contrasts varying in perceptual assimilation to the listener's native phonological system. *The Journal of the Acoustical Society of America*, *109*(2), 775–94.
Best, C. T., McRoberts, G. W. & Sithole, N. M. (1988). Examination of perceptual reorganization for nonnative speech contrasts: Zulu click discrimination by English-speaking adults and infants. *Journal of Experimental Psychology: Human Perception and Performance 14*(3), 345–60.
Best, C. & Tyler, M. (2007). Second language speech learning: the role of language experience in speech perception and production. *Nonnative and second-language speech perception: commonalities and complementarities*, 13–34.
Blumstein, S. E. & Myers, E. B. (2014). Neural Systems Underlying Speech Perception. *Oxford Handbook of Cognitive Neuroscience* (Oshsner, K., and Kosslyn, S., Eds., Vol. 2).
Blumstein, S. E. & Stevens, K. N. (1979). Acoustic invariance in speech production: Evidence from measurements of the spectral characteristics of stop consonants. *The Journal of the Acoustical Society of America*, *66*(4), 1001–1017.
Blumstein, S. E. & Stevens, K. N. (1980). Perceptual invariance and onset spectra for stop consonants in different vowel environments. *The Journal of the Acoustical Society of America*, *67*(2), 648–662.
Bosseler, A. N., Taulu, S., Pihko, E., Mäkelä, J. P., Imada, T., Ahonen, A. & Kuhl, P. K. (2013). Theta brain rhythms index perceptual narrowing in infant speech perception. *Frontiers in Psychology*, 4.

Bradlow, A. R. & Bent, T. (2008). Perceptual adaptation to non-native speech. *Cognition*, *106*(2), 707–29.

Bradlow, A. R., Pisoni, D. B., Akahane-Yamada, R. & Tohkura, Y. (1997). Training Japanese listeners to identify English /r/ and /l/: IV. Some effects of perceptual learning on speech production. *The Journal of the Acoustical Society of America*, *101*(4), 2299–2310.

Brawn, T. P., Nusbaum, H. C. & Margoliash, D. (2010). Sleep-dependent consolidation of auditory discrimination learning in adult starlings. *The Journal of Neuroscience: The Official Journal of the Society for Neuroscience*, *30*(2), 609–613.

Brouwer, S., Mitterer, H. & Huettig, F. (2012). Speech reductions change the dynamics of competition during spoken word recognition. *Language and Cognitive Processes*, *27*(4), 539–571.

Callan, A. M., Callan, D. E., Tajima, K. & Akahane-Yamada, R. (2006). Neural processes involved with perception of non-native durational contrasts. *Neuroreport*, *17*(12), 1353–1357.

Callan, D. E., Jones, J. A., Callan, A. M. & Akahane-Yamada, R. (2004). Phonetic perceptual identification by native- and second-language speakers differentially activates brain regions involved with acoustic phonetic processing and those involved with articulatory-auditory/ orosensory internal models. *Neuroimage*, 22(3), 1182–94.

Chandrasekaran, B., Yi, H.-G. & Maddox, W. T. (2014). Dual-learning systems during speech category learning. *Psychonomic Bulletin & Review*, *21*(2), 488–495.

Chang, E. F., Rieger, J. W., Johnson, K., Berger, M. S., Barbaro, N. M. & Knight, R. T. (2010). Categorical speech representation in human superior temporal gyrus. *Nature Neuroscience*, *13*(11), 1428–1432.

Chevillet, M. A., Jiang, X., Rauschecker, J. P. & Riesenhuber, M. (2013). Automatic phoneme category selectivity in the dorsal auditory stream. *The Journal of neuroscience: the official journal of the Society for Neuroscience*, *33*(12), 5208–5215.

Clahsen, H. & Felser, C. (2006). How native-like is non-native language processing? *Trends in Cognitive Sciences*, *10*(12), 564–570.

Clarke, C. (2000). Perceptual adjustments to foreign accented English. *Research on Spoken Language Processing Progress Report*, (24).

Clarke, C. M. & Garrett, M. F. (2004). Rapid adaptation to foreign-accented English. *The Journal of the Acoustical Society of America*, *116*(6), 3647.

D'Ausilio, A., Bufalari, I., Salmas, P. & Fadiga, L. (2012). The role of the motor system in discriminating normal and degraded speech sounds. *Cortex; a Journal Devoted to the Study of the Nervous System and Behavior*, *48*(7), 882–887.

D'Ausilio, A., Craighero, L. & Fadiga, L. (2012). The contribution of the frontal lobe to the perception of speech. *Journal of Neurolinguistics*, *25*(5), 328–335.

Davis, M. H. & Gaskell, M. G. (2009). A complementary systems account of word learning: neural and behavioural evidence. *Philosophical Transactions of the Royal Society B: Biological Sciences*, *364*(1536), 3773–3800.

Diekelmann, S. & Born, J. (2010). The memory function of sleep. *Nature Reviews. Neuroscience*, *11*(2), 114–126.

Dumay, N. & Gaskell, M. G. (2007). Sleep-associated changes in the mental representation of spoken words. *Psychological Science*, *18*(1), 35–39.

Earle, F. S. & Myers, E. B. (2014). Building phonetic categories: an argument for the role of sleep. *Frontiers in Psychology*, *5*, 1192.

Earle, F. S. & Myers, E. B. (2015a). Overnight consolidation promotes generalization across talkers in the identification of nonnative speech sounds. *The Journal of the Acoustical Society of America*, *137*(1), EL91.

Earle, F. S. & Myers, E. B. (2015b). Sleep and native language interference affect non-native speech sound learning. *Journal of Experimental Psychology: Human Perception and Performance, 41*(6), 1680.

Eimas, P. D., Siqueland, E. R., Jusczyk, P. & Vigorito, J. (1971). Speech perception in infants. *Science, 171*(968), 303–6.

Eisner, F. & McQueen, J. M. (2005). The specificity of perceptual learning in speech processing. *Perception & Psychophysics, 67*(2), 224.

Eisner, F. & McQueen, J. M. (2006). Perceptual learning in speech: Stability over time. *The Journal of the Acoustical Society of America, 119*(4), 1950.

Eisner, F., Melinger, A. & Weber, A. (2013). Constraints on the transfer of perceptual learning in accented speech. *Frontiers in Psychology, 4*, 148.

Fenn, K. M., Margoliash, D. & Nusbaum, H. C. (2013). Sleep restores loss of generalized but not rote learning of synthetic speech. *Cognition, 128*(3), 280–286.

Fenn, K. M., Nusbaum, H. C. & Margoliash, D. (2003). Consolidation during sleep of perceptual learning of spoken language. *Nature, 425*(6958), 614–616.

Flege, J. E. (1991). Age of learning affects the authenticity of voice-onset time (VOT) in stop consonants produced in a second language. *The Journal of the Acoustical Society of America, 89*(1), 395–411.

Flege, J. E., MacKay, I. R. & Meador, D. (1999). Native Italian speakers' perception and production of English vowels. *The Journal of the Acoustical Society of America, 106*(5), 2973–87.

Francis, A. L., Baldwin, K. & Nusbaum, H. C. (2000). Effects of training on attention to acoustic cues. *Perception and Psychophysics, 62*(8), 1668–80.

Francis, A. L. & Nusbaum, H. C. (2002). Selective attention and the acquisition of new phonetic categories. *Journal of Experimental Psychology: Human Perception and Performance, 28*(2), 349–66.

Fry, D. B., Abramson, A. S., Eimas, P. D. & Liberman, A. M. (1962). The Identification and Discrimination of Synthetic Vowels. *Language and Speech, 5*(4), 171–189.

Galantucci, B., Fowler, C. A. & Turvey, M. T. (2006). The motor theory of speech perception reviewed. *Psychonomic Bulletin & Review, 13*(3), 361–377.

Gaskell, M. G. & Dumay, N. (2003). Lexical competition and the acquisition of novel words. *Cognition, 89*(2), 105–32.

Golestani, N. & Zatorre, R. J. (2004). Learning new sounds of speech: reallocation of neural substrates. *Neuroimage, 21*(2), 494–506.

Golestani, N. & Zatorre, R. J. (2009). Individual differences in the acquisition of second language phonology. *Brain and Language, 109*(2–3), 55–67.

Guenther, F. H. & Gjaja, M. N. (1996). The perceptual magnet effect as an emergent property of neural map formation. *Journal of the Acoustical Society of America, 100*(2 Pt 1), 1111–21.

Guenther, F. H., Husain, F. T., Cohen, M. A. & Shinn-Cunningham, B. G. (1999). Effects of categorization and discrimination training on auditory perceptual space. *Journal of the Acoustical Society of America, 106*(5), 2900–12.

Hayes-Harb, R. (2007). Lexical and statistical evidence in the acquisition of second language phonemes. *Second Language Research, 23*(1), 65–94.

Healy, A. F. & Repp, B. H. (1982). Context independence and phonetic mediation in categorical perception. *Journal of Experimental Psychology: Human Perception and Performance, 8*(1), 68–80.

Hickok, G., Costanzo, M., Capasso, R. & Miceli, G. (2011). The role of Broca's area in speech perception: evidence from aphasia revisited. *Brain and Language, 119*(3), 214–220.

Hickok, G. & Poeppel, D. (2004). Dorsal and ventral streams: a framework for understanding aspects of the functional anatomy of language. *Cognition*, *92*(1–2), 67–99.

Hickok, G. & Poeppel, D. (2007). The cortical organization of speech processing. *Nature Reviews Neuroscience*, *8*(5), 393–402.

Holt, L. L. & Lotto, A. J. (2006). Cue weighting in auditory categorization: implications for first and second language acquisition. *The Journal of the Acoustical Society of America*, *119*(5 Pt 1), 3059–3071.

Jesse, A. & McQueen, J. M. (2011). Positional effects in the lexical retuning of speech perception. *Psychonomic bulletin & review*, *18*(5), 943–950.

Jongman, A., Wade, T. & Sereno, J. (2003). On improving the perception of foreign-accented speech. *Proceedings of the 15th international congress of phonetic sciences* (pp. 1561–1564).

Kraljic, T. & Samuel, A. G. (2005). Perceptual learning for speech: Is there a return to normal? *Cognitive psychology*, *51*(2), 141–178.

Kraljic, T. & Samuel, A. G. (2006). Generalization in perceptual learning for speech. *Psychonomic Bulletin & Review*, *13*(2), 262.

Kraljic, T. & Samuel, A. G. (2007). Perceptual adjustments to multiple speakers. *Journal of Memory and Language*, *56*(1), 1–15.

Kraljic, T. & Samuel, A. G. (2011). Perceptual learning evidence for contextually-specific representations. *Cognition*, *121*(3), 459–465.

Kraljic, T., Samuel, A. G. & Brennan, S. E. (2008). First impressions and last resorts: how listeners adjust to speaker variability. *Psychological Science*, *19*(4), 332–338.

Kuhl, P. K. (1991). Human adults and human infants show a "perceptual magnet effect" for the prototypes of speech categories, monkeys do not. *Perception and Psychophysics*, *50*(2), 93–107.

Kuhl, P. K. (2010). Brain Mechanisms in Early Language Acquisition. *Neuron*, *67*(5), 713–727.

Kuhl, P. K., Conboy, B. T., Coffey-Corina, S., Padden, D., Rivera-Gaxiola, M. & Nelson, T. (2008). Phonetic learning as a pathway to language: new data and native language magnet theory expanded (NLM-e). *Philosophical Transactions of the Royal Society of London, Series B, Biological Sciences*, *363*(1493), 979–1000.

Kuhl, P. K., Conboy, B. T., Padden, D., Nelson, T. & Pruitt, J. (2005). Early Speech Perception and Later Language Development: Implications for the "Critical Period." *Language Learning and Development*, *1*(3–4), 237–264.

Leech, R., Holt, L. L., Devlin, J. T. & Dick, F. (2009). Expertise with artificial nonspeech sounds recruits speech-sensitive cortical regions. *Journal of Neuroscience*, *29*(16), 5234–9.

Lee, Y.-S., Turkeltaub, P., Granger, R. & Raizada, R. D. S. (2012). Categorical speech processing in Broca's area: an fMRI study using multivariate pattern-based analysis. *The Journal of Neuroscience*, *32*(11), 3942–3948.

Liberman, A. M., Cooper, F. S., Shankweiler, D. P. & Studdert-Kennedy, M. (1967). Perception of the speech code. *Psychological Review*, *74*(6), 431.

Liberman, A. M., Harris, K. S., Hoffman, H. S. & Griffith, B. C. (1957). The discrimination of speech sounds within and across phoneme boundaries. *Journal of Experimental Psychology*, *54*(5), 358–68.

Liberman, A. M. & Mattingly, I. G. (1985). The motor theory of speech perception revised. *Cognition*, *21*(1), 1–36.

Liebenthal, E., Desai, R., Ellingson, M. M., Ramachandran, B., Desai, A. & Binder, J. R. (2010). Specialization along the left superior temporal sulcus for auditory categorization. *Cerebral Cortex*, *20*(12), 2958–2970.

Lisker, L. & Abramson, A. S. (1964). A cross-language study of voicing in initial stops: acoustical measurements. *Word, 20*, 384–422.

Lively, S., Logan, J. & Pisoni, D. (1993). Training Japanese listeners to indentify English /r/ and /l/. II: The role of phonetic environment and talker variability in learning new perceptual categories. *Journal of the Acoustical Society of America, 94*(3), 1242–1255.

Logan, J., Lively, S. & Pisoni, D. (1991). Training Japanese listeners to identify English/r/ and /l/: A first report. *Journal of the Acoustical Society of America, 89*(2), 874–886.

Maye, J., Werker, J. F. & Gerken, L. (2002). Infant sensitivity to distributional information can affect phonetic discrimination. *Cognition, 82*(3), B101–11.

McAllister, R., Flege, J. E. & Piske, T. (2002). The Influence of L1 on the Acquisition of Swedish Quantity by Native Speakers of Spanish, English and Estonian. *Journal of Phonetics, 30*(2), 229–258.

McCandliss, B. D., Fiez, J. A., Protopapas, A., Conway, M. & McClelland, J. L. (2002). Success and failure in teaching the [r]-[l] contrast to Japanese adults: tests of a Hebbian model of plasticity and stabilization in spoken language perception. *Cognitive Affective and Behavioral Neuroscience, 2*(2), 89–108.

McClelland, J. L., Fiez, J. A. & McCandliss, B. D. (2002). Teaching the /r/-/l/ discrimination to Japanese adults: behavioral and neural aspects. *Physioogy and Behavior, 77*(4–5), 657–62.

McQueen, J. M. & Huettig, F. (2012). Changing only the probability that spoken words will be distorted changes how they are recognized. *The Journal of the Acoustical Society of America, 131*(1), 509–517.

Miller, J. L. (1994). On the internal structure of phonetic categories: a progress report. *Cognition, 50*(1–3), 271–285.

Munro, M. J. & Derwing, T. M. (1995a). Processing time, accent, and comprehensibility in the perception of native and foreign-accented speech. *Language and Speech, 38 (3)*, 289–306.

Munro, M. J. & Derwing, T. M. (1995b). Foreign Accent, Comprehensibility, and Intelligibility in the Speech of Second Language Learners. *Language Learning, 45*(1), 73–97.

Myers, E. B. (2007). Dissociable effects of phonetic competition and category typicality in a phonetic categorization task: An fMRI investigation. *Neuropsychologia, 45*(7), 1463–73.

Myers, E. B. (2014). Emergence of category-level sensitivities in non-native speech sound learning. *Frontiers in Neuroscience, 8*, 238.

Myers, E. B., Blumstein, S. E., Walsh, E. & Eliassen, J. (2009). Inferior frontal regions underlie the perception of phonetic category invariance. *Psychological Science, 20*(7), 895–903.

Myers, E. B. & Mesite, L. M. (2014). Neural systems underlying perceptual adjustment to nonstandard speech tokens. *Journal of Memory and Language, 76*, 80–93.

Myers, E. B. & Swan, K. (2012). Effects of category learning on neural sensitivity to non-native phonetic categories. *Journal of Cognitive Neuroscience, 24*(8), 1695–1708.

Norris, D., McQueen, J. M. & Cutler, A. (2003). Perceptual learning in speech. *Cognitive Psychology, 47*(2), 204–238.

Peterson, G. E. & Barney, H. L. (1952). Control methods used in a study of vowels. *The Journal of the Acoustical Society of America, 24*, 175.

Polka, L., Colantonio, C. & Sundara, M. (2001). A cross-language comparison of /d /–/ð / perception: Evidence for a new developmental pattern. *The Journal of the Acoustical Society of America, 109*(5), 2190–2201.

Polka, L. & Werker, J. F. (1994). Developmental changes in perception of nonnative vowel contrasts. *Journal of Experimental Psychology: Human Perception and Performance, 20*(2), 421–35.

Pruitt, J. S., Jenkins, J. J. & Strange, W. (2006). Training the perception of Hindi dental and retroflex stops by native speakers of American English and Japanese. *The Journal of the Acoustical Society of America*, *119*(3), 1684–96.

Reinisch, E. & Holt, L. L. (2014). Lexically guided phonetic retuning of foreign-accented speech and its generalization. *Journal of Experimental Psychology. Human Perception and Performance*, *40*(2), 539–555.

Sanders, L. D. & Neville, H. J. (2003). An ERP study of continuous speech processing: II. Segmentation, semantics, and syntax in non-native speakers. *Cognitive Brain Research*, *15*(3), 214–227.

Schwartz, S., Maquet, P. & Frith, C. (2002). Neural correlates of perceptual learning: a functional MRI study of visual texture discrimination. *Proceedings of the National Academy of Sciences of the United States of America*, *99*(26), 17137–17142.

Scott, S. K. & Johnsrude, I. S. (2003). The neuroanatomical and functional organization of speech perception. *Trends in Neuroscience*, *26*(2), 100–7.

Sidaras, S. K., Alexander, J. E. D. & Nygaard, L. C. (2009). Perceptual learning of systematic variation in Spanish-accented speech. *The Journal of the Acoustical Society of America*, *125*(5), 3306.

Stevens, K. N. & Blumstein, S. E. (1978). Invariant cues for place of articulation in stop consonants. *Journal of the Acoustical Society of America*, *64*(5), 1358–68.

Sumner, M. (2011). The role of variation in the perception of accented speech. *Cognition*, *119*(1), 131–136.

Sundara, M., Polka, L. & Genesee, F. (2006). Language-experience facilitates discrimination of/d-/in monolingual and bilingual acquisition of English. *Cognition*, *100*(2), 369–388.

Swan, K. S. & Myers, E. B. (2013). Category labels induce boundary-dependent perceptual warping in learned speech categories. *Second Language research*, *29*(4), 391–411.

Tamminen, J. & Gaskell, M. G. (2008). Newly learned spoken words show long-term lexical competition effects. *Quarterly Journal of Experimental Psychology (2006)*, *61*(3), 361–371.

Trude, A. M., Tremblay, A. & Brown-Schmidt, S. (2013). Limitations on adaptation to foreign accents. *Journal of Memory and Language*, *69*(3), 349–367.

Ventura-Campos, N., Sanjuán, A., González, J., Palomar-García, M.-Á., Rodríguez-Pujadas, A., Sebastián-Gallés, N., Deco, G., et al. (2013). Spontaneous brain activity predicts learning ability of foreign sounds. *The Journal of Neuroscience*, *33*(22), 9295–9305.

Volaitis, L. E. & Miller, J. L. (1992). Phonetic prototypes: Influence of place of articulation and speaking rate on the internal structure of voicing categories. *Journal of the Acoustical Society of America*, *92*(2, Pt 1), 723–735.

Wade, T., Jongman, A. & Sereno, J. (2007). Effects of acoustic variability in the perceptual learning of non-native-accented speech sounds. *Phonetica*, *64*(2–3), 122–144.

Wang, Y., Sereno, J. A., Jongman, A. & Hirsch, J. (2003). fMRI evidence for cortical modification during learning of Mandarin lexical tone. *Journal of Cognitive Neuroscience*, *15*(7), 1019–27.

Weber-Fox, C. & Neville, H. (1996). Maturational Constraints on Functional Specializations for Language Processing: ERP and Behavioral Evidence in Bilingual Speakers. *Journal of Cognitive Neuroscience*, *8*(3), 231–256.

Weil, S. (2001). Foreign accented speech: Encoding and generalization. *Journal of the Acoustical Society of America*, *109*(5), 2473.

Werker, J. F. & Tees, R. C. (1984). Phonemic and phonetic factors in adult cross-language speech perception. *The Journal of the Acoustical Society of America*, *75*(6), 1866–78.

Werker, J. F. & Tees, R. C. (1999). Influences on infant speech processing: toward a new synthesis. *Annual Review of Psychology*, *50*, 509–535.

Witteman, M. J., Weber, A. & McQueen, J. M. (2013). Tolerance for inconsistency in foreign-accented speech. *Psychonomic Bulletin & Review*, *21*(2), 512–519.

Wong, P. C. M., Perrachione, T. K. & Parrish, T. B. (2007). Neural characteristics of successful and less successful speech and word learning in adults. *Human Brain Mapping*, *28*(10), 995–1006.

Xie, X. & Myers, E. B. (under review). Learning a talker or learning an accent: Acoustic similarity constrains generalization of foreign accent adaptation to new talkers.

Xie, X., Theodore, R. & Myers, E. B. (in press). More than a boundary shift: perceptual adaptation to foreign-accented speech reshapes internal structure of phonetic categories. *Journal of Experimental Psychology: Human Perception and Performance*.

Ylinen, S., Uther, M., Latvala, A., Vepsäläinen, S., Iverson, P., Akahane-Yamada, R. & Näätänen, R. (2010). Training the brain to weight speech cues differently: a study of Finnish second-language users of English. *Journal of Cognitive Neuroscience*, *22*(6), 1319–1332.

Sandra Kotzor, Allison Wetterlin and Aditi Lahiri
Symmetry or asymmetry: Evidence for underspecification in the mental lexicon

Abstract: We focus here on asymmetries which are part and parcel of phonological systems of natural language. We provide an overview of our assumptions concerning asymmetric representations, which are abstract and underspecificied, outlining the principles underpinning the *Featurally Underspecified Lexicon* (FUL; Lahiri & Reetz, 2002, 2010) and illustrating how questions regarding the specificity of lexical representations can be translated into experimental paradigms addressing processing issues. The second half of the chapter is dedicated to the discussion of experimental studies, covering segmental feature contrasts (place and manner) in consonants and vowels as well as duration contrasts in consonants. Experimental results from English and Bengali support our hypotheses that underspecified asymmetric representations lead to asymmetries in processing.

1 Introduction

Most phonological analyses assume some form of representation which is not akin to the surface form largely because assimilations or dissimilations, deletions or epentheses, optional or otherwise occur more often than not to alter the pronunciation of words. This is evident in morphophonological alternations (German *Tag* [taːk] ~ *Tage* [taːgə] 'day SINGULAR~PLURAL') as well as in purely phonological shapes of words which are inevitably articulated differently even by the same speaker (English *bottle* [bɒtl̩] ~ [bɒtʰɨl]; *mat* [mætʰ] ~ [mæt̚] ~ [mæʔ]; *different* [dɪfrənt] ~ [dɪfərɛnt]; Bengali [nɑːk] 'nose' ~ [nɑk-i] 'nose-ADJECTIVE' ~ [nɑːk=i] 'nose-ALSO'). The vowel length differences in Bengali, for instance, are due to the fact that monosyllabic prosodic words must have a long vowel. Consequently, although a clitic {=i} leads to a disyllabic word, it is attached to the prosodic word $((\text{nɑːk})_\omega = i)_\omega$ and hence the vowel is already long. As a result of the considerable variation in speech, one has become accustomed to frustrations in dealing with computerised dialogue systems requiring knowledge of our personal data such as

---

Sandra Kotzor, Faculty of Linguistics, Philology & Phonetics, University of Oxford;
School of Education, Oxford Brookes University
Allison Wetterlin, Department of Foreign Languages and Translation, Univeristy of Agder
Aditi Lahiri, Faculty of Linguistics, Philology & Phonetics, University of Oxford

DOI 10.1515/9783110422658-005

our names or date of birth. Spelling one's name with the usual alphabetic details such as "A for *Alpha*, D for *Delta*" is easier than pronouncing it normally. Articulating names and digits can easily lead to misperceptions, particularly when speaking to a machine.

Human brains are far better than computers at coping with variation in the speech signal and, despite the clamorous environment we live in, our comprehension system is remarkably efficient. Two extreme approaches to word recognition have been distinguished. One, where different phonetic exemplars of a word with perhaps details of the speaker are stored and the second, where the words are stored in an abstract form. The truth is probably somewhere in between but there can be little doubt that even with a full storage hypothesis, there must be some level of abstraction. The question which then arises is how abstract is abstract. Our model, FUL (*Featurally Underspecified Lexicon*, Lahiri & Reetz, 2002, 2010), was developed with the basic premise that phonological representations in the mental lexicon are crucially abstract and can even be underspecified. Such representations predict asymmetric processing, which, in turn, has an effect on language change.[1] We outline below a research programme which has been examining the effects of levels of phonological representations on processing. The phonological elements we have been investigating concern features relating to place and height, nasality, as well as phonological duration. We begin by laying out our assumptions regarding phonological representations and then discuss the role these representations play in the course of language comprehension.

2 Phonological representations in FUL

One fundamental assumption is that only features which contrast within a language play a role in lexical representation (cf. Dresher, 2009) and that place features are shared by consonants and vowels. [NASAL], for instance, is contrastive in English, but only for consonants not for vowels while the same feature is contrastive in Bengali for both vowels and consonants. Thus, if the feature appears contextually on the surface, it is not contrastive in so far as the lexical phonological representation is concerned. This has the consequence that the segment containing a feature may be part of the vocabulary of a language, but does not have a contrastive function in the representation. One such feature is [SPREAD GLOTTIS] for English; it appears on voiceless stops only in specific syllabic position, e.g.

---

[1] We assume that it is not 'languages' which change, but rather grammars and grammatical systems in the minds of speakers and listeners undergo change (Lahiri & Plank 2010).

syllable initial (Gussenhoven, 1986) and is thus not represented in the lexicon. On the other hand, the feature is required to contrast consonants in the underlying representation in Bengali, distinguishing phonemes such as /p pʰ/ and /b bʰ/. In the same vein, the strident fricatives [s] and [ʃ] occur in standard versions of Dutch, English and Bengali but they are contrastive only in English (Evers et al., 1998). In Bengali the underlying consonant is /ʃ/ while [s] occurs contextually when followed by [t̪] – [miʃ-i] ~ [miʃ-b-o] ~ [mis-t̪-o] 'mix-PRESENT.1P ~ FUTURE-1P ~ HABITUAL PAST-3P'. In Dutch, the opposite is the norm where /s/ is the underlying fricative and /ʃ/ is derived in the context of /j/; e. g., *ijs ~ ijsje* [ɛɪs] ~ [ɛɪʃə] 'ice cream ~ little ice cream'.

Second, not all features are specified in the underlying lexical representation. Underspecified features which have been proposed are [CORONAL] and [PLOSIVE] (see Lahiri 2015 for a discussion). One reason for this assumption is that that these features are available in all languages of the world and therefore in some sense redundant. This assumption has been controversial even with those who do assume underspecification. Dresher and colleagues, for instance, assume underspecification but not always for a specific feature (Compton & Dresher, 2011). Clements (2001) also assumed underspecification but proposed different levels where some features, like coronal, were underspecified but not always. Thus, for Dresher and Clements, languages may differ with respect to which features are active and visible in the phonology. From our perspective, other than the fact [CORONAL] and [PLOSIVE] are always underspecified, the active presence of other features will be dependent on whether they are contrastive in a particular language or not. For example, the feature which distinguishes /s/ from /ʃ/ is [HIGH] (see below). If these consonants do not contrast (as in Bengali or Dutch), the consonant /ʃ/ need not be specified in the underlying representation for this feature. However, [HIGH] plays an important role in English. Recall that consonants and vowels share place features and a partial feature tree is given in (1) to illustrate how this feature-sharing works.

(1) PLACE in FUL

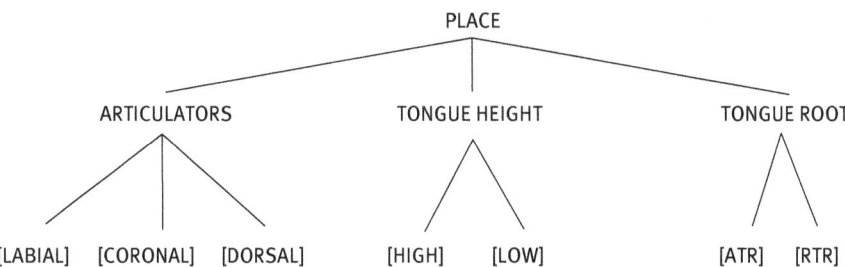

Examples:

[CORONAL]	[i e ɛ y œ]	[t d θ t̪ ɖ s ʃ]
[LABIAL]	[y u o ɔ]	[p f w]
[DORSAL]	[a ɯ]	[k x]
[HIGH]	[i ɪ]	[ʃ t̪ ɖ]
[LOW]	[æ ɑ]	[t̪ ḍ ṣ]
[ATR]	[i y e]	
[RTR]	[ɪ ʊ ɛ]	

Third, no features are dependent on others. Thus [CORONAL] has no dependents such as [anterior] or [distributed]. Contrasts within the [CORONAL] feature are handled by other related features such as [HIGH] and [LOW]. The following contrastive fricatives in English illustrate how different [CORONAL] fricatives are distinguished without dependent features.

(2) Feature contrasts of fricatives in English

	θ	s	ʃ
CORONAL	√	√	√
HIGH			√
LOW	√	√	
STRIDENT		√	√

It should also be noted, however, that not all phonetic segments will have the same phonological feature contrasts across languages. This is particularly true for vowels; [ɔ], for instance, is [LOW] in Bengali (cf. Lahiri, 2000a) and patterns together with [æ] but is definitely not low in English or German. Similarly, in Turkish, phonetically mid vowels such as [o] and [ɛ] pattern along with the low vowel [a] for the purposes of height harmony (Kabak, 2011; Lahiri, 2000b).

The same lack of isomorphism is observed in consonants. In English, for instance, /θ/ is not marked as [STRIDENT]. This is evident from various morphophonological patterns such as the regular plural which induces an epenthetic schwa when a noun ends with a [STRIDENT] fricative, but not with a non-strident; eg. *moths* [θs] but *buses* [bʌsəz]. On the other hand, in Tahlatan, the harmony patterns (cf. (3)) suggest that /θ s ʃ tʃ dʒ/ are all [STRIDENT] (Lahiri & Reetz, 2010): within a word, adjacent obstruents specified for [STRIDENT] must agree in TONGUE HEIGHT features. Thus, the phonology may not consistently pattern with the phonetics.

(3) Tahlatan harmony

u[θ]idʒɛ	u[ʃ]idʒɛ	we are called	[θ] [dʒ] > [ʃ] [dʒ]
mɛθɛ[s]ɛθ	mɛθɛ[θ]ɛθ	I'm wearing (on feet)	[s] [θ] >[θ] [θ]
ya[s]tɬetʃ	ya[ʃ]tɬetʃ	I'm singing	[s] [tʃ] > [ʃ] [tʃ]

Nevertheless, in language comprehension and speech recognition, the auditory system must extract the information from the phonetic signal and map this information on to a lexical representation. Our model, FUL, makes explicit claims about both the representation and the mapping. Since the representation is abstract and underspecified, the mapping is hardly assumed to be perfect. Thus, in addition to a *match* (where the signal agrees with the representation) and a *mismatch* (where the signal conflicts with the representation), there is the possibility of a *no-mismatch*, which is a tolerance relationship. Since the first two cases are obvious, we will concentrate on the *no-mismatch*. There are three main consequences of the introduction of a no-mismatch relationship. First, if we assume that [CORONAL] is unspecified and the signal extracts [DORSAL], then a larger cohort of words is activated since there is no *mismatch* although there is also no perfect *match*. Thus, if one is interested in the notion of competition, an unspecified feature leads to more competition. Second, although a feature can be unspecified in the lexicon, it can be extracted if it is needed for the phonetic output. Consequently, [CORONAL] can be extracted which can then, of course, mismatch with [DORSAL]. As a result, an asymmetry is immediately postulated. We claim that this asymmetry is in fact fundamental to the recognition process. If contrast sensitivity is asymmetric, then it is easier for the perceptual system to correctly detect, for instance, a phoneme such as /g/ after /ŋ/ rather than the opposite, viz. /ŋ/ after /g/. In other words, the idea is that the overall detection rate should be better in a situation where the contrast sensitivity is **not** symmetric. And of course, a pre-requisite for a sensitivity to asymmetric contrasts is that not all features are equally specified, which is the crux of FUL.

In a range of experimental studies (cf. Lahiri 2012 for a review), we examine the central tenet of FUL that, irrespective of whether the variants are allophonic (so entirely predictable as in the case of American English flaps; Pitt, 2009) or neutralizing (i. e., the contrast is neutralized as in the case of assimilations of phonemes), the representation will assist in resolving the variation. Thus, in an assimilatory context, the nasal consonant in *rain* is underspecified for its place of articulation feature [CORONAL], that is, it is not stored in the mental representation. A crucial difference between FUL and other models is that the latter do not expect any asymmetries during perception and comprehension based on feature specifications. Asymmetries in recognition can be governed by lexical frequency

(Pierrehumbert, 2016) and cohorts and the uniqueness point (Zwitserlood & Marslen-Wilson, 1989). Under such assumptions, a word like *tennis* will be recognised much faster than *tenet* since the former is about 10 times as frequent as the latter. Equally, *sclerosis* will be recognised faster than *scrutiny* since the former has a much smaller cohort. Based on CELEX, the uniqueness point of *sclerosis* is [sklə] with a cohort of two at the point of [skl]. In contrast, *scrutiny*'s uniqueness point is [skrutɪn] with a cohort of 115 when counted from [skr]. FUL, however, suggests that if a feature is unspecified, its parallel features will be tolerated during comprehension. An example of a set of matching assumptions is given in (4) using place and manner features.

(4) Sample feature mapping: signal to lexicon

Signal	*Matching*	Representation
[CORONAL]	MISMATCH	[DORSAL]
[NASAL]	MISMATCH	[STRIDENT]
[LABIAL]	NO-MISMATCH	[CORONAL]
[DORSAL]	NO-MISMATCH	[CORONAL]
[STRIDENT]	MISMATCH	[NASAL]
[LOW]	MISMATCH	[HIGH]

Thus, in terms of lexical activation, if a feature in the signal is unspecified, and a corresponding feature conflicts with it, there is a *mismatch* and the relevant phoneme will not be activated. A feature-based, rather than phoneme-based, cohort is activated, a sample of which is given in (5).

(5) Activation of cohort: spoken word *beet* [biːt] and *boot* [buːt]

UR	[b	iː/uː	t]	Surface	/b	iː/uː	t/
	OBSTR	SON	OBSTR		OBSTR	SON	OBSTR
	CONS	VOW	CONS		CONS	VOW	CONS
	LAB	COR/DOR	COR		LAB	–/DOR	–
		HIGH				HIGH	

(i) [b]   **bee, beet, bail, boot, book, pea, pool, pin**
(ii) [iː] **bee, beet, bail,** ~~boot, book,~~ **pea,** ~~pool,~~ **pin**
(iii) [t] **bee, beet,** ~~bail, boot, book, pea, pool,~~ **pin**

(iv) [b]   **bee, beet, bail, boot, book, pea, pool, pin**
(v) [uː]   **bee, beet, bail, boot, book,** ~~pea,~~ **pool, pin**
(vi) [t]   **bee, beet,** ~~bail,~~ **boot,** ~~book,~~ **pea,** ~~pool, pin~~

The example above considers a sample of words which may be activated as the signal is perceived. This is very similar to Marslen-Wilson's Cohort model (Zwitserlood & Marslen-Wilson, 1989) except that it depends on features of individual phonemes rather than the phonemes as a whole. The difference between *boot* and *beet* lies in the ARTICULATOR features. On perceiving [b], the activated cohorts are the same; note, however, that words with /p/ are also in the cohort since there is no mismatching in [VOICE]. In comparison, for a phoneme-based cohort, no word with a different phoneme would be activated and only words beginning with /b/ would be considered. Moving on to the next phoneme, since [CORONAL] from the surface of the next phoneme /i/ will mismatch with [DORSAL] in the underlying representation of /u/ in *boot* but not vice versa, on perceiving [buː] ((5v), 7 words), a larger cohort is activated than for [biː] ((5ii), 5 words); i. e. all words with [CORONAL] vowels, such as *bee, beat, bail, pin* are still activated when [buː] is perceived. Once the final consonant is heard, given that it is an [OBSTRUENT] and also [CORONAL], the final sonorants as well as all CV words are deactivated, leaving two words in (5vi) and only one in (5iii).

A further point to note is that the mental lexicon and the cohort of words play a significant role in constraining available word choices. A sequence such as [zʊ] would lead to a cohort of two (with a perfect match) along with around six (monomorphemic) words beginning with [sʊ] (*no-mismatch*). [nʊ] has a cohort of one while [mʊ] has two words with perfect match in its cohort plus [nʊ]'s cohort. Underspecificied representation entails that hearing fully specified features by definition results in the activation of larger cohorts. Thus, all phonemes beginning with [DORSAL] must activate the no-mismatching [CORONAL] cohort but not vice versa.

In the case of length contrasts, the representation is not based on features; instead duration is represented on a skeletal or timing tier (cf. Hayes, 1989; Kotzor et al., 2015). This representation is also reflected in a processing asymmetry, particularly for consonants. Here, vowels and consonants have asymmetric representations: a short vowel has one mora and a long vowel has two moras while a long consonant has a single mora but a short consonant has no moraic representation. However, it should be noted that in most Germanic languages, the vowel length contrast goes hand in hand with an ATR/RTR contrast where long vowels have the feature [ATR]. An idealised representation of phonological length contrast is given in (6).

(6) Representation of phonological length

```
μ    μμ        μ
|    \/        |
a    aː    p   pː
```

We have experimentally explored the notion of symmetry and asymmetry with a variety of phonological features including PLACE features such as [LABIAL, DORSAL, CORONAL], TONGUE HEIGHT features [HIGH, LOW] as well as other features such as [NASAL, STRIDENT, PLOSIVE]. We have primarily contrasted symmetry vs. asymmetry, where symmetry can be realised on the basis of matching features *or* mismatching features. That is, identical features will by default match, while conflicting features such as [STRIDENT/NASAL] (see (4)) will mismatch. Asymmetry will occur only if a particular feature has been unspecified where it will be in a *nomismatch* relationship with the opposing feature; e.g. [CORONAL] is underspecified and the other place features will not mismatch with it, but it itself will mismatch with features such as [DORSAL] (cf. (4)). For phonological length contrasts, however, we have examined only consonantal length in Bengali and in Swiss German.

In what follows, we briefly discuss the experimental paradigms we have used and then provide a summary of the types of experiments which have supported the symmetry and asymmetry in processing reflecting the proposed representations.

3 Experimental methods to investigate phonological representations

In order to experimentally investigate the validity of the central tenet of FUL introduced above, a number of different experimental paradigms and methods have been employed which, taken together, provide varied sources of support for underspecified lexical representations and processing asymmetries.

3.1 Behavioural paradigms

One of the primary means of investigation used in our research is a cross-modal lexical decision task using mispronunciations. Mispronunciations have been used successfully in a number of studies with both adults and children (among others Bailey & Plunkett, 2002; Bölte & Coenen, 2000; Mani & Plunkett, 2010; Roberts et al., 2013) and have been an extremely useful tool in probing the nature of phonological detail in lexical representations. Mispronunciations are used in priming tasks where the prime in a related prime-target combination (e.g. sonnet – POEM) is replaced with a mispronunciation (e.g. *sommet – POEM) to determine whether an incorrectly pronounced prime will still result in facilitation of the recognition of the target. If the listener is able to use the mispronounced prime to activate the original word (in this case *sonnet*), this should result in priming while, if they are unable to do so, no facilitation for the target word will be observed. The degree of featural difference between the real word and its mispronunciation can be varied according to the hypotheses regarding the underspecification of certain features (e. g. [CORONAL]). Thus, if the medial coronal consonant in a word such as the above *sonnet* is replaced with **sommet*, this should lead to priming since the bilabial nasal in the signal would not mismatch with the underspecified nasal of the real word while the reverse manipulation (*baggage* to **baddage*) will not facilitate the response to the target *suitcase* since the coronal plosive in the signal mismatches with the specified representation of the dorsal plosive in *baggage* (cf. Roberts et al., 2013). These mispronunciation studies have also been carried out with duration manipulations where a geminate consonant or a long vowel was replaced with a singleton or short vowel respectively to investigate the representation of duration in the lexicon (see section 5 in this chapter).

In addition to semantic priming, further methods used to shed light on lexical representations include form priming as well as fragment form priming to trace how much information needs to be available to the listener (especially in the case of the geminate duration experiments) to be able to make an accurate assessment of what has been heard. Forced-choice identification experiments were also used to gather evidence on which type of information, surface cues or underlying representations, listeners primarily use to distinguish between minimally different stimuli such as nasal and oral vowels (cf. 4.3 in this chapter).

Taken in combination, these behavioural methods allow for different angles on the same central question of the phonological specificity of lexical representations and enable us to draw conclusions which are based on a variety of phenomena as well as multiple experimental paradigms.

3.2 Electrophysiological experiments

To complement the behavioural methods described above, several of the paradigms were translated into EEG experiments. The main methods employed were lexical decision tasks with semantic priming to elicit a difference in the N400 and mismatch negativity experiments to tap into pre-attentive processing of featural and durational contrasts. The semantic priming experiments using mispronunciations (featural and durational) were designed to probe the facilitation effect of words which were mispronounced in certain, strictly controlled ways. If a mispronunciation is still able to lead the listener to activation of the real word prime, the EEG experiments would show a reduced N400 effect as seen for regular semantic priming paradigms (e. g. Kutas & Hillyard, 1980).

The mismatch negativity (MMN) experiments, on the other hand, tap into a less conscious phase of processing and provide valuable insights into the early stages of lexical processing and whether certain featural mismatches, for example, result in responses of differing magnitude. The MMN is an automatic change detection paradigm which, when a change in stimulus is registered by the processing system, results in a large negative deflection in ERP at about 180-250ms after the onset of the stimulus. Subjects hear a string of similar sounds (standards) with different sounds (deviants) interspersed, often at a ration of 85/15 or similar. It is well attested that phonemic differences (e. g. a change from [a] to [ɔ] in English) would result in a large MMN component while an allophonic change would not (MMNm, Kazanina et al., 2006). The MMN has been used with simple acoustic differences (duration, pitch, loudness) but has also been very successfully used with a variety of linguistic stimuli (for an overview, see Näätänen et al., 2007) and is generally proposed to be linked to the availability of a central sound representation of the stimuli. Thus, if a change is very noticeable (e. g. according to FUL a *mismatch* such as between a [CORONAL] deviant and a [LABIAL] standard), a larger MMN is expected. In terms of featural underspecification, MMNs are still expected for any kind of phonemic difference but the magnitude of the response may be contingent on the *match/mismatch* status of any given standard-deviant pair with certain pairs (*no-mismatches*) resulting in reduced MMN responses compared to others (*mismatch* conditions).

One additional use of this methodology is the fact that the stimuli can either be single sounds or words. This allows the investigation of the question of independence between the representation of phonological properties and lexical items.

Using several behavioural and electrophysiological paradigms and methods provides a more solid foundation for the investigation of the representations in the lexicon and the phenomenon of underspecification. It allows for a multi-dimensional approach which will, in the end, result in a more complete picture than a more unilateral set of experiments.

4 Processing of feature contrasts

This section presents experimental evidence for CORONAL underspecification in both consonants and vowels as well as an investigation of the representation of the feature [NASAL] in vowels in Bengali. Since the languages we have been working with (English, German, Dutch, Bengali, Swedish, Norwegian) tend to have three features under the ARTICULATOR node, we have focused on the features CORONAL, DORSAL, and LABIAL.

4.1 Coronal underspecification in consonants

The very first experimental study where we proposed underspecfication was a gating study on the nasal ~ non-nasal vowel contrast in Bengali and English (see 4.3). The hypothesis was that, since Bengali has nasal vowel phonemes, these vowels would be specified for [NASAL] while any other contextual nasalisation would not be specified. Thus [kãdʰ] would contain an underlying vowel specified for nasality while the surface [kãn] from /kan/ would be unspecified. The results suggested that any nasality from the signal, whether from [VN] or [ṼC] would elicit only Ṽ responses and hardly any VN responses suggesting that the specified nasal was a better match. That is, even if the nasality in a [VN] word was *acoustically less* than a 'real' nasal, the underlying Ṽ were preferred (Lahiri & Marlsen-Wilson, 1992). Later, after the FUL model was developed (Lahiri & Reetz, 2002), a series of experiments with different methodologies was undertaken to examine place asymmetries.

Since one of the reasons for assuming underspecification was the occurrence of directional asymmetries in assimilations (where CORONAL consonants were more likely to assimilate than DORSAL or LABIAL), the first set of experiments began with asymmetries in coda consonants such as comparing *Bahn* 'train' and *Baum* 'tree' with their opposite variants. In semantic priming experiments, we found that mispronounced variants **Baun* did not activate *Baum* but **Bahm* did activate *Bahn* (Lahiri & Reetz, 2002). However, Gaskell and colleagues (Gaskell & Marslen-Wilson, 1998; Snoeren & Gaskell, 2007) argued that the reason why **browm* activated *brown*, but **crean* did not activate **cream* was because listeners are exposed to assimilated variants and would be familiar with them. That is, brow[m][b]*ay* would be heard by listeners in normal pronunciation which would make it more acceptable. However, FUL's hypotheses were more general and assumed that the underspecification was not position specific. Consequently, unless there was a particular phonological exception, [CORONAL] would be unspecified in all word positions, initial, medial and final; no assimilation could be expected in word initial or medial (intervocalic) position.

These hypotheses led to a further series of experiments where the crucial consonants were in medial or initial positions. Here we used both behavioural and electrophysiological techniques in German (Friedrich et al., 2006, 2008; Cornell et al., 2011, 2013) and in English. For example, for English, we considered medial place asymmetries comparing word pairs like *sonnet* vs. *image* (Roberts et al., 2014). The hypothesis was that if /n/ was underspecified for place but /m/ was not, then the mispronounced word **sommet* would still activate *poem* (synonymous with *sonnet*) but **inage* should not activate a word related to *image* such as *picture*. These hypotheses were borne out. In a semantic priming study, **inage* failed to prime *picture*, but **sommet* primed *poem*. Furthermore, in an EEG study, **inage* invoked a high N400 while **sommet* was not significantly different from its real word counterpart *sonnet*. Similar asymmetries were found in other EEG (with MMN) and behavioural studies. In German, for instance, using nonsense syllables such **edi* and **ezi*, we found that MMNs for /d/ and /z/ were entirely symmetrical (since [STRIDENT] and [NASAL] mismatch) while /g/ and /d/ show asymmetric MMNs since [CORONAL] mismatches [DORSAL] but not vice versa (Cornell et al., 2013).

4.2 Place and height mismatch in vowels

An early study (Eulitz & Lahiri, 2004) provided the first pieces of evidence for underspecification from a neurobiological perspective using an MMN study with German vowel stimuli which differed in the specification of place features. If one assumes a fully specified lexicon, a reversal of standards and deviants in a mismatch negativity study should result in responses of equal magnitude in all cases as each sound is fully specified and would thus mismatch with the other sounds to the same degree as the acoustic distance between the stimuli remains constant. In an underspecified lexicon, this reversal of standards and deviants may, depending on the exact specifications of the sounds, result in an asymmetry where one direction elicits a greater MMN response (a *mismatch*) than the other (a *no-mismatch*). Eulitz & Lahiri (2004) contrasted the features [CORONAL], [DORSAL] and [LABIAL] using the German vowels /e/ ([CORONAL]), /ø/ ([CORONAL]; [LABIAL]) and /o/ ([LABIAL]; [DORSAL]) and found strong support for FUL as the same vowel pairs showed asymmetrical MMN responses depending on the specification of phonological features in the underlying representation. As the underlying form of the standard /ø/, for example, is underspecified for place, it does not conflict with the surface signal of the deviant /o/ which is specified for [LABIAL]. In the reverse situation, however, the surface form of the [CORONAL] /ø/ as a deviant conflicts with the underlying [LABIAL] representation of the standard /o/ as [CORONAL], while not specified, is nevertheless extracted from the acoustic signal. This results in a *mismatch* which generates a larger and earlier MMN response.

A further, more recent, study on place and height features in English vowels (Kotzor et al., 2016) provides additional evidence for processing asymmetries resulting from underspecified representations. The aim of this study was to compare listeners' automatic responses to two differently represented feature sets: in addition to using the asymmetric place representations between [CORONAL] and [DORSAL] vowels /ɛ/ and /ɔ/, a pair of vowels where both members are fully specified for height (/ɪ/ and /æ/ which are [HIGH] and [LOW] respectively) was also selected. A second question addressed in this study was whether the asymmetry observed in earlier studies using individual vowels would remain constant when these vowels appear in words and nonwords. By altering the lexical status of the items the vowels are presented in, conclusions can be drawn as to the independence of the representation of sounds.

Table 1: Design and predictions

	Experiment 1				Experiment 2			
DEV SR	sit [HIGH]	sat [LOW]	*sif [HIGH]	*saf [LOW]	get [COR]	got [DOR]	*gef [COR]	*gof [DOR]
STD UR	sat [LOW]	sit [HIGH]	*saf [LOW]	*sif [HIGH]	got [DOR]	get [ ]	*gof [DOR]	*gef [ ]
MMN predictions	MMN	MMN	MMN	MMN	MMN	reduced MMN	MMN	reduced MMN

The stimuli in this study were two pairs of English ablaut verbs, *get-got* and *sit-sat*, with one differing only in place (*get-got* [CORONAL]/[ ] – [DORSAL]) and the other in vowel height (*sit-sat* [HIGH] – [LOW]). Each pair was complemented by a matching nonword pair: **gef-*gof* and **sif-*saf* to investigate the effect of lexical status. We used a standard oddball paradigm (15 % deviants) and each item was presented once as the standard and once as the deviant with block order randomized across participants (see Table 1 for details). Four tokens of each stimulus were cross-spliced from recordings by a female Southern British English speaker and the only variation between these tokens was the naturally occurring variation in the vowel while one version of each consonant was used.

Following the predictions FUL makes regarding place and height features, we should expect to see the following pattern of results. In the height conditions, the MMN responses should be of equal magnitude regardless of the stimulis' standard/deviant status since both [HIGH] and [LOW] vowels are fully specified for vowel height. Thus, when a [HIGH] vowel deviant is heard after a [LOW] vowel standard, this will result in a *mismatch* (and therefore an early MMN response of high magnitude) and the same should be seen for the reverse case. The place difference, however, is expected to create a different pattern as the coronal /ɛ/ in *get* and **gef* is underspecified for place. Here, the same predictions as in the Eulitz & Lahiri (2004) study discussed above apply: if a [DORSAL] deviant (*got/*gof*) is heard after underspecified standards (*get/*gef*), the MMN response should be of lower amplitude since this results in a *no-mismatch* as the surface form of the deviant does not mismatch with the underspecified underlying representation of the standard. The reverse case, on the other hand, would be a *mismatch* as the surface information of the coronal deviant (*get/*gef*) would mismatch with the underlyingly dorsal standard (*got/*gof*). In terms of the effect of lexical status, FUL would not predict a difference between words and nonwords since the representation of the vowels is considered independent of lexical items. If [CORONAL] was specified in the lexicon, a symmetrical pattern of MMN amplitudes of equal latency and magnitude would be expected in all conditions.

The data shows strong support for FUL as the predictions made by the model are borne out. The vowel height pair *sit-sat* results in MMN amplitudes of equal size regardless of which member of the pair appears as the standard and which as the deviant. The same results are also found for the corresponding nonword pair **sif-*saf*. The data for the place feature pair shows a difference between the two directions of presentation. In blocks with a coronal (underspecified) standard (i. e. *get* or **gef*), we see a significantly lower MMN amplitude than in those blocks where the standard is fully specified. This confirms the results from earlier studies and, in addition, opens up the discussion of the effect of lexical status in phonological processing.

4.3 Processing of nasal vowels

In addition to the investigations into features such as [CORONAL] and [HIGH]/[LOW], a study on nasal vowels shows a similar pattern of results for the feature [NASAL]. Unlike the feature contrasts investigated in the experiments described above, nasality can be a result of the underlying representation of the vowel or a consequence of regressive assimilation from a following nasal consonant (e. g. Bengali [bãd^h] 'dam' vs. [bãn] 'flood'). Many languages use nasality contrastively which enables us to consider the question whether surface cues (i. e. any nasality in the signal) or underlying representations (only nasality which is represented in the lexicon) guide listeners' perception of nasal vowels.

There have been several proposals regarding the representation of nasality in the lexicon with some arguing for an equipollent pair of features ([+NASAL] and [-NASAL]; Chomsky & Halle, 1968: 316) while others propose a privative feature [NASAL] (Lahiri & Marslen-Wilson, 1992; Lahiri & Reetz, 2002, 2010). There have also been proposals which differentiate between languages which possess underlying nasal vowels and those where only contextualized nasality occurs (Cohn, 1993; Trigo, 1993). These proposals claim those languages which do have an underlying contrast represent nasality using an equipollent set of features while in languages without such a contrast, a privative feature is used. In light of these different theoretical proposals, the central question concerns the representation of nasality in the lexicon. In addition, we were also aiming to determine whether listeners are equally sensitive to surface and underlying cues or whether these properties are treated differently in the recognition process.

The experiments reported on here were conducted with native speakers of Bengali, a language with an underlying nasal vowel contrast. This allowed for the creation of triplets of words with the same vowel in three different versions: oral (CVC; [tʃal] 'uncooked rice'), contextually nasalized (CVN; [tʃan] 'bath') and underlyingly nasal (CṼC; [tʃãd] 'moon'). Furthermore, since some combinations are not attested in the language and to see how listeners reacted when they were constrained by the lexicon, two sets of doublets were used as stimuli; one where no CVN was attested (e. g. [dʒʰal] 'spicy' – [dʒʰãp] 'jump') and one without a CṼC word (e. g. [tin] 'three' – [til] 'sesame'). The experiment was a cross-modal forced-choice task with auditory fragment primes and visually presented full-word targets. Subjects were presented with the CV segment of Bengali CVC monosyllables and were asked to identify which of the targets the fragment corresponded to.

If nasality is indeed represented by a privative feature [NASAL], we would expect faster response latencies and lower error rates for conditions where the prime is a nasal vowel (either underlyingly or contextually nasalized) and the target is a CṼC word compared to all other conditions. However, if an equipollent representation is correct, we would also expect to see faster latencies and greater accuracy for those cases where the prime is an oral vowel and the target is either a CVC or a CVN word since both vowels would be represented as [-NASAL].

The results in both doublet experiments support a privative feature [NASAL] rather than an equipollent set. Participants were both significantly faster and more accurate when responding to a nasal vowel prime which could be matched to a CṼC target while all other conditions were similar in accuracy and response latencies. The results of the triplet experiment also supported the privative representation in both response latencies and errors and illustrated that any surface nasality in the prime would be mapped (very quickly) on a CṼC target if one was available. If there is no such target available, listeners seem to use surface cues to find the best possible match which could be seen in a preference of CVN targets over CVC targets after a CṼ(C) prime.

5 Processing and representation of consonant duration – evidence from Bengali

Following on from the discussion of featural contrasts above, this section will introduce several experiments investigating the processing and representation of consonantal duration. Experimental evidence from Bengali, a language with a well-established geminate-singleton contrast, provides evidence for a privative moraic representation of duration which leads to a processing asymmetry reminiscent of those found for featural underspecification (e. g. for [CORONAL]).

Bengali, like many of the world's languages, has a productive word-medial duration contrast where almost all consonants can occur as either singletons or geminates (e. g. [pata] 'leaf' vs. [pat:a] 'whereabouts'). While duration is not a phenomenon on the featural level but rather a structural one, there seem to be certain similarities the questions asked about its representation regarding the detail of specification in the lexicon. Specific predictions about the processing of durational properties have not been put forward. In a series of behavioural and neurolinguistic experiments, we have begun to explore the representation of the geminate-singleton contrast.

5.1 Consonant duration

Duration, unlike featural contrasts, is not characterized by a presence or absence of a certain type of information in the acoustic signal but rather by the length of time this information is presented for. In addition, durations of long and short consonants vary widely across the world's languages and are also dependent on the context they appear in as well as on phenomena such as speech rate. This makes the geminate-singleton contrast a different type of distinction which is intrinsically variable and therefore requires a degree of flexibility in its representation. Often, humans are considered to perceive sounds categorically rather than discriminating on the most detailed level reducing this variability to a small number of distinct phonological categories. This is said to be the case for the geminate-singleton contrast across languages (Hankamer, Lahiri & Koreman, 1989; Phillips et al., 2000; Raizada & Poldrack, 2007; Reetz & Jongman, 2009). As mentioned above, there are large differences between languages in terms of both absolute differences of singleton and geminate consonants and relative differences and in some languages the duration of vowels and consonants is interdependent.

Bengali is a language with word-medial geminates only but in this position, the geminate-singleton contrast is very common and the majority of consonants can be found as both singletons and geminates. Furthermore, consonant duration in Bengali is independent of the duration of the preceding vowel which makes the language well-suited for an experimental investigation of the duration contrast. Word-medial geminates are always heteromorphemic but are considered a single unit rather than a sequence of two identical segments. This position is supported by the fact that geminates cannot, for example, be broken up through epenthesis (cf. for example Kenstowicz and Pyle, 1973) while a sequence of two identical consonants can.

As far as the representation of duration in phonological theory is concerned, several proposals have been put forward. For the purpose of our research here, three will be considered: a featural approach proposing an equipollent set of features ([+LONG] and [-LONG], X-slot theory with a single slot for a singleton and two for a geminate and a moraic approach which posits a mora for a geminate while a singleton does not have any additional specification.

As is evident from these three standpoints, one of the central questions, similar to the case of the nasal vowels, is whether duration is represented in a privative or equipollent manner. That is, whether both long and short consonants are specified for duration in their lexical representation or whether one, most likely the singleton, is underspecified and serves as the default.

The three approaches lead to different predictions regarding the outcome of any experimental study. The featural approach as well as the X-slot option should result in a symmetric result while the account based on mora theory would expect a processing asymmetry to be evident in the data.

5.2 Experimental evidence

A series of experiments using mispronunciations of Bengali medial consonants was designed to test these hypotheses. Six lexical decision tasks with form and semantic priming (Kotzor et al., 2015) and two EEG experiments (one N400 study and one MMN study) were conducted with native speakers of Bengali. All tasks use mispronunciation and the rationale behind the design is identical to that in the experiments used to investigate coronal underspecification (cf. 4.1). All lexical decision tasks were cross-modal with auditory primes and visual targets. In the first two experiments, the primes were disyllabic Bengali words with either a singleton or geminate where a change in consonant duration would result in a non-word (e. g. [ʃona] 'gold' to *[ʃon:a] or [ʃun:o] 'zero' to *[ʃuno]) while the targets were semantically related words (e. g. [rupo] 'silver'). Experiments 3–6 were form priming experiments using the CVC segment of the primes from the first two experiments (e. g. /ʃon/ or */ʃon:/ and /ʃun:/ or */ʃun/). In two of the experiments (3 and 4), only the consonant duration of the medial consonant was included in the fragment while in the subsequent two experiments (5 and 6) the first two glottal pulses of the vowel were also added to determine whether the additional information would result in greater ease of processing since it allows the listener to make an unambiguous decision about the duration status of the medial consonant. See Table 2 for a summary of stimuli and predictions.

Table 2: Examples of experimental stimuli and predictions for lexical decision tasks

	Prime	Target	Behavioural predictions	N400 predictions
Experiment 1	[ʃona] 'gold' *[ʃon:a]	[rupo] 'silver'	facilitation facilitation	reduced N400 reduced N400
Experiment 2	[ʃun:o] 'zero' *[ʃuno]	[kʰali] 'empty'	facilitation no facilitation	reduced N400 no reduced N400
Experiments 3 & 5	[ʃon] / [ʃonᵥ] *[ʃon:]/ *[ʃon:ᵥ]	[ʃona]	facilitation facilitation	
Experiments 4 & 6	[ʃun:] / [ʃun:ᵥ] *[ʃun] / *[ʃunᵥ]	[ʃun:o]	facilitation no facilitation	

All behavioural results showed a pattern consistent with our predictions based on the moraic theory proposal discussed above. If a listener heard a singleton real word which was mispronounced as a geminate, this prime still activated the real word and its semantic relation. This could be seen in the facilitation shown for mispronounced primes in Experiments 1, 3 and 5 which did not differ significantly from that following real word primes. In those cases, however, where the listeners heard a real word geminate mispronounced as a singleton, no facilitation was observed for the mispronunciations in the semantic priming task (Experiment 2) while the two form priming tasks (Experiments 4 and 6) did show a degree of priming (most likely due to the complete featural overlap between prime and target) but this effect was significantly weaker compared to the degree of facilitation shown for real word primes. It seems that providing too much durational information is less detrimental to comprehension than not providing enough.

In terms of the moraic account, this can be explained in analogy to a featural underspecification approach. Since the contrast between geminates and singletons is represented privatively, when a singleton is mispronounced as a geminate, the additional mora which is present in the acoustic input does not mismatch with the underlying representation since the singleton is not specified for duration. In the reverse scenario, the short duration in the signal conflicts with the underlying representation of the geminate real word which requires an additional mora that cannot be constructed based on the information from the signal. Therefore, the singleton mispronunciation does not successfully activate the geminate real word.

A further two studies were conducted using EEG to determine whether the results obtained from the behavioural studies would be confirmed by neurolinguistic evidence. An N400 study (Roberts et al., 2014) based on Experiments 1 and

2 (semantic priming tasks) showed an identical pattern where the N400 amplitude for short real words mispronounced as long patterns with the responses to semantically related real word items while the geminate real words mispronounced as singletons fails to result in an attenuated N400 response. A mismatch negativity study using a standard oddball paradigm contrasting real geminate and singleton words with mispronounced singletons and geminates also provided additional support for the fact that the mispronounced geminate is accepted in place of the real word while the singleton mispronunciation of a geminate is not. As the MMN probes pre-attentive processing, it is interesting to see that this effect is already evident very early on in the comprehension process and does not seem to be dependent on strategic processing.

While duration is not a contrast at the featural level, the processing asymmetries observed in our data are strikingly similar to those found in cases where one feature is underspecified. It thus follows that duration is likely represented privatively with the long consonant specified for duration (in the case of Bengali with an additional mora) while the singleton is unspecified. More research into different manifestations of duration contrasts, e. g. vowel duration, and duration contrasts in other languages is necessary to be able to firmly establish the precise nature of the representational basis of duration contrasts in order to be able to integrate these into an underspecification model.

6 Lessons learned

Misperceptions and mispronunciations are not infrequent in the languages of the world. In addition, no matter how hard we try, no individual can ever produce a word in an identical fashion twice. Given this variation, we have three options to choose from in terms of mapping from the signal to lexical representations: (i) all variants are stored and they then have prototypes which still are fully specified; (ii) representations are abstract and underspecified, ensuring that the mental lexicon does a great deal of work in constraining the choices; (iii) a hybrid between the two. The third is possibly true but we need to define precisely what is abstract and what is not in order to be able to test it rigorously in experiments. We chose the second hypothesis based on facts from language change as well as synchronic phonological patterns. The central idea was that, if representations are sparse and not fully specified, there is more chance of resolving variation. The experimental evidence presented in this chapter shows that we are not too far off the mark. Processing symmetries as well as asymmetries, which point to asymmetric representations, have been found in a number of experiments for a variety of featural contrasts (e. g. [CORONAL] vs. [DORSAL] and [LABIAL]; [HIGH] vs. [LOW]; [STRIDENT] vs. [NASAL]). Asymmetric representation of consonantal length contrast also leads to processing asymmetries. Frequency as well as talker specificity undoubtedly play a role in language comprehension. Nevertheless, our results suggest that there is a coherent underlying structure which both allows and constrains variability. As has become evident, it is not a question of separating symmetry from asymmetry; rather, both are necessary and more research is required to examine these principles on a broader crosslinguistic basis.

Acknoweldgements: This research has been funded by the European Research Council (Grant: FP7-IST-269670; PI A. Lahiri). The ERC team, who contributed equally to the research presented here, includes the authors as well as Adam C. Roberts.

References

Bailey, T. & Plunkett, K. (2002). Phonological Specificity in Early Words. *Cognitive Development*, *17*(2), 1267–1284.
Bölte, J. & Coenen, E. (2000). Domato primes paprika: Mismatching words activate semantic and phonological representations. *Proceedings of the workshop on Spoken Word Access Processes (SWAP)*. MPI for Psycholinguistics, Nijmegen, The Netherlands.
Chomsky, N. & Halle, M. (1968). *The Sound Pattern of English*. New York, NY: Harper & Row.
Clements, G. N. (2001). Representational economy in constraint-based phonology. In T. A. Hall (ed.), *Distinctive feature theory*, Berlin: Mouton de Gruyter, 71–146.
Cohn, A. (1993). *Nasalisation in English: phonology or phonetics? Phonology*, *10*(1), 43–81.
Compton, R. & Dresher, B. E. (2011). Palatalization and "Strong i" across Inuit Dialects. *Canadian Journal of Linguistics/Revue canadienne de linguistique*, *56*, 203–228.
Cornell, S. A., Lahiri, A. & Eulitz, C. (2011). "What you encode is not necessarily what you store": Evidence for sparse feature representations from mismatch negativity. *Brain Research*, *1394*, 79–89.
Cornell, S. A., Lahiri, A. & Eulitz, C. (2013). Inequality across consonantal contrasts in speech perception: evidence from mismatch negativity. *Journal of Experimental Psychology: Human Perception and Performance*, *39*(3), 757–772.
Dresher, B. E. (2009). *Contrastive hierarchy in phonology*. Cambridge: Cambridge University Press.
Eulitz, C. & Lahiri, A. (2004). Neurobiological Evidence for Abstract Phonological Representations in the Mental Lexicon during Speech Recognition. *Journal of Cognitive Neuroscience*, *16*(4), 577–583.
Evers, V., Reetz H. & Lahiri, A. (1998). Crosslinguistic acoustic categorization of sibilants independent of phonological status. *Journal of Phonetics*, *26*, 345–370.
Fikkert, P. & Levelt, C. C. (2008). How does place fall into place? The lexicon and emergent constraints in the developing phonological grammar. In P. Avery, B. E. Dresher & K. Rice (eds), *Contrast in phonology: Perception and Acquisition*, Berlin: Mouton, 231–270.

Friedrich, C. K, Eulitz, C. & Lahiri, A. (2006). Not every pseudoword disrupts word recognition: an ERP study. *Behavioral and Brain Functions*, *2*, 1–36

Friedrich, C. K., Lahiri, A. & Eulitz, C. (2008). Neurophysiological Evidence for Underspecified Lexical Representations: Asymmetries With Word Initial Variations. *Journal of Experimental Psychology: Human Perception and Performance*, 34(6), 1545–1559.

Gaskell, M. G. & Marslen-Wilson, W. D. (1998). Mechanisms of phonological inference in speech perception. *Journal of Experimental Psychology: Human Perception and Performance*, 24, 380–396.

Gussenhoven, C. (1986). English plosive allophones and ambisyllabicity, *Gramma* 10, 119–41.

Hankamer, J., Lahiri, A. & Koreman, J. (1989). Perception of consonant length: voiceless stops in Turkish and Bengali. *Journal of Phonology*, *17*, 283–298.

Hayes, B. (1989). Compensatory Lengthening in Moraic Phonology. *Linguistic Inquiry*, *20*, 253–306.

Kabak, B. (2011). Turkish vowel harmony. In: M. van Oostendorp, C. Ewen, B. Hume & K. Rice (eds), *The Blackwell Companion to Phonology*, Wiley-Blackwell, 2831–2854.

Kazanina, N., Phillips, C. & Idsardi, W. (2006). The influence of meaning on the perception of speech sounds. *PNAS*, *103*(30), 11381–11386.

Kenstowicz, M. & Pyle, C. (1973). On the phonological integrity of geminate clusters. In: M. Kenstowicz & C. Kisseberth (eds), *Issues in phonological theory*, The Hague, The Netherlands: Mouton, 27–43.

Kotzor, S., Wetterlin, A., Roberts, A. C. & Lahiri, A. (2015). Processing of phonemic consonant length: Semantic and fragment priming evidence from Bengali. *Language and Speech*, 1–30.

Kotzor, S., Zhou, B., Alter, K. & Lahiri, A. (2016). Place and height mismatch in vowels: evidence from an MMN study. Poster presented at the *Annual Conference of the Society of the Neurobiology of Language*, London, UK (August 17-20th 2016).

Kuhl, P. K. & Miller, J. D. (1978). Speech perception by the chinchilla: Voiced–voiceless distinction in alveolar plosive consonants. *Science*, *190*, 69–72.

Kutas, M. & Hillyard, S. A. (1980). Reading senseless sentences: Brain potentials reflect semantic incongruity. *Science*, *207*, 203–205.

Lahiri, A. & Hankamer, J. (1988). The timing of geminate consonants. *Journal of Phonetics*, *16(3)*, 327–338.

Lahiri, A. & Marslen-Wilson, W. D. (1992). Lexical processing and phonological representation. In R. D. Ladd & G. Docherty (eds), *Papers in Laboratory Phonology II: gesture, segment, prosody*, Cambridge: Cambridge University Press, 229–254.

Lahiri, A. (2000a). Hierarchical restructuring in the creation of verbal morphology in Bengali and Germanic: evidence from phonology. In A. Lahiri (ed.), *Analogy, Levelling, Markedness*, Berlin: Mouton, 71–123,

Lahiri, A. (2000b). Phonology: Structure, Representation and Process. In L. Wheeldon (ed.), *Language Production*, Cambridge: Psychology Press, 165–225.

Lahiri, A. & Reetz, H. (2002). Underspecified recognition. In C. Gussenhoven & N. Warner (eds), *Laboratory Phonology VII*, Berlin, Germany: Mouton de Gruyter, 637–677.

Lahiri, A. & Reetz, H. (2010). Distinctive Features: Phonological underspecification in representation and processing. *Journal of Phonetics, 38*, 44–59.

Lahiri, A. & Plank, F. (2010). Phonological phrasing in Germanic: the judgement of history, confirmed through experiment. *Transactions of the Philological Society, 108:3*, 370–398.

Lahiri, A. (2012). Asymmetric phonological representations of words in the mental lexicon. In A. C. Cohn, C. Fougeron & M. K. Huffman (eds), *The Oxford Handbook of Laboratory Phonology*, Oxford: Oxford University Press, 146–161.

Lahiri, A. (2015). Change in word prososdy: stress and quantity. In P. Honeybone & J. Salmons (eds), *The Oxford Handbook of Historical Phonology*, Oxford: Oxford University Press, 219–244.

Mani, N. & Plunkett, K. (2010). Does size matter?: Graded sensitivity to vowel mispronunciations of familiar words. *Journal of Child Language, 38*, 606–627.

Näätänen, R. (2001). The perception of speech sounds in the human brain as reflected by the mismatch negativity (MMN) and its magnetic equivalent (MMNm). *Psychophysiology, 38*, 1–21.

Näätänen, R., Paavilainen, P., Rinne, T. & Alho, K. (2007). The mismatch negativity (MMN) in basic research of central auditory processing: A review. *Clinical Neurophysiology, 118*, 2544–2590.

Phillips, C., Pellathy, T., Marantz, A., Yellin, E., Wexler, K., Poeppel, D., McGinnis, M. & Roberts, T. (2000). Auditory cortex accesses phonological categories: an MEG mismatch study. *Journal of Cognitive Neuroscience, 12*(6), 1038–1055.

Pierrehumbert, J. (2016). Phonological representation: Beyond abstract versus episodic. *Annual Review of Linguistics, 2016*(2), 33–53.

Pitt, M. A. (2009). How are the pronunciation variants of spoken word recognized? A test of generalization to newly learned words. *Journal of Memory and Language, 61*(1), 19–36.

Raizada, R. D. S. & Poldrack, R. A. (2007). Selective Amplification of Stimulus Differences during Categorical Processing of Speech. *Neuron, 56*(4), 726–740.

Reetz, H. & Jongman, A. (2009). *Phonetics: Transcription, Production, Acoustics and Perception*. London, UK: Wiley-Blackwell.

Ridouane, R. (2010). Geminates at the junction of phonetics and phonology. In C. Fougeron, B. Kuhnert, M. Imperio & N. Vallee (Eds.), *Papers in Laboratory Phonetics 10*. Berlin, Germany: Mouton de Gruyter, 61–90.

Roberts, A. C., Wetterlin, A. & Lahiri, A. (2013). Aligning mispronounced words to meaning: Evidence from ERP and reaction time studies. *The Mental Lexicon 8*(2), 140–163.

Roberts, A. C., Kotzor, S., Wetterlin, A. & Lahiri, A. (2014). Asymmetric processing of durational differences – electrophysiological investigations in Bengali. *Neuropsychologia, 58*, 88–98.

Snoeren, N. D. & Gaskell, M. G. (2007). Computational modeling of assimilated speech: Cross-linguistic evidence. In D. S. McNamara & J. G. Trafton (eds), *Proceedings of the 29th Annual Cognitive Science Society*, Austin, TX: Cognitive Science Society, 1509–1514.

Trigo, R. L. (1993). The inherent structure of nasal segments. In M. K. Huffman & R. A. Krakow (eds). *Nasals, Nasalisation, and the Velum*, Phonetics & Phonology (Volume 5), New York: Academic Press, 369–400.

Zwitserlood, P. & Marslen-Wilson, W. D. (1989). The locus of the effects of sentential-semantic contexts in spoken-word processing. *Cognition, 32*, 25–64.

Julia R. Drouin, Nicholas R. Monto and Rachel M. Theodore
Talker-specificity effects in spoken language processing: Now you see them, now you don't

Abstract: A fundamental goal of research in the domain of speech perception has been to describe how listeners resolve the lack-of-invariance problem in order to achieve stable word recognition. Here we review work from our laboratory and others that has examined the representational nature of prelexical and lexical knowledge by considering the degree to which listeners customize the mapping from the acoustic signal to meaning on a talker-specific basis. One central finding is that while talker-specificity effects in speech perception are observed frequently, they are not absolute, and seem to be influenced by rich interactions within the cognitive and language architectures. We consider these findings with respect to their implications for abstract and episodic accounts of spoken word recognition.

1 Introduction

One remarkable feat of human speech perception is listeners' ability to create stable linguistic representations, despite substantial variation in the acoustic-phonetic signal produced for any given speech segment. As a case in point, the acoustic pattern for a given consonant or vowel reflects coarticulatory characteristics from one context to another. Research by Liberman et al. (1954) examined productions of the syllables /di/ and /du/ and revealed that while both contain acoustic patterns consistent with articulatory gestures of the /d/ phoneme, the /d/ production manifests in different acoustic forms depending on the syllable

---

Julia R. Drouin, Department of Speech, Language, and Hearing Sciences, University of Connecticut
Nicholas R. Monto, Department of Speech, Language, and Hearing Sciences, University of Connecticut
Rachel M. Theodore, Department of Speech, Language, and Hearing Sciences, University of Connecticut, Connecticut Institute for the Brain and Cognitive Sciences, University of Connecticut

DOI 10.1515/9783110422658-006

context. Specifically, they observed differences in second formant transitions, where in the /di/ context the transition rises and in the /du/ context the transition falls to reflect the final /u/. Thus, while the production of the /d/ stop consonant shows acoustic energy consistent with the vocal tract occlusion required to produce this stop consonant, the input for the perceptual system is markedly different due to coarticulatory influences. Termed the lack of invariance problem, this finding demonstrates that there is no one-to-one correspondence between the acoustic-phonetic signal and any particular phoneme. However, despite this lack of invariance, listeners robustly map acoustic variation to discrete phonetic categories.

In addition to coarticulatory factors, a primary contributor to the lack of invariance problem observed in speech perception comes from talker variability. Previous research has shown that different acoustic forms from different talkers may correspond to the same percept (Dorman, Studdert-Kennedy & Raphael, 1977; Peterson & Barney, 1952). Thus, speakers of a given language show great between-talker variability, where productions vary extensively from one talker to the next to reflect a talker's acoustic-phonetic signature. Further, talkers also show extensive within-talker variability where their own productions of a specific phoneme may vary from one production to the next.

Despite such rampant talker variability in the acoustic signal of speech, listeners reliably extract meaning from talkers that they have never before encountered. However, given enough experience with a talker's voice, listeners show processing benefits for familiar compared to unfamiliar talkers. This forms a central theoretical problem in the speech perception domain: What mechanisms and representations support listeners' ability to both comprehend a novel speaker of the language *and* capitalize on systematic phonetic variability leading to familiar talker benefits in spoken language processing? This question forms the basis of this chapter.

We begin by describing literature documenting talker differences in phonetic properties of speech. We then review literature from our lab and others' that has examined perceptual adaptation to talker variability, both at the segmental and lexical levels of speech processing. Following, we discuss evidence suggesting that there are bi-directional links between linguistic processing and voice recognition. Finally, we conclude by considering how theoretical models of human speech perception can account for these effects.

2 Talker differences in phonetic properties of speech

Talkers vary on a range of acoustic parameters including pitch, fundamental frequency, and vocal quality – parameters that have collectively been referred to as indexical variation. However, these are not the only features that differentiate one speaker from another. Research in the speech production domain has revealed that talkers show systematic differences in the acoustic-phonetic parameters used to mark phonemic contrasts. That is, talkers not only differ in indexical properties, but they also differ in how they implement phonetic properties of speech. One such parameter is voice-onset-time (VOT). VOT is an articulatory feature for word-initial stop consonants and is measured as the time between the release of the occlusion necessary for stop consonant production and the subsequent onset of vocal fold vibration. VOT is an important feature of stop consonants in the English language as it marks the voicing distinction between stop consonants with the same place of articulation, such as the /b/ – /p/ contrast for bilabial stop consonants. Though this relative VOT distinction marks the voicing contrast across speakers, the absolute VOTs produced for a given stop consonant systematically vary among individual talkers. Allen, Miller & DeSteno (2003) examined word-initial VOTs of monosyllabic words produced by eight different talkers. After controlling for other contextual features on VOT production including speaking rate and place of articulation, they found a significant amount of variation in VOT that reflected systematic differences between talkers. That is, some talkers produced characteristically longer VOTs than other talkers.

Evidence of talker-specificity for VOT production was also reported by Theodore, Miller & DeSteno (2009). Recall that in Allen et al. (2003) talker differences in VOT were examined after controlling for contextual factors on VOT production. Theodore et al. (2009) examined whether talkers differ in these contextual influences proper. Specifically, they examined whether the effect of speaking rate and place of articulation on VOT vary across speakers of American English. Previous research has shown that VOT is robustly influenced by both of these factors. Consider first speaking rate. As speaking rate slows, and words become long, so too do VOTs produced for a given stop consonant (e. g., Volaitis & Miller, 1992). Now consider place of articulation. As place moves from front-to-back in the vocal tract, VOTs systematically increase (e. g., Cho & Ladefoged, 1999; Lisker & Abramson, 1964). Theodore et al. (2009) examined whether talkers differ in VOT production not only when these factors are controlled, but also whether these contextual influences are themselves talker-specific.

In our first experiment (Theodore et al., 2009), we used a magnitude production procedure to elicit many productions of the syllable /ti/ from 10 native monolingual speakers of American English. The productions were elicited to span a wide range of speaking rates as would be expected as someone altered their speaking rate to be very fast, perhaps due to excitement, or very slow, due to speaking clearly. For each token, VOT and syllable duration (as a metric of speaking rate) were measured. For each talker, a linear function relating VOT to syllable duration was calculated, and the slope of this function was used as an indicant of the effect of speaking rate on VOT. Hierarchical linear modeling (HLM) was used to examine whether there was significant variability in the talkers' slopes, and the results confirmed that this was indeed the case. That is, the effect of speaking rate on VOT was talker-specific. Moreover, the results of the HLM showed that at a given speaking rate, talkers also showed systematic differences in VOT, replicating findings from Allen et al. (2003).

The second experiment examined potential talker-specificity of the place of articulation effect on VOT. Using the same procedures as describe above, production of the syllables /pi/ and /ki/ were elicited from a different group of 10 talkers. Again, the effect of speaking rate on VOT was calculated by determining the slope of the function relating VOT to syllable duration. The results confirmed that for both the /pi/ and /ki/ syllables, the effect of speaking rate on VOT again varied across talkers. However, the results did not show any evidence indicating that the effect of place of articulation varied across talkers. That is, for all talkers, the VOTs of the /ki/ syllables were displaced towards longer VOTs compared to the /pi/ syllables, but the magnitude of this displacement did not significantly vary across the 10 speakers. Thus, unlike the effect of speaking rate, the effect of place of articulation on VOT was not talker-specific. As we describe below, these findings point to specific predictions regarding the type of experiences listeners may need in order to adapt to talker differences in VOT.

Talker differences in phonetic properties of speech have also been observed for vowels (e. g., Peterson & Barney, 1952) and other consonants. For example, Newman, Clouse & Burnham (2001) examined productions of the /s/ and /ʃ/ fricatives among a group of talkers. They found that there was extensive variability in their speech productions, such that some talkers had relatively distinct phonemic categories, where examination of frication centroid and skewness clearly indicated two speech sound categories. However, other talkers presented with overlapping /s/ and /ʃ/ categories. Further, they found that perception of these fricatives was largely influenced by the stability of the talker's productions. That is, more variable speech productions were perceived as more ambiguous than talkers with more consistent productions. Also, Newman and colleagues (2001) observed that listeners who encountered talkers with more variable productions had slower response times, compared to listeners who encountered talkers with consistent productions, suggesting that consistency in production plays a role in how listeners categorize sounds from a given talker.

Collectively, findings from the speech production literature demonstrate that talkers show systematic differences in how they implement phonetic properties of speech. These findings challenge the long-standing view that differences in talker's voices are limited to indexical variation, such as the fundamental frequency associated with rate of vocal fold vibration. Because talkers also differ in how they implement phonetic properties of speech, the very input to the auditory system that allows listeners to derive meaning in spoken language processing, suggests that a strict delineation between indexical and phonetic variation is not possible. Moreover, as we describe below, the perceptual system may track this type of phonetic variation and use it to customize speech processing on a talker-specific basis.

3 Talker-specificity for speech sound perception

One key theoretical problem in the speech perception domain is describing how listeners are able to extract reliable linguistic information from a highly variable acoustic speech signal. We have previously described some variation in the acoustic signal that can be attributed to talker differences in speech production. The talker differences in speech production reviewed above represent one type of talker variation that does not lead to ambiguity in phonetic category membership. However, there are other forms of variation that may manifest as extremely ambiguous, such as in the case of foreign-accented speech or disordered speech. In this section we will review findings that have demonstrated striking talker-specificity for both ambiguous and unambiguous acoustic variation. A growing body of research in the speech perception literature has shown that listeners can use talker specific phonetic variability to modify speech processing for that talker. Previous research has also suggested that listeners may use this talker specific-phonetic variability to assist in word recognition (e. g., Nygaard et al., 1994). However, relatively little is known about the specific mechanisms the listener implements to do so.

One way that listeners may accommodate such variation by recruiting lexical knowledge. Lexically-informed perceptual learning is one mechanism that listeners may implement to accommodate variation across a range of talkers. This type of learning allows the listener to make relatively long-lasting changes in the perceptual system in response to a changing environment by using lexical information to adjust speech sound categories (Goldstone, 1998; Norris et al., 2003). Listeners process the acoustic speech stream in a categorical manner to maintain perceptual constancy. However, speech sound categories, like other cognitive and perceptual categories, have a graded internal structure with some members of the category being more representative than others (Kuhl, 1991; Miller & Volaitis, 1989; Samuel, 1982). Because of this, it is unclear whether the listener only learns information about a specific talker characteristic and thus only adjusts internal category structure or if it involves a more comprehensive restructuring of phonetic categories. Previous research has suggested that the nature of the variation – whether it constitutes clearly defined category membership or whether it is ambiguous – influences whether listeners modify internal category structure or comprehensively adjust the phonetic category boundary. We begin by describing perceptual accommodation of within-category phonetic variation and then describe findings for ambiguous, between-category phonetic variation.

3.1 Talker-specificity for within-category variation

Recall that VOT is one phonetic property of speech for which talkers show systematic individual variation. Research has examined whether listeners are able to track such talker variability in VOT. Allen & Miller (2004) exposed listeners to two different talkers during a training and identification period. In the training period, listeners were exposed to the words "dime" and "time," each produced by two female talkers. The voiceless alveolar stop /t/ was manipulated such that the VOTs of the "time" stimuli were relatively long in one talker and relatively short in the other. That is, the speech was manipulated such that in one condition talker one had long VOTs and talker two had short VOTs and a different set of listeners hearing the opposite pattern of VOT exposure. During test, listeners were presented with the long and short VOT variants from the same talkers that they heard during training and were asked to select the production that was most representative of one of the talkers. The results were consistent with their experience during training. That is, listeners who heard long VOTs from talker one and short VOTs from talker two consistently identified the long VOT variant as more representative of talker one and the short VOT variant as more representative of talker two. Interestingly, this effect also persisted in a novel word condition where listeners were able to transfer knowledge of one talker's characteristic production of a specific stop consonant in a new phonetic environment (i. e. "time" to "town"). This suggests that listeners were learning how the talker implemented the /t/ category and were able to generalize rather than limiting their learning to only the specific training exemplars. Allen & Miller (2004) suggested that listeners may benefit from talker-specific experiences as a way to bootstrap their sensitivity to fine-grained acoustic-phonetic features. These results further support the notion that listeners can account for this lack of invariance problem in speech, and suggest that even minimal exposure to a talker's voice can help the listener reshape their phonetic categories and be better equipped to process subsequent productions.

Previous research lends supports to the idea that listeners can use relatively limited exposure to a production in a specific context and generalize to other phonetic contexts (Allen & Miller, 2004), however it is unclear how far this generalizes. To address this, Theodore & Miller (2010) investigated whether generalization extends beyond one given stop consonant. In a training phase, they exposed listeners to two female talkers, "Annie" and "Laura," and heard each talker produce the token "pain." Critically, one group of participants heard Annie produce short VOTs and Laura long VOTs, while the other group of participants heard Annie produce long VOTs and Laura produce short VOTs. In both training conditions, listeners were exposed to the corresponding variant of the voiceless "pain" and its voiced counterpart "bane," produced by each talker. On each trial, participants were asked to identify both the talker and the initial consonant of each stimulus. At test, listeners were given the name of a talker on the screen and were asked to choose the corresponding production of "pain" that was most representative of that voice, thus providing a replication of Allen & Miller (2004). In session 2, the test procedure was identical except that listeners were tested on a novel lexical item, either "cane" or "coal." Their results showed that, in both cases, listeners robustly generalized knowledge learned during training to a novel place of articulation. In other words, listeners were sensitive to characteristic VOTs for not only the token presented in training, but also for the novel word that varied in either place of articulation and phonetic context. Strikingly, the generalization observed in Theodore & Miller (2010) was complete in that learning was not attenuated for the novel word compared to the training word.

This line of research illustrates that listeners are able track systematic talker-specific variation for individual properties of speech, which provides a logical precursor for examining mechanisms that may support talker-specificity at higher levels of linguistic processing. It is well known that listeners process variability in the acoustic speech stream in a categorical manner, which facilitates perceptual constancy. However, speech sound categories, like other cognitive and perceptual categories, have a graded internal structure with some members of the category being more representative than others. That is, though some tasks suggest that category membership is an all-or-nothing phenomenon, other tasks have demonstrated that members of individual phonetic categories show rich variation in category goodness. That listeners can account for talker differences in phonetic properties of speech raises the possibility that they can use this information to restructure phonetic categories on a talker-specific basis, either by shifting category boundaries or by a reorganization of internal category structure. To examine this possibility, Theodore, Myers & Lomibao (2015b) examined talker-specific influences on phonetic category structure. In a training phase, they exposed two groups of listeners to the speech of two female talkers, referred to as "Joanne" and "Sheila." Both groups heard Joanne and Sheila produce the words "gain" and "cane." Critically, one group of listeners heard Joanne produce the word initial /k/ with short VOTs and Sheila produce word initial /k/ with long VOTs, while the other group of participants heard the opposite pattern of VOT exposure. Following this, all participants were tested in three different tasks using Joanne's voice. In the first test, participants were asked to listen to two productions of "cane," one produced with short VOT and the other produced with long VOT. They were asked to identify which production was most representative of Joanne's voice. In the second test, participants were tested on a VOT continuum ranging from "gain" to "cane" and were asked to rate the goodness of each item as a member of the /k/ category. In the third test, participants heard the same VOT continuum and were asked to identify whether the initial consonant was a /g/ or /k/.

The results from Theodore et al. (2015b) are as follows. First, the findings from Allen & Miller (2004) were replicated in that listeners who heard Joanne produce /k/ with short VOTs selected the short-VOT version of Joanne's voice when presented with the short-VOT and long-VOT pair. Second, experience with Joanne's voice promoted a comprehensive reorganization within the /k/ category such that the best exemplars of the /k/ category differed between the two training groups. Specifically, those who had heard Joanne produce long VOTs during training rated the long VOT members of the /k/ category as better exemplars of /k/ compared to listeners who heard Joanne produce short VOTs during training. This finding suggests that one mechanism for accommodating talker differences in speech production is to alter internal category structure in line with experience with a talker's voice. Strikingly, their results showed no evidence that listeners shifted the voicing boundary between /g/ and /k/ as a function of experience during training. In other words, talker-specificity for the type of unambiguous talker variability examined in this study was accommodated within the category proper, leaving the boundary intact. As we review in the following section, this type of adjustment may differ when the talker-specific phonetic variation to be learned does in fact consist of ambiguous productions that are not clearly defined category members.

3.2 Talker-specificity for between category variation

As previously highlighted, talker-specific changes to internal category structure can occur for well-defined productions. However, some types of acoustic variability occurs as a result of highly ambiguous speech. Previous research has suggested that listeners use lexical information to retune phonetic category boundaries, particularly when encountering productions that vary significantly and fall outside a category boundary. Norris, McQueen & Cutler (2003) manipulated /s/ and /f/ fricatives such that Dutch listeners were exposed to an ambiguous phoneme midway between an /s/ and /f/ during a lexical decision training task. In this task, listeners were biased into hearing the ambiguous fricative either in the context of /s/-final Dutch words like "naaldbos," creating the interpretation of the ambiguous blend as an /s/ based on lexical context, or /f/-final Dutch words like "witlof," creating the interpretation of the ambiguous blend as an /f/ based on lexical context. After exposure, they tested both groups of participants on a continuum ranging from more /f/-like to more /s/-like and found that listeners in the /f/-biasing condition categorized more items as an "f" and listeners in the /s/-biasing condition categorized more items as an "s." They concluded that listeners, with very little exposure to variation, were able to use lexical knowledge to guide the way they accommodate an ambiguous signal. Critically, this type of learning did not occur when the ambiguity was embedded in non-words, indicating a strong role for lexical information in guiding perceptual retuning.

Furthermore, Eisner & McQueen (2005) examined talker-specificity of this type of perceptual learning. They exposed Dutch listeners to one female talker. In a training phase listeners were exposed to talker with deviant fricative productions that were created by blending /f/ and /s/ sounds in a perceptually ambiguous manner. In one condition, participants were always exposed to the ambiguous sound in the context of /f/-final words, whereas in another condition participants were always exposed to the ambiguous sound in the context of /s/-final words. The listeners then categorized a continuum of tokens ranging from more /f/- like to more /s/-like and were asked to categorize items as either /f/ or /s/. They found listeners in an /f/- biased training group categorized more items as /f/, whereas listeners in an /s/-biased training group categorized more items as /s/. Critically, Eisner & McQueen (2005) found that these changes at the category boundary did not appear when the listener was tested on a novel talker, unless the ambiguous fricative from the novel talker was embedded into the training stimuli, suggesting that the lexically-informed perceptual learning adjustment was applied on a talker-specific basis.

Other research has aimed to extend findings from Eisner & McQueen (2005) and Norris et al. (2003) by examining whether the source of variation leads to differences in how the listener deals with these inconsistencies. Previous research has shown that the source of the variation plays a key role in determining how such variation is handled by the perceptual system. Kraljic, Brennan & Samuel (2008) examined this by exposing one group of participants to an audiovisual domain and another group of participants to an audio-only domain. In the audio-only group, one group of participants heard an ambiguous phoneme midway between /s/ and /ʃ/. The ambiguous blend was inserted into real words that contained either an /s/, creating the interpretation of that ambiguous sound as an /s/, or into words containing an /ʃ/, creating the interpretation of that ambiguous sound as an /ʃ/. For example, participants in an /s/-biasing condition heard words like "dinosaur" where the medial /s/ was replaced with the ambiguous sound. Conversely, participants in the /ʃ/-biasing condition heard words like "crucial" where the medial /ʃ/ was replaced with the ambiguous sound. In the audiovisual condition one group of participants heard ambiguous /s/ and /ʃ/ pronunciations while presented with a visual of a speaker with a pen in her mouth during such productions, while the other group of listeners saw the speaker without a pen in her mouth during the ambiguous productions. Following exposure, they tested participants on a continuum of sounds ranging from more /s/-like to more /ʃ/-like; participants were asked to categorize the tokens as either /s/ or /ʃ/. They observed a learning effect in the audio-only condition, and in the audiovisual condition, they only observed a learning effect in the second group of listeners, those who did not see the speaker with a pen in her mouth during the production of the ambiguous phoneme. However, the group who did see the speaker with a pen in her mouth did not exhibit a learning effect. Kraljic et al. (2008) posited that the perceptual system did not recalibrate for under such conditions because the ambiguity could be attributed to external contextual factors and that when such factors are at play lexically-informed perceptual learning does not occur, thus pointing at some constraints for this type of learning.

Other work has extended these findings by examining what type of exposure might constrain the perceptual learning process. Kraljic & Samuel (2011) used a similar training paradigm as Kraljic et al. (2008), where listeners were exposed to an ambiguous token midway between /s/ and /ʃ/ inserted into either /s/ or /ʃ/-biasing contexts. However, in one group of participants, listeners heard a block of non-standard tokens, followed by a block of standard tokens, where both standard and non-standard productions were recorded from the same talker. Another group of participants heard the opposite pattern of exposure where they listened to a block of standard tokens first, followed by a block of non-standard productions. Following this, both experimental groups were tested on a continuum of sounds ranging from more /s/-like to more /ʃ/ -like to measure categorization responses and compared listeners in both exposure conditions. They found that when participants were first exposed to the ambiguity, listeners in the first group, they showed a lexically-guided perceptual learning effect. However, this was not observed in those who were first exposed to standard pronunciations, followed by non-standard productions. These results suggest that the perceptual system is selective with respect to modifying category boundaries such that simple talker mispronunciations, as is the case of some non-standard productions following standard productions, do not lead to comprehensive perceptual adjustments. These results suggest that listeners are selective on when to robustly reorganize category boundaries.

Collectively, results from these studies suggest that the listener can learn and track different phonetic properties of speech on a talker-by-talker basis, such that they can learn acoustic characteristics features specific to an individual talker. The mechanisms that the listener uses to account for this variability includes tracking within-category variation and adjusting internal category structure so that some productions are weighted as more representative than others. However, the type of variation is also an important factor that plays a role in the how the perceptual system adjusts. For acoustic variation that is relatively unambiguous in nature, the perceptual system may adjust within the category, leaving the boundary region intact. Conversely, when the variation is deviant and ambiguous in nature, listeners may shift category boundaries and/or within the category. In sum, this literature suggests that the specific type of acoustic variation plays a role in the mechanisms listeners use to achieve talker-specificity in spoken language processing.

Such input-driven constrains on perceptual learning for talker variability would predict that when listeners accommodate talker productions that are ambiguous, they may do so by modifying the category boundary, as has been shown in previous research (e. g., Norris et al., 2003), but without concomitantly modifying internal category structure. Current research from our laboratory is examining this question to observe whether learning an ambiguous fricative limits the listener to restructuring only at the category boundary, or whether this type of learning also results in changes in internal category structure (Drouin, Theodore & Myers, 2016). In this study, listeners were exposed to an ambiguous fricative midway between an /s/ and /ʃ/ during a lexical decision training task. Critically, some listeners heard the ambiguous fricative in items like "Tennessee," where the middle /s/ sound was replaced with the ambiguous blend, creating the interpretation of such an ambiguous sound as an /s/. Conversely, some listeners heard the ambiguous fricative in items like "ambition," where the middle /ʃ/ sound is replaced with the ambiguous blend, creating the interpretation of the ambiguous sound as an /ʃ/. Following training, listeners were asked to listen to a continuum of sounds ranging from more /ʃ/-like to more /s/-like, and were asked to rate how good, or representative the token is of either an /ʃ/ (experiment 1), or an /s/ (experiment 2). Using a scale from one to seven, listeners ranked each token as either an excellent or poor exemplar of either fricative. This task allowed us to examine changes occurring within the category boundary. Following this, listeners were asked to listen to the same continuum of sounds, however this time listeners make a judgment on category boundary, where they decided whether the token sounded more like /s/ or /ʃ/. This task allowed us to examine changes at the category boundary as a function of training.

In experiment 1, listeners who rated the items as /ʃ/, we observed a change both at the category boundary and within the category. However for those participants in experiment 2, listeners who rated the items as /s/, we observed a change only at the category boundary, but no evidence that exposure during training shifted internal category structure. We posit that this difference reflects the distributional properties of the acoustic signal presented during the exposure phase; the /s/ and /ʃ/ tokens presented to the /ʃ/-bias group formed two distinct distributions with the modified /ʃ/ tokens showing minimal deviation from the naturally-produced tokens. In contrast, the /s/ and /ʃ/ tokens presented to the /s/-bias group formed two distributions with considerable overlap; moreover, the /s/ tokens for these listeners showed considerable deviation from the natural /s/ productions. Thus, we hypothesize that the difference we observed for the /s/ and /ʃ/ categories in terms of whether learning pervades internal category structure reflects interactions between top-down, lexically-driven perceptual learning and bottom-up learning that is driven by distributional information in the speech signal proper (e. g., Clayards et al., 2008; Kleinschmidt & Jaeger, 2015). On-going research aims to test this hypothesis.

4 Talker-specificity for lexical processing

In addition to talker-specificity effects for segmental perception, described above, there is a large body of evidence indicating that adaptation to talker-specific phonetic variability pervades higher-levels of linguistic processing. Specifically, research has shown a talker-familiarity effect for word recognition, which raises the possibility that lexical representations can be modified to represent talker-specific phonetic variation. Research indicates that listeners experience a host of comprehension benefits for familiar compared to unfamiliar talkers, suggesting that efficient language comprehension relies on integrating acoustic information about talker identity and the linguistic message (e. g., Goldinger, 1996). One of these benefits is increased intelligibility of the spoken message when listening to a familiar talker compared to an unfamiliar talker (Nygaard, Sommers & Pisoni, 1994). Nygaard et al. (1994) trained participants to learn to recognize ten talkers over a nine-day training period. At the end of this nine-day period, listeners transcribed words produced by the talkers presented during training and by novel talkers. The results showed that participants had increased comprehension for the trained compared to the novel talkers, suggesting that lexical knowledge had been modified to reflect experience with the talkers' voices presented during training. This talker familiarity benefit in terms of intelligibility has been shown for both isolated words and sentences (Nygaard & Pisoni, 1998). Moreover, the talker familiarity benefit generalizes to novel utterances, which suggests that the comprehension benefits observed at the lexical level reflect knowledge of how talkers' implement individual phonological segments and not specific words. Other talker comprehension benefits observed at the lexical level include decreased processing time for familiar compared to unfamiliar talkers (Clarke & Garrett, 2004) and decreased resource allocation for familiar compared to unfamiliar talkers (Mullenix, Pisoni & Martin, 1989).

This familiar talker benefit demonstrated in adults has also been shown in school-aged children (Levi, 2014). In this study, 41 native English-speaking children aged 7–12 were trained on 6 female bilingual German-English speakers for five days. A baseline measurement of spoken word recognition was obtained prior to training, which consisted of the child listening to a series of words (spoken by the 6 female voices they were to be trained on) and asked to repeat back the word that they heard. After explicit training on these 6 voices, children demonstrated a significant improvement in their ability to identify highly familiar words spoken by these familiar talkers (Levi, 2014). Additionally, children who performed the poorest at baseline (who were also the youngest subjects) demonstrated the greatest magnitude of improvement from pre- to post-test, indicating that talker familiarization may actually facilitate spoken language processing for children during this critical time of language acquisition.

Evidence for talker-specificity in the lexicon also comes from findings in the memory literature. Specifically, listeners show better recognition memory for words when voice in held constant between initial and subsequent presentations (Goldinger, 1998). This finding has been replicated many times, and has been interpreted as evidence that lexical representations are rich in phonetic detail, including that associated with individual talkers' voices (Church & Schacter, 1994; Schacter & Church, 1992; Palmeri et al., 1993; Theodore et al., 2015b).

Recent findings have lead to the development of the time-course hypothesis, which posits that talker-specificity effects in spoken word recognition arise relatively late in processing, compared to more allophonic-specificity effects, which are considered to be more generalized across speakers of a given language. McLennan, Luce & Charles-Luce (2003) examined the time-course of specificity effects for talker variability and allophonic variability using a repetition-priming paradigm. Their results show that both sources of variability revealed specificity effects, as measured by increased priming, but that the two types of specificity effects differed in their time course. Specifically, allophonic specificity effects emerged when processing was fast and talker specificity effects emerged when processing was relatively slower. These data were interpreted as the consequence of increased time needed to process the episodic information associated with talker variability (McLennan & Luce, 2005). Additional support for this account was provided using a recognition memory paradigm where one group of listeners heard typical speech and a different group of listeners heard dysarthric speech (Mattys & Liss, 2008). Talker-specificity effects were not observed for typical speech, where processing times were fast, but were observed for dysarthric speech, where processing times were relatively slower.

Theodore, Blumstein & Luthra (2015a) examined an alternative account to the emergence of talker-specificity effects. Recall that the time-course hypothesis states that talker-specificity effects only emerge when processing time is slow, reflecting the increased time needed to activate lower-frequency episodic information. In previous examinations of the time-course hypothesis, processing time was manipulated via task difficulty such that slow processing times were associated with a "hard" task and fast processing times were associated with an "easy" task. Given findings demonstrating that task difficulty can shift attention during encoding (e. g., Craik & Tulving, 1975), we tested the possibility that attention during encoding, and not processing time, could predict when talker-specificity effects would emerge during lexical retrieval.

In Theodore et al. (2015a), we reported three recognition memory experiments. In all experiments, listeners completed an encoding phase, in which a series of words was presented over headphones, followed by a recognition phase, in which words were again presented over headphones and listeners were asked to indicate if the item had been presented during training or not. Critically, some words were presented in the same voice during encoding and recognition, and some words were presented in different voices during the two phases. With this design, a talker-specificity effect manifests as higher hit rate at recognition for words presented in the same voice compared to words presented in different voices.

In the first experiment, attending during encoding was differentially manipulated for two groups of listeners. One group was directed to attend to the word and press a button to advance to the next trial; the other group was directed to identify the talker gender on each trial. The recognition phase was identical for both groups – they indicated whether each item had been presented during training. The results shows that those who attended to talker had increased hit rate at recognition as well as faster response times to same talker trials compared to those who attended to lexical characteristics. Critically, there was no difference in processing time at recognition between the groups. Thus attention during encoding, and not processing time at retrieval, determined the presence of talker-specificity effects. In the second experiment attention was again manipulated during retrieval. Participants either made a syntactic decision or the same talker decision as describe above. Again, talker-specificity effects at recognition only emerged for those who attended to talker during encoding, even those in the syntactic condition showed slower response times at recognition. The third experiment aimed to hold attention during retrieval constant, and focused on lexical characteristics, but manipulated processing time at retrieval with some listeners performing the recognition task in quiet and others performing it in the context of background noise. Neither group showed a talker-specificity effect at recognition, even though processing times were extremely slow for those performing the task in noise. Collectively, these results suggest that attention during encoding is the critical predictor of lexical specificity effects, even when pitted against processing time (Theodore et al., 2015a).

5 Language-specificity effects on voice recognition

As reviewed above, experience with a talker's voice promotes talker-specific changes in spoken language processing. Listeners track talker differences in phonetic properties of speech and restructure the mapping to linguistic categories as a consequence of experience with a talker's voice. Moreover, listeners show increased word recognition and recognition memory for words as a consequence of talker familiarity, indicating that the talker-specific influences on spoken language processing pervade the lexical network. Strikingly, a separate body of evidence suggests that just as experience with a talker's voice influences linguistic processing, so too does linguistic ability influence voice recognition. Specifically, listeners show heighted voice recognition in the native compared to a non-native language, suggesting that linguistic experience facilitates identifying speakers of that language (Goggin et al., 1991; Perrachione & Wong, 2007). Given this evidence, models of spoken language processing must specify which aspect of linguistic expertise and experience contribute to the native-language benefit for voice recognition. There is some evidence indicating that the putative factor is phonological knowledge. Previous research has found a native language benefit for talker discrimination, even when participants are exposed to speech that is time-reversed in their native language (Fleming et al., 2014), thus pointing to a strong role of sub-lexical mechanisms in this process.

Converging evidence comes from studies that examined clinical populations with phonological deficits. One clinical population that presents with a deficit in phonological awareness is individuals with dyslexia. Perrachione et al. (2011) examined talker identification ability in adults with and without dyslexia for native and non-native languages. Their results found that the adults with dyslexia performed equally as poor in both native and non-native languages, where the adults without dyslexia showed a native language benefit. This pattern of performance has also been found in children, however children with dyslexia also showed a native language benefit (Perea et al., 2014). Other evidence in support of a phonological influence on voice recognition comes from Bregman & Creel (2014), who examined talker identification in Korean-English bilinguals, where one group learned English early in life and the other group learned English late in life. They found that the group of bilinguals who had learned English early in life showed faster learning rates for English talkers compared to those who had learned English late in life, suggesting that phonological ability facilitates talker identification. Taken together, these results suggest that one aspect of linguistic competence, phonological ability, mediates talker identification and comprehension.

However, other research indicates the native language benefit may be supported by experiences that precede phonological competence. Specifically, 7-month-old infants show a native language benefit for voice discrimination, which is earlier than even primitive phonological competency has been developed (Johnson et al., 2011). This finding raises the possibility that the native language benefit for voice recognition may even bootstrap subsequent language acquisition.

While the previously described literature examined talker identification in impaired readers with dyslexia, work by Kadam, Orena, Theodore & Polka (2016) aimed to examine whether these effects held when examining talker identification as a function reading ability in an unimpaired population. Kadam et al. (2016) categorized participants as either average or advanced readers based on performance for a standardized assessment battery of reading and reading sub-skills. Listeners were then exposed to eight different talkers, four native English talkers and four native French talkers. Listeners participated in familiarization, training, and test tasks, which were blocked by language. The familiarization task served as a passive learning task, during which listeners associated a talkers voice with a cartoon face. During the training task, listeners were presented two previously seen cartoon faces along with a spoken sentence. Listeners were tasked with selecting the correct "face" for each sentence and feedback was provided after their response. The training phase ended when listeners correctly matched 85 % of the voices to their respective face in a given training block. The test phase consisted a similar face-voice matching task; but no feedback was provided at test. The results showed that advanced readers required less exposure learn the talkers' voices compared the average readers, and that the advantage gained by heightened reading ability held during the test phase.

The findings reviewed above provided converging evidence that linguistic ability and voice recognition are fundamentally intertwined in spoken language processing. With respect to the findings from Kadam et al. (2016), differences between the two groups of readers emerged for the native speech, consistent with the hypothesis that phonological ability facilitates voice recognition. However, the two reading groups also differed with respect to the non-native voices. This latter finding raises the possibility that some non-phonological factor may in fact be leading to improved performance on both phonological and voice recognition tasks. Future work is aimed at examining this possibility.

6 Conclusions

In this chapter, we have discussed a key theoretical problem in the speech perception domain: How do listeners achieve reliable linguistic perception given that there is no one-to-one mapping between the acoustic signal and any given phoneme? We have reviewed findings from one contributor to this lack of invariance problem, that of talker variability. Many studies have demonstrated that talkers differ in phonetic properties of speech. Moreover, listeners are able to track these differences and customize speech processing to reflect talker-specific productions. Findings from studies that have examined two types of talker variability – ambiguous productions and clearly defined productions – point to a system that is conservative in the degree to which modifications are made. When the productions are clearly defined category members, listeners adjust internal category structure to reflect a talker's characteristic productions, while leaning the category boundary intact. However, when the talker's productions are so deviant that they fall ambiguous between categories, listeners robustly shift category boundaries to the degree that it is licensed by the lexicon. Just as experience with a talker's voice facilitates linguistic processing, so too does experience with language facilitate voice recognition. These findings point to constraints on models of spoken language processing, though of course future research is needed in order to determine if the these patterns hold across more exhaustive examinations.

Abstract theories of spoken word recognition posit that listeners filter out aspects of speech that are non-linguistic in order to capture more consistent aspects of the signal. Doing so provides a system that is robust to variation, including talker variation, and can easily describe how the system is capable of gleaning meaning from the speech of novel talkers. In contrast, episodic theories of spoken word recognition posit that listeners retain information about every aspect of the speech signal for every unique utterance presented to them. With respect to talker-specificity, episodic theories would suggest that listeners retain specific information unique to each utterance made by each encountered talker. This class of model provides an elegant way of describing talker-specificity effects, but requires some level of abstraction (e. g., averaging across exemplars) to describe how listeners recognize words produced by novel talkers. In order to fully account for how listeners are able to readily interpret information provided from an intensely variable signal, while still retaining the information necessary to identify individual sources, a combination of abstract and episodic processing is necessary.

One way that abstract and episodic models may be bridged comes from the domain of dynamic system theories. Attractor dynamics and the formation of attractor basins are rooted in dynamic systems theory. Briefly, dynamic systems theory posits that systems have attractor states, behaviors that they prefer, and repeller states, behaviors that they are repelled from (Hale & Koçak, 2012). This theory can be used to describe many different systems, one of the most iconic being phase coupled oscillators (Kuramoto, 1984). Breakspear, Heitmann & Daffertshofer (2010) provided a neural application of this theory, where they treat neurons as oscillators and utilize a modified Kuramoto model (Kuramoto, 1984) to describe how neurons "talk" to one another in groups. Dynamic systems theory provides an additional way to model problems found in speech perception.

Vallabha & McClelland (2007) utilize attractor dynamics (in the form of attractor basins) to model the /r-l/ problem in speech perception. The /r-l/ problem in speech perception pertains to the difficulty that Japanese listeners have when learning English as a second language. Native Japanese speakers have a profound difficulty in perceiving the difference between the /r/ and /l/ phonemes in English (Logan, Lively & Pisoni, 1991). Vallabha and McClelland (2007) used attractor basins created in topographic input maps in order to model this phenomenon in speech perception. In their model, attractor basins are formed during training and are representative of phonemic categories acquired during development (i. e., language learning). These basins are created via the similarity of the input. This degree of input similarity is what determines the strength of the attractor basins. If the system is presented with inputs that are highly similar, a strong, but rather narrow basin will be formed. If the inputs presented are highly dissimilar, a weak, but rather wide basin will be formed. The peak of the attractor basin can be considered the exemplar of the given input. Inputs to the system after the attractor basins are formed get categorized according to which basin they are closer to. The model presented by Vallabha and McClelland (2007), had difficulty in perceiving the difference between English /r/ and /l/ phonemes because their input fell inside of the Japanese /ɾ/ phoneme.

The use of attractor basins provides a way to tie together abstract and episodic theories of spoken language recognition. It is possible that when we process spoken language, we make use of a currently available episodic acoustic trace, which acts as input to each level of the language hierarchy. As this trace gets sequentially inputted into each level, it gets attracted to abstracted exemplars, formed during language acquisition. One can consider the episodic trace as a marble and the abstracted attractor basins as funnels at each level of the language hierarchy. The marble will pass through the funnels that it falls closer to. This structure would allow variation in the input to be recognized as perceptually equivalent. When multiple talkers are introduced to the system, listeners may be able to associate deviance within their constructed attractor basins to specific talkers. A listener may rely on cues from the episodic acoustic information to subsequently alter the strength of their abstracted attractor basins at each level. Dynamic attractor basins would allow for easy recognition and familiarity with talker increases. Deeply entrenched attractor basins would allow for easy recognition when presented items with certain qualities, but would not allow for easy recognition otherwise. Entrenched attractor basins could explain why listeners are much better at identifying talkers in their native language when compared to a foreign (non-native) language. Level of entrenchment may explain why this can be attenuated by long-term exposure to the non-native language.

References

Allen, S. J. & Miller, J. L. (2004). Listener sensitivity to individual talker differences in voice-onset-time. *Journal of the Acoustical Society of America 115*(6), 3171–3183.
Allen, S. J., Miller, J. L. & DeSteno, D. (2003). Individual talker differences in voice-onset-time. *Journal of the Acoustical Society of America 113*(1), 544–552.
Breakspear, M., Heitmann, S. & Daffertshofer, A. (2010). Generative models of cortical oscillations: neurobiological implications of the Kuramoto model. *Frontiers in Human Neuroscience* 4. 190. doi:10.3389/fnhum.2010.00190 (published 11 November 2010).
Bregman, M. R. & Creel, S. C. (2014). Gradient language dominance affects talker learning. *Cognition 130*(1), 85–95.

Clarke, C. M. & Garrett, M. F. (2004). Rapid adaptation to foreign-accented English. *Journal of the Acoustical Society of America 116*(6), 3647–3658.

Cho, T. & Ladefoged, P. (1999). Variation and universals in VOT: evidence from 18 languages. *Journal of phonetics 27*(2), 207–229.

Church, B. A. & Schacter, D. L. (1994). Perceptual specificity of auditory priming: implicit memory for voice intonation and fundamental frequency. *Journal of Experimental Psychology: Learning, Memory, and Cognition 20*(3), 521–533.

Clayards, M., Tanenhaus, M. K., Aslin, R. N. & Jacobs, R. A. (2008). Perception of speech reflects optimal use of probabilistic speech cues. *Cognition 108*(3), 804–809.

Craik, F. I. M. & Tulving, E. (1975). Depth of processing and the retention of words in episodic memory. *Journal of Experimental Psychology: General 104*(3), 268–294.

Dorman, M. F., Studdert-Kennedy, M. & Raphael, L. J. (1977). Stop-consonant recognition: Release bursts and formant transitions as functionally equivalent, context-dependent cues. *Perception & Psychophysics 22*(2), 109–122.

Drouin, J. R., Theodore, R. M. & Myers, E. B. (2016). Lexically guided perceptual tuning of internal phonetic category structure. *Journal of the Acoustical Society of America 140*, EL307–EL313.

Eisner, F. & McQueen, J. M. (2005). The specificity of perceptual learning in speech processing. *Perception & Psychophysics 67*(2), 224–238.

Fleming, D., Giordano, B. L., Caldara, R. & Belin, P. (2014). A language-familiarity effect for speaker discrimination without comprehension. *Proceedings of the National Academy of Sciences 111*(38), 13795–13798.

Goggin, J. P., Thompson, C. P., Strube, G. & Simental, L. R. (1991). The role of language familiarity in voice identification. *Memory & Cognition 19*(5), 448–458.

Goldinger, S. D. (1996). Words and voices: Episodic traces in spoken word identification and recognition memory. *Journal of Experimental Psychology: Learning, Memory, and Cognition 22*(5), 1166.

Goldinger, S. D. (1998). Echoes of echoes? An episodic theory of lexical access. *Psychological Review 105*(2), 251–279.

Goldstone, R. L. (1998). Perceptual learning. *Annual review of psychology 49*(1), 585–612.

Hale, J. K. & Koçak, H. (2012) [1991]. *Dynamics and bifurcations*. Vol. 3. Springer Science & Business Media.

Johnson, E. K., Westrek, E., Nazzi, T. & Cutler, A. (2011). Infant ability to tell voices apart rests on language experience. *Developmental Science 14*(5), 1002–1011.

Kadam, M. A., Orena, A. J., Theodore, R. M. & Polka, L. (2016). Reading ability influences native and non-native voice recognition, even for unimpaired readers. *Journal of the Acoustical Society of America, 139*(1), EL6–EL12.

Kleinschmidt, D. F. & Jaeger, F. T. (2015). Robust speech perception: Recognize the familiar, generalize to the similar, and adapt to the novel. *Psychological Review, 122*(2), 148–203.

Kraljic, T., Samuel, A. G. & Brennan, S. E. (2008). First impressions and last resorts how listeners adjust to speaker variability. *Psychological Science 19*(4), 332–338.

Kraljic, T. & Samuel, A. G. (2011). Perceptual learning evidence for contextually-specific representations. *Cognition, 121*(3), 459–465.

Kuhl, P. K. (1991). Human adults and human infants show a "perceptual magnet effect" for the prototypes of speech categories, monkeys do not. *Perception & Psychophysics 50*(2), 93–107.

Kuramoto, Y. (1984). *Chemical Oscillations, Waves, and Turbulence*. Mineola, NY: Dover Publications.

Levi, S. V. (2014). Individual differences in learning talker categories: The role of working memory. *Phonetica 71*(3), 201–226.

Liberman, A. M., Delattre, P. C., Cooper, F. S. & Gerstman, L. J. (1954). The role of consonant-vowel transitions in the perception of the stop and nasal consonants. *Psychological Monographs: General and Applied 68*(8), 1–13.

Lisker, L. & Abramson, A. S. (1964). A cross-language study of voicing in initial stops: Acoustical measurements. *Word 20*(3), 384–422.

Logan, J. S., Lively, S. E. & Pisoni, D. B. (1991). Training Japanese listeners to identify English/r/ and/l: A first report. *Journal of the Acoustical Society of America 89*(2), 874–886.

Mattys, S. L. & Liss, J. M. (2008). On building models of spoken-word recognition: When there is as much to learn from natural "oddities" as artificial normality. *Perception & Psychophysics 70*(7), 1235–1242.

McLennan, C. T., Luce, P. A. & Charles-Luce, J. (2003). Representation of lexical form. *Journal of Experimental Psychology: Learning, Memory, and Cognition 29*(4), 539–553.

McLennan, C. T. & Luce, P. A. (2005). Examining the time course of indexical specificity effects in spoken word recognition. *Journal of Experimental Psychology: Learning, Memory, and Cognition 31*(2), 306–321.

Miller, J. L. & Volaitis, L. E. (1989). Effect of speaking rate on the perceptual structure of a phonetic category. *Perception & Psychophysics 46*(6), 505–512.

Mullennix, J. W., Pisoni, D. B. & Martin, C. S. (1989). Some effects of talker variability on spoken word recognition. *Journal of the Acoustical Society of America 85*(1), 365–378.

Newman, R. S., Clouse, S. A. & Burnham, J. L. (2001). The perceptual consequences of within-talker variability in fricative production. *Journal of the Acoustical Society of America 109*(3), 1181–1196.

Norris, D., McQueen, J. M. & Cutler, A. (2003). Perceptual learning in speech. *Cognitive Psychology 47*(2), 204–238.

Nygaard, L. C. & Kalish, M. L. (1994). Modeling the effect of learning voices on the perception of speech. *Journal of the Acoustical Society of America 95*(1), 2873–2873.

Nygaard, L. C. & Pisoni, D. B. (1998). Talker-specific learning in speech perception. *Perception & Psychophysics 60*(3), 355–376.

Palmeri, T. J., Goldinger, S. D. & Pisoni, D. B. (1993). Episodic encoding of voice attributes and recognition memory for spoken words. *Journal of Experimental Psychology: Learning, Memory, and Cognition 19*(2), 309–328.

Peterson, G. E. & Barney, H. L. (1952). Control methods used in a study of the vowels. *Journal of the Acoustical Society of America 24*(2), 175–184.

Perea, M., Jiménez, M., Suárez-Coalla, P., Fernández, N., Viña, C. & Cuetos, F. (2014). Ability for voice recognition is a marker for dyslexia in children. *Experimental Psychology 24*(1), 480–487.

Perrachione, T. K. & Wong, P. C. M. (2007). Learning to recognize speakers of a non-native language: Implications for the functional organization of human auditory cortex. *Neuropsychologia 45*(8), 1899–1910.

Perrachione, T. K., Del Tufo, S. N. & Gabrieli, J. D. E. (2011). Human voice recognition depends on language ability. *Science 333*(6042), 595.

Samuel, A. G. (1982). Phonetic prototypes. *Perception & Psychophysics 31*(4), 307–314.

Schacter, D. L. & Church, B. A. (1992). Auditory priming: Implicit and explicit memory for words and voices. *Journal of Experimental Psychology: Learning, Memory, and Cognition 18*(5), 915–930.

Theodore, R. M. & Blumstein, S. E. & Luthra, S. (2015a). Attention modulates specificity effects in spoken word recognition: Challenges to the time-course hypothesis. *Attention, Perception, and Psychophysics 77*(5), 1674–1684.

Theodore, R. M., Myers, E. B. & Lomibao, J. A. (2015b). Talker-specific influences on phonetic category structure. *Journal of the Acoustical Society of America 138*(2), 1068–1078.

Theodore, R. M., Miller, J. L. & DeSteno, D. (2010). Characteristics of listeners' sensitivity to talker-specific phonetic detail. *Journal of Acoustical Society of America 128*(4), 2090–2099.

Theodore, R. M., Miller, J. L. & DeSteno, D. (2009). Individual talker differences in voice-onset-time: Contextual influences. *Journal of the Acoustical Society of America 125*(6), 3974–3982.

Vallabha, G. K. & McClelland, J. L. (2007). Success and failure of new speech category learning in adulthood: Consequences of learned Hebbian attractors in topographic maps. *Cognitive, Affective & Behavioral Neuroscience 7*(1), 53–73.

Volaitis, L. E. & Miller, J. L. (1992). Phonetic prototypes: Influence of place of articulation and speaking rate on the internal structure of voicing categories. *Journal of the Acoustical Society of America 92*(2), 723–735.

Chao-Yang Lee
Processing acoustic variability in lexical tone perception

Abstract: A fundamental question in speech perception is how listeners cope with various sources of acoustic variability to retrieve linguistic representations. In a series of studies, we explored the roles of stimulus and listener characteristics in lexical tone perception. In particular, we examined the effects of reduced acoustic input, contextual variation, noise, and speaker variability on Mandarin tone perception by native listeners, non-native listeners, and musicians. The findings show that reduced acoustic input, contextual variation, and noise disrupt non-native tone perception disproportionately. Speaker variability, on the other hand, appears to affect native and non-native tone perception similarly. Musicians have an advantage over non-musicians in tone perception, but the advantage is in identifying contour tones, not level tones. Taken together, these findings suggest that not all sources of acoustic variability affect lexical tone perception equally, and listener characteristics play a significant role in tone perception. Specifically, non-native tone perception is particularly susceptible to acoustic variability only when syllable-internal tonal information is compromised. The advantage of musicians in tone identification is most likely attributed to their superior ability to track F0 contours rather than detecting relative F0 height.

1 Introduction

Speech perception involves extracting information from the acoustic signal to uncover linguistic representations. Although there are many sources of variability in the acoustic signal, neurologically intact listeners rarely have trouble understanding spoken language. Therefore, a fundamental issue in speech perception is to understand how listeners process acoustic variability to retrieve speakers' intended sounds. The process can be explicated by examining sources of acoustic variability (e. g., speaker differences) and characteristics of listeners (e. g., native vs. non-native listeners). In this chapter, I will discuss a series of

Chao-Yang Lee, Division of Communication Sciences and Disorders, Ohio University Athens

studies conducted in my lab on how acoustic variability is processed in lexical tone perception by listeners with various characteristics.

In lexical tone languages, tones are functionally analogous to consonants and vowels. That is, lexical tones can distinguish words just as segmental structure does. Ample research has established that fundamental frequency (F0) is the primary acoustic correlate of lexical tone (Howie, 1976; Abramson, 1978; Gandour & Harshman, 1978; Tseng, 1981). In Mandarin Chinese, for example, monosyllabic words can be distinguished by F0 variations over a syllable. As an example, the syllable *ma* with Tone 1 (a high-level tone) means "mother"; *ma* with Tone 2 (a mid-rising tone) means "hemp"; *ma* with Tone 3 (a low-dipping tone) means "horse"; and *ma* with Tone 4 (a high-falling tone) means "scorn." Figure 1 shows examples of the four tones. In addition to F0, secondary cues such as duration and amplitude contour also contribute to tone perception (Abramson, 1972; Blicher, Diehl & Cohen, 1990; Whalen & Xu, 1992; Liu & Samuel, 2004). Nonetheless, when F0 information is available, it remains the most powerful cue for tonal distinctions. More specifically, F0 height and F0 direction are the two major dimensions used by listeners to identify tones, and the weight assigned to F0 height and F0 direction varies depending on a listener's language experience (Gandour, 1983).

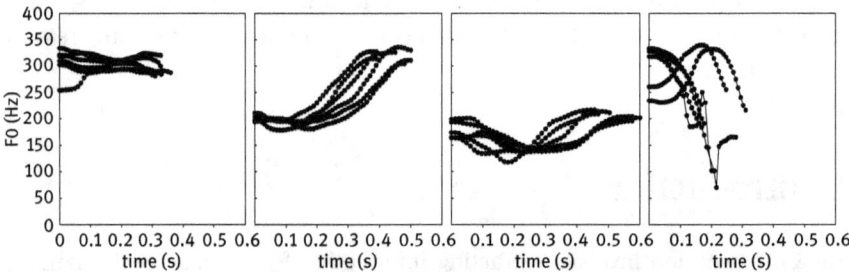

Figure 1: F0 contours of the Mandarin tone stimuli used in Lee, Tao, and Bond (2008). From left to right: Tone 1, Tone 2, Tone 3, and Tone 4.

As tone languages account for the majority of known languages in the world (Laver, 1994), investigating tone perception may provide further insights to the nature of speech perception. Since lexical tone and segmental structure involve distinct acoustic correlates, findings from segmental perception may not necessarily generalize to tone perception. Previous research has focused on identifying acoustic correlates for specific tonal contrasts (Gårding, Kratochvil, Svantesson & Zhang, 1986; Shen & Lin, 1991; Shen, Lin & Yan, 1993). In contrast, little is known about the effects of acoustic variability or adverse conditions on tone perception.

In addition, how listeners with various characteristics deal with acoustic variability in tone perception has not been systematically investigated. For example, does acoustic variability affect native and non-native tone perception in the same way? Do musicians enjoy an advantage in lexical tone perception because of their substantial exposure to musical pitch? The overarching question to be discussed in this chapter is: How do different sources of acoustic variability affect tone perception by listeners with various characteristics? I will first discuss how various sources of acoustic variability affect tone perception, focusing on their effects on native and non-native tone perception. I will then discuss the role of musical training in the perception of lexical tones.

2 Tone identification from reduced acoustic input and context

As noted, F0 is the primary acoustic correlate of tone, meaning tonal information is carried primarily by the vowel of a syllable. If a substantial portion of the vowel is missing, tonal information should be compromised significantly. Gottfried & Suiter (1997) tested this prediction by constructing four types of consonant-vowel stimuli: intact, center-only (initial six and final eight glottal periods were silenced), silent-center (all but the initial six and final eight periods were silenced), and onset-only (all but the initial six periods were silenced). The results showed that native listeners made few identification errors except for the initial-only syllables. Remarkably, although the majority of the syllable was missing from the silent-center stimuli, tone identification from these syllables was as accurate as in intact and center-only stimuli. These results suggest that the listeners are able to integrate information from both the initial and the final portions of a syllable to identify tones, just like listeners are able to identify vowels from silent-center syllables by using dynamic spectral information (e. g., Strange, Jenkins & Johnson, 1983).

Gottfried & Suiter (1997) also explored the contribution of tonal context by presenting the stimuli in isolation or in the context of a following syllable. The results showed that the pattern of identification confusions changed substantially depending on context. For example, in isolation, onset-only Tone 4 (a high-falling tone) was often misidentified as Tone 1 (a high-level tone) because both tones have a relatively high F0 onset. When the context was present, the Tone 4 – Tone 1 confusion largely disappeared, suggesting the listeners were able to use contextual information to disambiguate the two tones. In particular, the F0 offset of the two tones (relatively low for Tone 4 but high for Tone 1) carries over to the context, resulting in distinct F0 onsets in the following syllable. The higher accuracy with context present indicates that native listeners were able to use the low F0 onset in the context as evidence for Tone 4 in the stimuli.

Lee, Tao & Bond (2008) extended Gottfried & Suiter (1997) by using reaction time as an additional response measure. They also elaborated on the manipulation of the tonal context. Like Gottfried & Suiter (1997), Mandarin syllables were digitally processed to generate four types of stimuli: intact, silent-center, center-only, and onset-only (Figure 2). The syllables were recorded in two carrier phrases such that the offset of the carrier tone and the onset of the stimulus tone were either a match or mismatch in F0. The stimuli were presented in the original carrier phrases, excised from the carrier phrases, or excised and cross-spliced with another carrier phrase. The accuracy results replicated Gottfried and Suiter (1997): silent-center tones were identified as accurately as intact and center-only tones. The reaction time measure, however, revealed that silent-center tones took longer to be identified than intact and center-only tones, indicating that reduction of acoustic input still incurred a processing cost. There were no effects of cross splicing or match/mismatch with the carrier tone. However, in the cross-spliced context, syllables originally produced with a matching carrier tone were identified faster and more accurately, suggesting the native listener's sensitivity to contextual tonal variations.

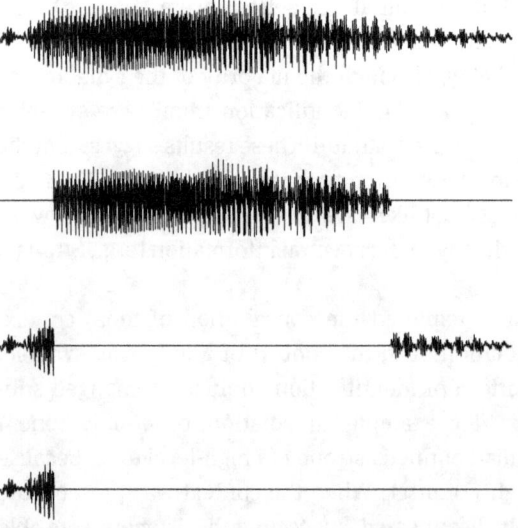

Figure 2: From top down: intact, center-only, silent-center, and onset-only stimuli used in Lee, Tao & Bond (2008) and Lee, Tao & Bond (2010a).

These two studies showed that native listeners are able to use syllable-internal tonal information to reconstruct tones and contextual information to infer tone identity. These findings suggest that native listeners' knowledge of tonal contour and tonal coarticulation helps them to compensate for reduced acoustic input and contextual variations. Will non-native listeners be able to cope with acoustic variability in the same way, or will they be affected by acoustic variability disproportionately because of their imperfect knowledge of the target language? Gottfried & Suiter (1997) showed that while native listeners were able to integrate the initial and final portions of silent-center stimuli to identify tones, non-native listeners were not able to do so as accurately. Furthermore, when the stimuli were presented in context, non-native listeners were not able to take advantage of the context to infer tone identity. The confusion matrix analyses in Gottfried & Suiter (1997) also revealed a number of differences between the native and non-native listeners. The native listeners made few errors except in the onset-only condition, where the common confusions involved tones sharing a similar F0 onset. In contrast, non-native listeners made more errors that were unusual for the native listeners. Gottfried & Suiter (1997) speculated that native listeners were able to make more effective use of acoustic information other than F0, such as the presence of creaky voice quality commonly present in Tone 3 (a low-dipping tone).

Lee, Tao & Bond (2010a) extended their 2008 study by evaluating tone identification by non-native perception of fragmented tones. These non-native listeners had Mandarin experience ranging from one to three years of formal instruction in a classroom setting. Contrary to the native perception results, non-native listeners did not identify the silent-center stimuli as accurately as intact and center-only stimuli, suggesting that non-native listeners could not use the F0 onset and offset information as effectively to reconstruct tones. In addition, the non-native listeners did not show evidence of using coarticulatory information from the context. Taken together, it appears non-native listeners are primarily using syllable-internal F0 information to identify tones, whereas native listeners are able to their knowledge of dynamic information from the F0 onset/offset, secondary cues, and contextual variation to reconstruct tone identity from reduced acoustic input.

3 Processing Speaker Variability and Noise in Tone Perception

The studies discussed in the previous section support the idea that tone perception by non-native listeners is particularly susceptible to acoustic variability. This makes intuitive sense, as non-native listeners do not possess the knowledge of the target language to the same degree as native listeners. However, there are many sources of acoustic variability. Do all sources affect non-native tone perception disproportionately?

Lee, Tao & Bond (2009) investigated the individual and joint effects of speaker variability, context, and reduced acoustic input on Mandarin tone identification. The literature on segmental processing indicates that adapting to different speakers demands cognitive resources. In particular, responses to multiple-speaker stimuli are usually less accurate and more time-consuming than responses to single-speaker stimuli (Creelman, 1957; Mullennix, Pisoni & Martin,

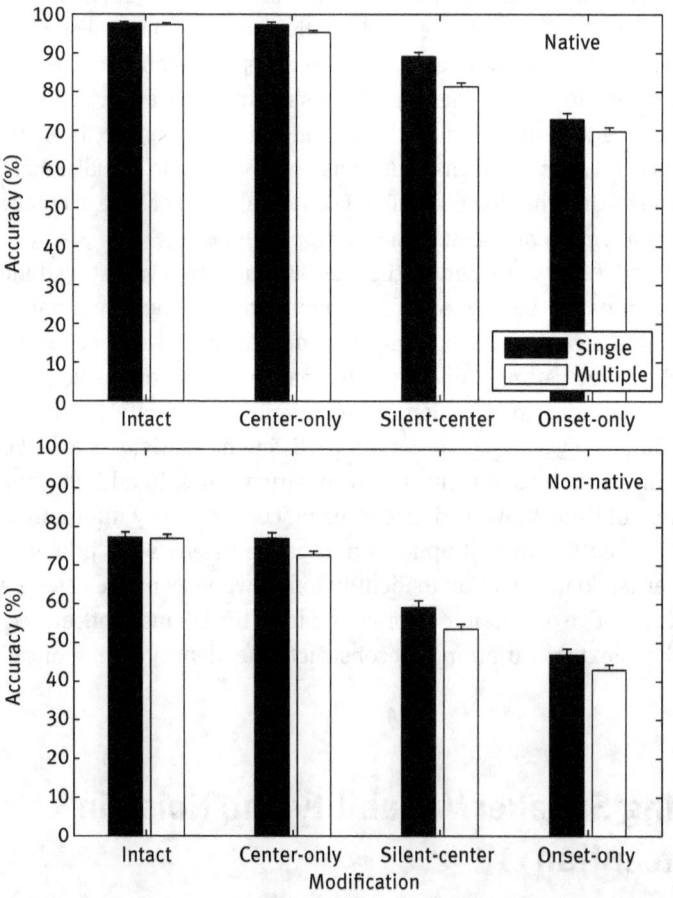

Figure 3: Accuracy of identification of single- and multiple-speaker tones by native and non-native listeners in Lee, Tao & Bond (2010a). Error bar indicates standard error.

1989; Nusbaum & Morin, 1992; Summerfield & Haggard, 1973; Verbrugge, Strange, Shankweiler & Edman, 1976). In Lee et al. (2009), Mandarin syllables produced by single versus multiple speakers were digitally processed to generate intact, silent-center, center-only, and onset-only stimuli. The stimuli were presented in isolation or with a precursor carrier phrase. Native and non-native listeners were put under time pressure to identify the stimulus tones. As expected, the results showed higher identification accuracy in the single-speaker presentation compared to multi-speaker presentation. However, the magnitude of the speaker variability effect was comparable between native and non-native listeners (Figure 3). In other words, non-native listeners were not affected disproportionately by the demand of multiple speakers in the stimuli. This result contrasts with the effect of reduced acoustic input and tonal context, which affected non-native tone perception disproportionately.

To further explore this unexpected finding, Lee, Tao & Bond (2010b) manipulated the degree of speaker variability by using stimulus sets blocked by speaker and mixed across speakers. Previous studies on tone perception showed that the mixed-speaker set is more challenging than the blocked-speaker set for tone identification (Wong & Diehl, 2003; Zhou, Zhang, Lee & Xu 2008). In addition to speaker variability, Lee et al. (2010b) also mixed speech-shaped noise with the stimuli to examine the effect of noise on tone identification. The question asked in Lee et al. (2010b), then, was whether speaker variability and noise, two of the most common adverse conditions in speech perception, would be disproportionately challenging for non-native listeners. Monosyllabic Mandarin words produced by three male and three female speakers were presented with five levels of signal-to-noise ratios (quiet, 0, −5, −10, and −15 dB) in two presentation formats (blocked by speaker and mixed across speakers) to listeners with various Mandarin experience (native, first-year, second-year, third year, and fourth-year students). Figure 4 shows the results. As expected, stimuli blocked by speaker yielded higher accuracy and shorter reaction time. Native listeners outperformed non-native listeners as expected, but the additional demand of processing mixed-speaker stimuli, did not compromise non-native performance more than native performance. Noise also disrupted identification performance as expected, but it did not compromise non-native identification more than native identification. It appears that speaker variability and noise behave differently from other sources of acoustic variability as they did not affect non-native tone identification disproportionately.

The lack of disproportionate effects of speaker variability and noise on non-native tone perception reported by Lee et al. (2010b) could have been due to a methodological issue. In particular, the stimuli were embedded in a carrier phrase, which was included to ensure that the participants could hear the tones against a heavy background noise. Although the carrier phrase was relatively short, it could have provided sufficient information about speakers, which could have neutralized the processing difference between native and non-native listeners. Furthermore, a follow-up analysis showed that when listeners were divided according to baseline performance instead of duration of Mandarin exposure, a significant noise level by baseline performance interaction emerged, suggesting disproportionate noise effect depending on Mandarin proficiency.

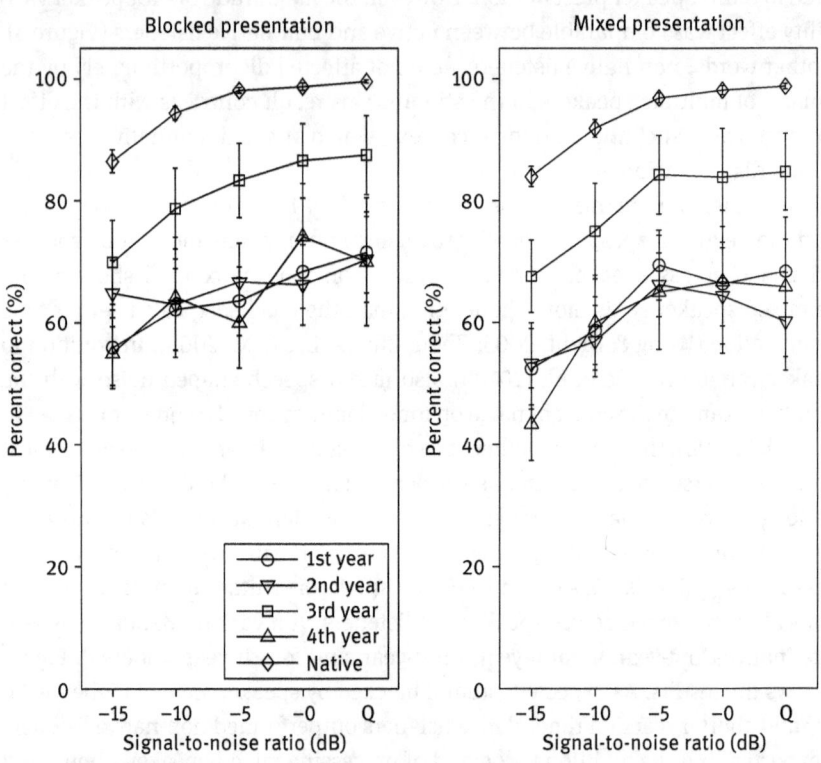

Figure 4: Accuracy of Mandarin tone identification as a function of speaker variability (blocked/mixed presentation), noise level (quiet to −15 dB SNR), and listener background (native and 1–4 years of instruction) in Lee, Tao & Bond (2010b). Error bar indicates standard error.

To address these two possibilities, Lee, Tao & Bond (2013) used multi-speaker stimuli embedded in speech-shaped noise. The stimuli were presented to native and non-native listeners in two formats: blocked by speaker and mixed across speakers. In contrast to Lee et al. (2010b), the stimuli were presented without a carrier phrase, and listeners were grouped by baseline performance instead of years of Mandarin instruction. The results (Figure 5) showed that the mixed-speaker presentation did not affect non-native listeners disproportionately, suggesting that speaker variability did not pose a special challenge to non-native listeners. In contrast, noise affected the listener groups disproportionately. Contrary to expectation, it was the listeners with higher proficiency that were more affected by noise. It was speculated that the less proficient listeners could not identify tones well in the easy, baseline conditions initially, so the extent to which their performance could be reduced became more constrained.

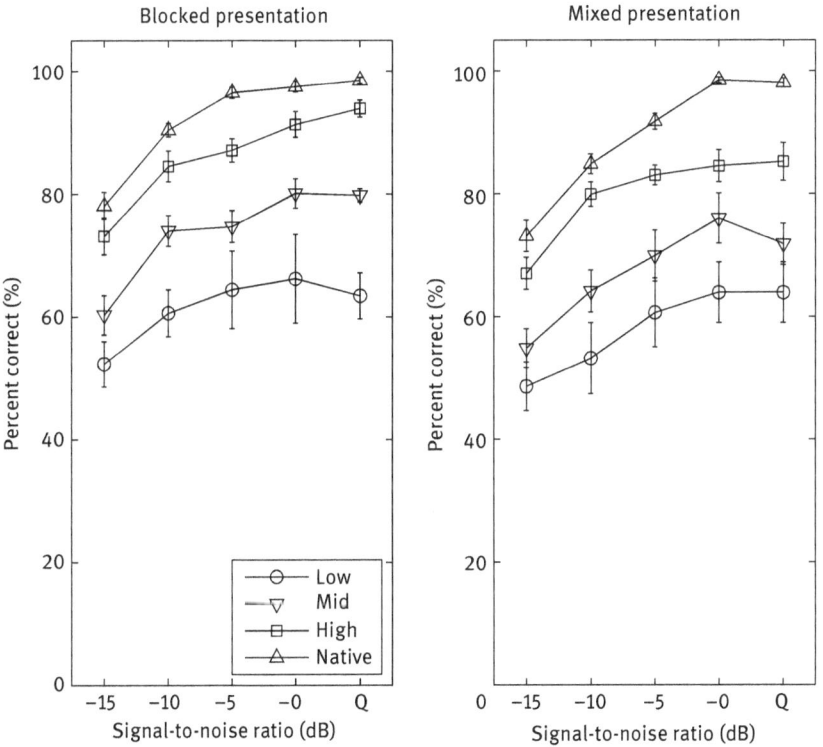

Figure 5: Accuracy of Mandarin tone identification as a function of speaker variability (blocked/mixed presentation), noise level (quiet to −15 dB SNR), and listener background (native and level of proficiency) in Lee, Tao & Bond (2013). Error bar indicates standard error.

Taken together, this series of studies on processing acoustic variability showed that not all sources of acoustic variability are equally disruptive to native and non-native tone perception. Most of the adverse conditions compromised non-native tone perception disproportionately (reduced acoustic input, contextual variation, and noise), whereas speaker variability affected native and non-native tone perception similarly. It appears that non-native tone perception is compromised disproportionately only when syllable-internal, canonical F0 information is removed or altered. This observation is consistent with the proposal that non-native listeners rely primarily on syllable-internal, canonical information for tone identification, whereas native listeners are able to use their knowledge of tonal coarticulation and contextual tonal variation (e. g., Xu, 1994) to compensate for the loss of F0 information. Consequently, when syllable-internal, canonical F0 information is reduced (as in fragmented tones) or altered (as in tones excised from original tonal context), non-native tone perception is disrupted disproportionately. In contrast, speaker variability does not affect non-native tone perception disproportionately because speaker variability does not remove or alter syllable-internal, canonical F0 information.

The noise effect also challenges the proposal that the source of disproportionate non-native difficulty with noise is not at a relatively low level of processing, such as identifying segmental phonemes from isolated syllables (Bradlow & Alexander, 2007; Cutler, Weber, Smits & Cooper, 2004). The idea is that disproportionate non-native difficulties usually do not surface when the stimuli are relatively simple and do not involve complex linguistic processing. Rather, non-native difficulties with noise accumulate across all levels of spoken language comprehension. The results from Lee et al. (2013), however, showed that non-native tone perception could be affected disproportionately even when the stimuli are relatively simple (i. e. isolated tones). To explore whether the disproportionate noise effect only applied to tonal but not segmental contrasts, Lee, Zhang, Li, Tao & Bond (2012) examined Mandarin fricative perception by native and non-native listeners. Multi-speaker Mandarin fricative stimuli were presented to native and non-native listeners blocked by speaker and mixed across speakers. The stimuli were also mixed with speech-shaped noise to create five levels of signal-to-noise ratios. The results showed that noise affected non-native fricative identification disproportionately. In contrast, the effect of speaker variability was again comparable between the native and non-native listeners. In other words, noise could affect non-native speech perception disproportionately even when the stimuli are relatively simple and do not involve complex linguistic processing.

4 Tone identification from brief acoustic input: Detecting F0 height

One notable finding from the studies on reduced acoustic input is the relatively high identification accuracy from onset-only stimuli by native listeners. Unlike silent-center stimuli, where listeners may be able to use interpolation between F0 onset and offset to reconstruct the tonal contour, onset-only stimuli do not allow such reconstruction. Yet identification accuracy in the studies that included onset-only stimuli was substantially higher than chance (25 %). Confusion patterns showed that listeners were able to identify whether the fragment starts with a relatively high (Tones 1 or 4) or low (Tones 2 or 3). This finding raised an interesting question about processing speaker variability. Since F0 range varies across speakers, a phonologically high tone produced by a male speaker could be acoustically equivalent to or even lower than a phonologically low tone produced by a female speaker. On the other hand, a given tone produced by two speakers could be acoustically distinct. Intuitively, judgment of the relative F0 height of a tone has to be made with reference to a speaker's F0 range. This observation is supported by research showing that tone perception is contingent on the perceived F0 range of a speaker. Leather (1983) examined identification of Mandarin tones that were synthesized to be lexically ambiguous. The tone stimuli were presented in carrier phrases produced by two speakers. The results showed that stimuli with identical absolute F0 contours were identified as different tones depending on which speaker was heard, indicating the use of perceived range information in tone perception. This finding was replicated by Moore & Jongman (1997), who showed that Mandarin tone stimuli with identical F0 patterns were perceived as high tones in a low F0 carrier phrase produced by one speaker, but as low tones in a high F0 carrier phrase produced by another speaker. Wong & Diehl (2003) examined identification of Cantonese level tones embedded in carrier phrases produced by seven speakers. The results showed that the same target tones were identified differently depending on which carrier phrase was used.

It is clear from these studies that context provides important information about speaker F0 range. Listeners can use contextual information to interpret tones just as they do in interpreting vowels (e. g., Ladefoged & Broadbent, 1957). Therefore, removing context should make it difficult to estimate speaker F0 range. The absence of context should particularly compromise identification of level tones, whose contrasts rely solely on relative F0 height. Wong & Diehl (2003) examined identification of three Cantonese level tones that were produced by seven speakers and presented in isolation. The results showed that tone identification was more accurate when the stimuli were blocked by speaker (80 %) than when they were mixed across speakers (49 %). As expected, identification performance was compromised by the mixed-speaker stimuli (Creelman, 1957; Zhou, Zhang, Lee & Xu, 2008). However, the fact that identification accuracy still exceeded chance (33 %) in both conditions indicates that the absence of context does not make F0 height judgment impossible. It also indicates that there are syllable-internal cues to relative F0 height. However, because listeners in the experiment heard the stimulus set 12 times, they could have become familiar with the F0 range of the speakers through repeated exposure.

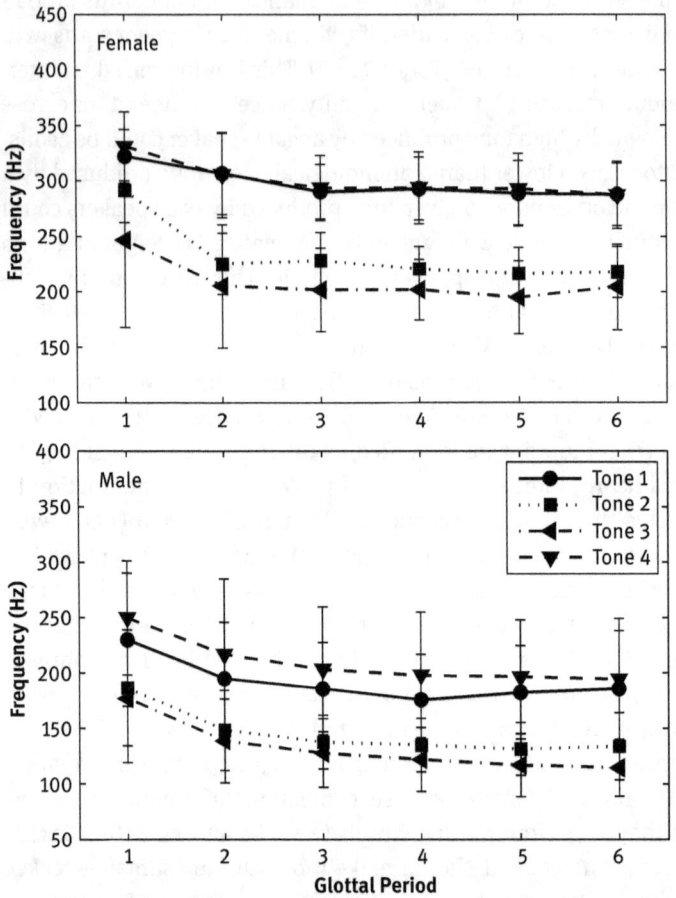

Figure 6: F0 contours of the onset-only stimuli used in Lee (2009). Each data point is an average of 16 female or male speakers. Error bar indicates standard error.

To rule out the familiarity account, Lee (2009) recorded Mandarin /sa/ syllables with four tones produced by 16 female and 16 male speakers. The syllables were digitally processed such that only the fricative and first six glottal periods of the vowel remained, effectively neutralizing F0 contour contrasts among the tones (Figure 6). These multi-speaker, level-F0 stimuli (i. e., no F0 contour cues) were presented in isolation (i. e., no contextual cues) with each stimulus being presented just once (i. e., no familiarity cues). Despite the absence of those cues typically considered necessary for speaker normalization, listeners were able to identify the intended tones with above-chance accuracy. This finding was replicated by Lee & Lee (2010) using listeners with musical training. Lee's (2009) acoustic analyses further revealed contrasts between the high- and low-onset tones in F0, duration, and two voice quality measures (F1 bandwidth and spectral tilt). Correlation analyses also showed that F0 covaried with the voice quality measures and that tone classification based on F0 height correlated with the voice quality measures. Since the same acoustic measures consistently distinguished female from male stimuli, Lee (2009) proposed that speaker gender detection may be the basis for the F0 height judgment performance.

Lee, Dutton & Ram (2010) evaluated the gender detection proposal by asking listeners to judge speaker gender from the same set of stimuli used in Lee (2009). The results showed that gender identification accuracy was above chance, suggesting that the ability to judge F0 height from these stimuli is likely due to successful identification of speaker gender as a precursor. Specifically, listeners identify speaker gender based on voice quality. They then exploit the covariation between F0 and voice quality for relative F0 height estimation. Once the gender decision is made, pitch class templates stored in memory that are gender-specific can be invoked to compare to the stimulus. Listeners may calibrate their judgments according to the templates, which reflect typical F0s for female and male speakers that listeners have experienced throughout their lives. It has been noted that pitch class templates can be acquired from exposure to prevalent speaking F0s of a linguistic community (Dolson, 1994). If so, F0 height of a tone stimulus could be inferred with the templates as a reference frame.

The ability to estimate relative F0 height without speaker normalization cues has also been reported for non-tone language listeners. Honorof & Whalen (2005) showed that English listeners were able to locate an F0 reliably within a speaker's F0 range without context or prior exposure to a speaker's voice. Isolated vowel tokens, produced by 20 English speakers with varying F0s, were presented to listeners to judge where each token was located in the speakers' F0 ranges. The results showed significant correlations between the perceived F0 location and the actual location in the speakers' F0 ranges, indicating that the listeners were able to estimate relative F0 height. It was speculated that covariation between F0 and voice quality might have contributed to the identification performance, although this hypothesis was not directly tested in the study.

The potential role of voice quality in F0 height estimation was evaluated by Bishop & Keating (2012). Their first experiment replicated Honorof & Whalen's (2005) finding that listeners' perceived F0 locations correlated with speakers' actual F0 locations, confirming that the listeners were able to estimate relative F0 height without cues typically present for speaker normalization.

Statistical modeling showed that F0 was the single most important predictor for the F0 estimation performance. By contrast, acoustic measures of voice quality contributed only minimally to F0 estimation. The second experiment showed that listeners were able to identify speaker gender from the same set of stimuli. Statistical modeling again showed that F0 was the most important predictor for the gender identification performance. In contrast, voice quality contributed to gender identification to a greater extent than it did to F0 height estimation. It was concluded that listeners form expectations about F0s for average male and female speakers through experience, and that they rely on absolute F0 to determine speaker gender, which in turn contributes to relative F0 estimation. That is, voice quality contributes to F0 estimation only indirectly through gender identification.

The contribution of gender identification to relative F0 estimation, however, was questioned by Honorof & Whalen (2005). Listeners were asked to judge speaker gender from isolated vowels spoken by 20 English male and female speakers with overlapping F0s. The listeners performed above chance, but showed a bias toward hearing high F0s as female and low F0s as male when stimulus F0s were near range extremes. There was no strong evidence for a contribution of voice quality, weakening the argument that voice quality is used to identify speaker gender. The authors suggested that the gender identification results are best explained by the listeners' primary reliance on absolute F0 and secondary reliance on formants or vocal tract information.

Findings from these English-based studies have provided important information about processing speaker variability in nonlinguistic F0 distinctions. However, it is not clear whether these conclusions would generalize to processing speaker variability in tone languages, in which F0 distinctions can be lexically contrastive. Although Lee (2009) and Lee et al. (2010) provided evidence for the role of voice quality and gender identification in relative F0 estimation, the conclusion is weakened by the fact that Mandarin tones do not involve contrasts that rely solely on F0 height. Three of the four Mandarin tones are contour tones. Therefore, listeners can use the contours to infer F0 range, i. e., they do not need to rely on F0 height to identify tonal contrasts. A more stringent test of the ability to estimate relative F0 height without speaker normalization cues will be to use a tone language that has intrinsic level-tone contrasts.

To that end, Lee, Lee & Shr (2011) examined perception of Taiwanese tones. Taiwanese is a tone language with seven lexical tones, two of which are level tones (high-level and mid-level) contrasting only in F0 height. In the study, the two level tones, produced by 30 male and female speakers, were presented in isolation (Figure 7). The results showed that native listeners were able to identify the tones with above-chance accuracy, indicating that they were able to estimate relative F0 height without cues typically considered necessary for speaker normalization. This finding was replicated by Lee, Lekich & Zhang (2014) with English-speaking musicians and non-musicians. Both groups of listeners were able to identify tone height above chance, but contrary to the native listeners, the non-native listeners could do so only for tones at the extremes of the speakers' overall vocal range. Taken together, the ability to identify pitch height in lexical tones appears to involve calibrating acoustic input according to gender-specific, internally stored pitch templates.

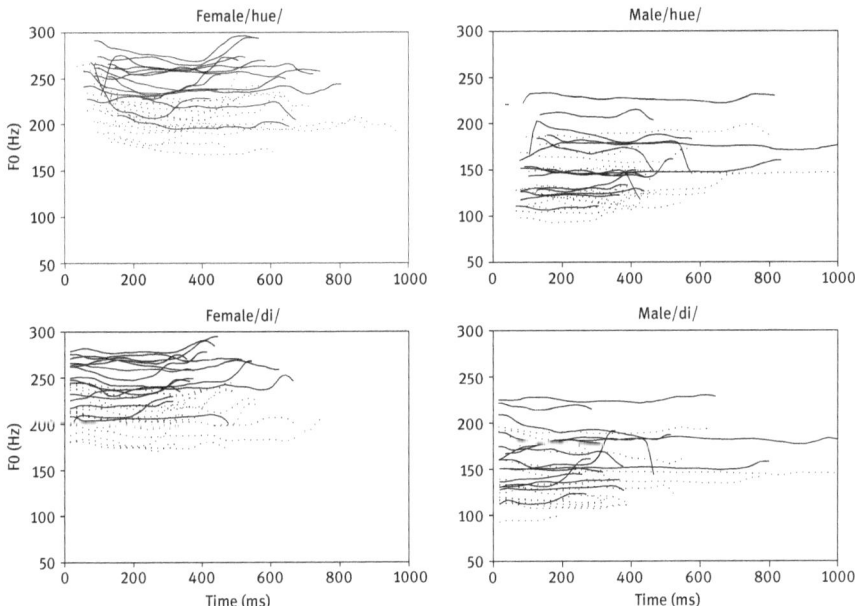

Figure 7: F0 contours of Taiwanese level-tone stimuli produced by 15 female and 15 male speakers used in Lee, Lee & Shr (2011) and Lee, Lekich & Zhang (2014). Solid lines represent high-tone stimuli and dotted lines represent mid-tone stimuli.

5 Role of music training in lexical tone perception

Since pitch perception is important to identifying both musical pitch and lexical tones, an intriguing question is whether processing musical pitch and lexical tones involves the same cognitive mechanism (Patel, 2008). In a series of studies on the music-tone relationship, we examined two questions: First, is musical pitch processing associated with lexical pitch processing? If so, musicians should outperform non-musicians in lexical tone identification. Second, is absolute pitch, or the ability to produce or name a musical note without a reference pitch, implicated in lexical pitch processing (Deutsch, 2006)? If so, musicians with absolute pitch should outperform those without absolute pitch in lexical tone perception.

Lee and Hung (2008) examined Mandarin tone identification by 36 English-speaking musicians and 36 non-musicians without prior knowledge of Mandarin or other tone languages. The stimuli included Mandarin /sa/ syllables produced with the four Mandarin tones by 16 female and 16 male speakers. We presented intact syllables, silent center syllables (in which 70% of the syllable center was removed; only the onset consonant, beginning 15% and ending 15% of the voiced portion of the syllable remained in the stimuli) and onset-only syllables (in which only the onset consonant and beginning 15% of the voiced portion of the syllable remained in the stimuli). The purpose of using the truncated syllables was to assess how listeners could use reduced acoustic information to retrieve tone identity.

The results (Figure 8) showed that English-speaking musicians outperformed non-musicians in this task, although the advantage diminished as the amount of F0 information was reduced. In particular, the musicians' advantage was 24% for intact syllables, 18% for silent-center syllables, and only 3% for onset-only syllables. Interestingly, since listeners heard each stimulus only once and the stimuli were quite brief and presented in isolation, typical cues for speaker normalization (such as F0 contour, external context, and familiarity with speakers) were not available in these multi-speaker stimuli. Nonetheless, some onset-only tones could still be identified even when the truncated tones were without these typical cues for speaker normalization, suggesting that the listeners were able to detect pitch height as a way to identify the tones.

In addition to the Mandarin tone identification task, we also gave the musicians a musical note identification task. Three sets of synthesized piano, viola, and pure tones were presented for identification without a reference pitch. These notes range from C3 to B5 and were 500 ms long. Consecutive notes were separated by more than at least one octave to prevent participants from using relative pitch for identification. The participants responded by notating the notes that they had heard on a staff paper. The results (Figure 9) showed that none of the musicians met the criterion for absolute pitch, defined as 85% or higher accuracy in identifying the piano notes (Deutsch, Henthorn, Marvin & Xu, 2006). When we calculated correlations between performance in Mandarin tone identification and musical note identification, none of the correlations were statistically significant, suggesting the two abilities are not associated.

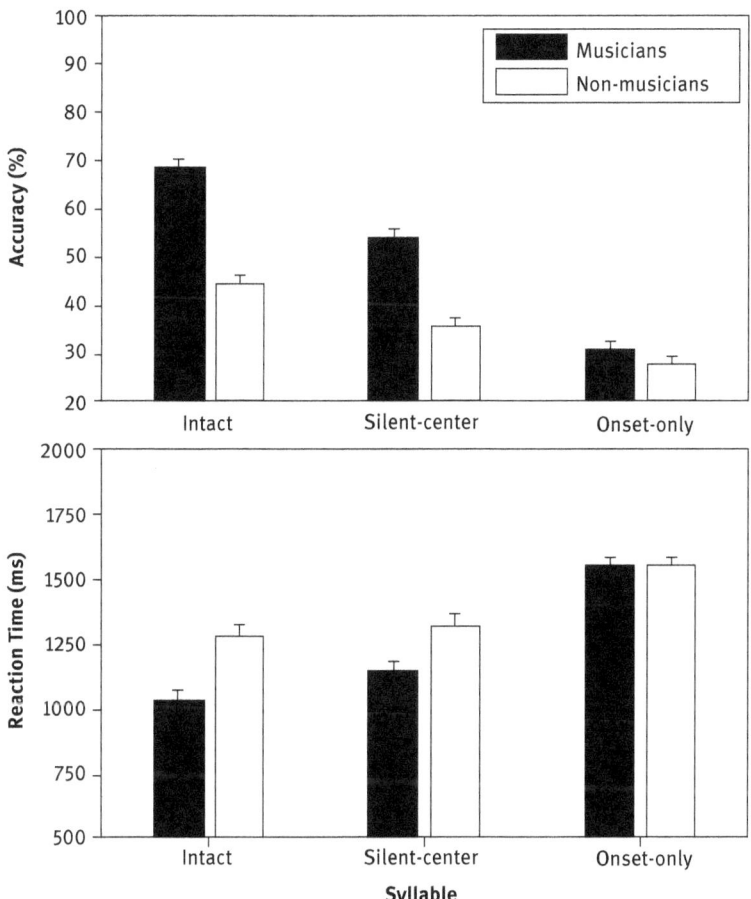

Figure 8: Accuracy and reaction time of Mandarin tone identification by English-speaking musicians and non-musicians in Lee & Hung (2008). Error bar indicates standard error.

In sum, even though the musicians outperformed the non-musicians in Mandarin tone identification, we did not find evidence that the advantage comes from the ability to identify musical notes without a reference pitch. However, since none of the musician participants in the study actually possessed absolute pitch, it is not known whether a significant correlation would emerge for musicians with absolute pitch.

Since higher occurrence of absolute pitch has been reported in musicians speaking a tone language (Deutsch, Henthorn & Dolson, 2004; Deutsch et al., 2006), we turned to Mandarin-speaking musicians in the next study. Lee and Lee (2010) examined Mandarin tone identification and musical note identification by

72 Mandarin-speaking musicians recruited in Taiwan. In the Mandarin tone task, we presented onset-only /sa/ syllables. Unlike Lee & Hung (2008), intact and silent-center syllables were not included because previous studies have shown that native listeners could identify them very well (Gottfried & Suiter, 1997; Lee et al., 2008). Furthermore, given our purpose in exploring the use of pitch height in lexical tone identification, the lack of distinct F0 contour in the onset-only tones would be optimal. The results (Figure 10) showed that the Mandarin-speaking musicians could identify some onset-only tones above chance without typical cues of speaker normalization, just as their non-musician counterparts did (Lee, 2009).

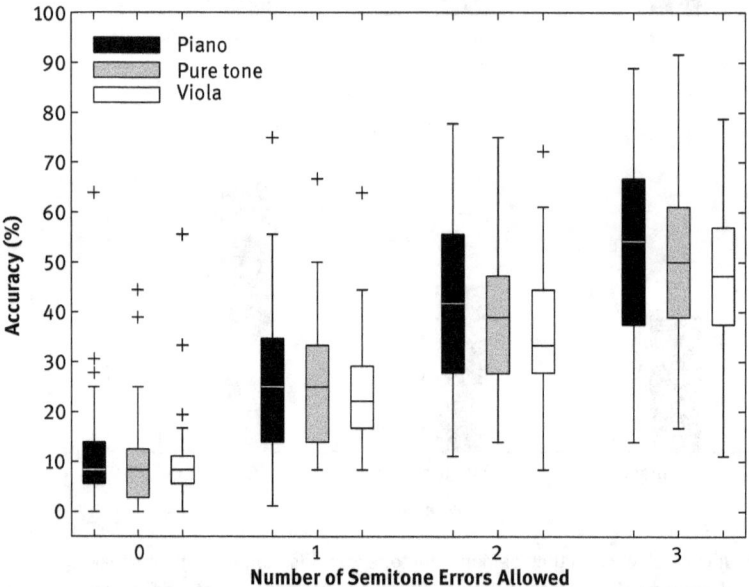

Figure 9: Box plot showing the accuracy of musical note identification for piano, pure tone, and viola stimuli in Lee and Hung (2008). The central mark is the median, the edges of the box are the 25th and 75th percentiles, the whiskers extend to the most extreme data points not considered to be outliers, and outliers are indicated by "+".

In the musical note identification task, 72% of the Mandarin-speaking musicians met the criterion for absolute pitch, which contrasted sharply with the data from English-speaking musicians in Lee & Hung (2008) (Figure 11). However, when we calculated correlations between performance in Mandarin tone identification and musical note identification, there were still no significant correlations whether we included all musicians or just those with absolute pitch. In other words, we still did not find evidence for the association between absolute pitch and lexical tone perception, even though this sample of musicians included individuals with absolute pitch.

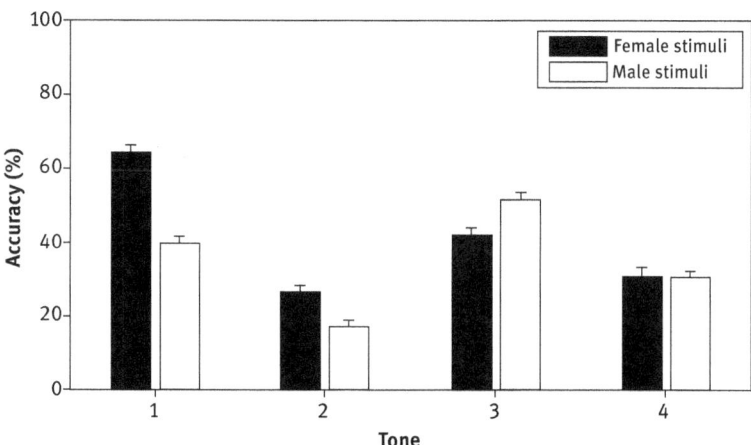

Figure 10: Accuracy of Mandarin onset-only tone identification by Mandarin-speaking musicians in Lee and Lee (2010). Error bar indicates standard error.

Although the onset-only Mandarin tones were analogous to the stimuli used in the musical note identification task in that they are truncated to include only a single, flat F0, the Mandarin tones themselves are contour in nature. That means the contrast among the four Mandarin tones can be judged based solely on F0 contour without reference to pitch height. Our next goal, therefore, was to identify a language with canonical level tones, where pitch height has to be identified in order to identify tonal contrasts. In Lee, Lee & Shr (2011), we used the two level tones in Taiwanese, which, unlike Mandarin contour tones, contrast in pitch height only. In the Taiwanese tone identification task, the syllables /hue/ ("flower" with a high tone and "meeting" with a mid tone) and /di/ ("pig" with a high tone and "chopsticks" with a mid tone) were recorded by 15 female and 15 male speakers of Taiwanese. Forty-three Taiwanese-speaking musicians were recruited to complete a Taiwanese word identification task and a musical note identification task. The results (Figure 12) showed that listeners could identify tone height above chance without typical cues of speaker normalization. In the musical note identification task, 65% of the listeners met the criterion for absolute pitch. However, when we calculated correlations between performance in Mandarin tone identification and musical note identification, there were still no significant correlations between the two sets of performance measures.

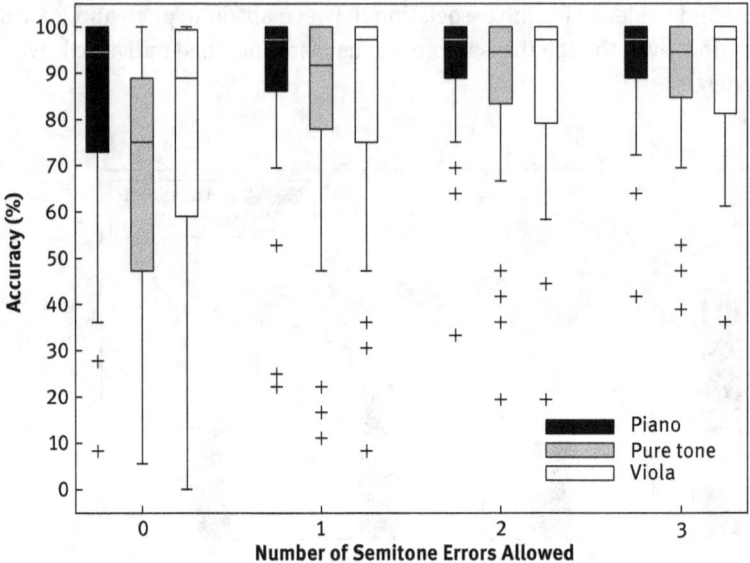

Figure 11: Box plot showing the accuracy of musical note identification for piano, pure tone, and viola stimuli in Lee & Lee (2010).

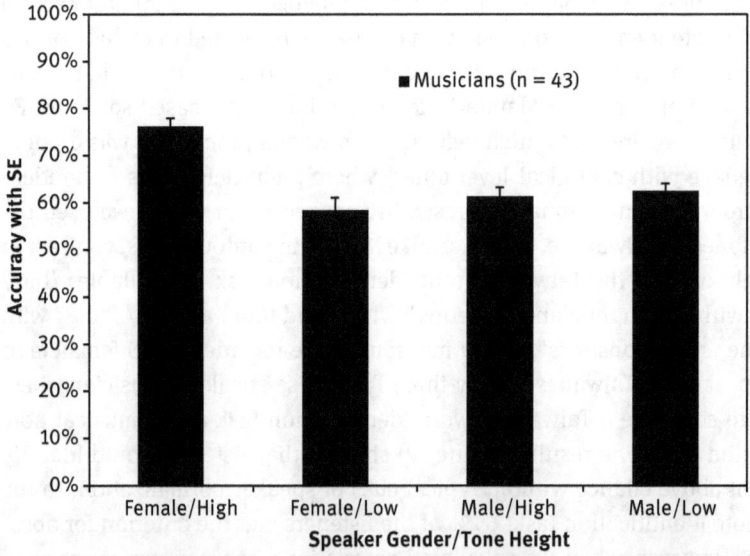

Figure 12: Accuracy of Taiwanese level tone identification by Taiwanese-speaking musicians in Lee, Lee & Shr (2011). Error bar indicates standard error.

Lee, Lekich & Zhang (2014) examined Taiwanese tone identification by 36 English-speaking musicians and 36 non-musicians without prior knowledge of Taiwanese or other tone languages. The results (Figure 13) showed that the musicians achieved higher identification accuracy than the non-musicians in this task, although the advantage was minimal. In particular, for mid tones, the musicians outperformed the non-musicians by 4%. For high tones, the musicians in fact did not have any advantage. This result replicated the finding on the identification of onset-only Mandarin stimuli reported in Lee & Hung (2008). In addition, both the musicians and non-musicians achieved above-chance accuracy only for tones at extremes of the speakers' pitch range. That is, they were able to identify high tones produced by female speakers and mid tones produced by the male speakers, but not mid tones produced by female speakers and high tones produced by the male speakers. As for musical note identification, none of the English-speaking musicians possessed absolute pitch (Figure 14). None of the correlations turned out significant between measures of Taiwanese tone identification and measures of musical note identification.

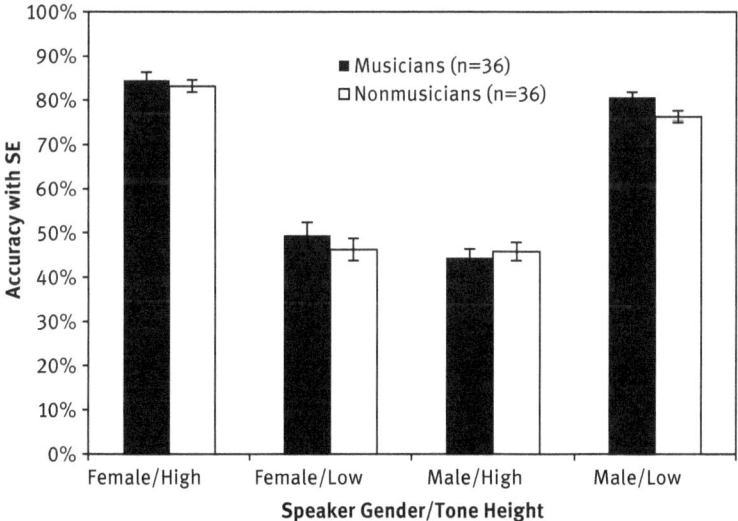

Figure 13: Accuracy of Taiwanese level tone identification by English-speaking musicians and non-musicians in Lee, Lekich & Zhang (2014). Error bar indicates standard error.

Taken together, findings from these four studies showed that musicians had an advantage in lexical tone identification over non-musicians, but the advantage was greater for contour tones than level tones. For level tones, listeners who do not speak a tone language achieved above-chance accuracy only for tones at extremes of speakers' pitch range. The percentage of absolute pitch was substantially higher in tone-speaking musicians, but there was no evidence of correlation between lexical tone identification and absolute pitch, irrespective of tone language experience.

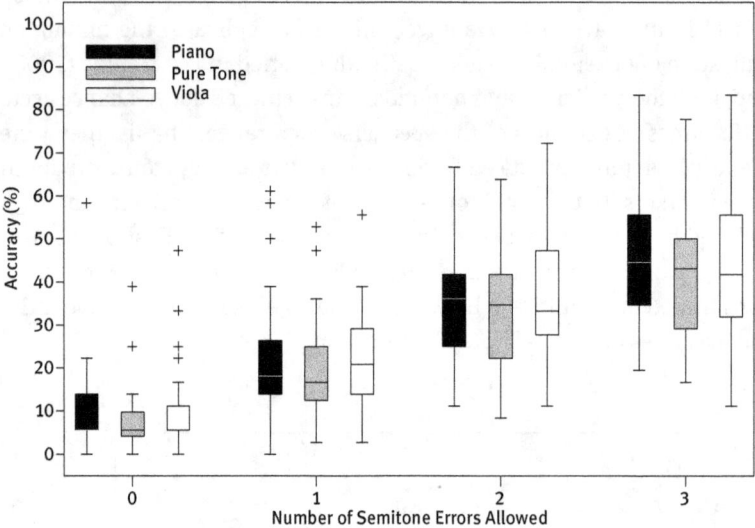

Figure 14: Box plot showing the accuracy of musical note identification for piano, pure tone, and viola stimuli in Lee, Lekich & Zhang (2014).

How do these findings answer the two questions raised earlier? First, we found evidence that musical pitch processing is associated with lexical pitch processing, as shown by the musicians' superior performance in the lexical tone identification task. However, the advantage of musicians over non-musicians in lexical tone identification seems to be attributed to their ability to track pitch movement rather than to detect pitch height. In particular, when contour information was reduced, the advantage was reduced (Lee & Hung, 2008). When no contour information was available, as in the case of level tones, the musicians' advantage became minimal compared to non-musicians (Lee, Lekich & Zhang, 2014). Furthermore, none of the English-speaking musicians possessed absolute pitch. All of these sources of evidence suggest that the ability to detect pitch height is not the underlying reason for the musicians' advantage. Rather, the advantage most likely arises from the ability to track pitch contours.

Second, we did not find evidence for the association between absolute pitch and lexical tone identification. In none of the four studies did we find a significant correlation between performance in lexical tone identification and performance in musical note identification. This conclusion applies to both musicians with absolute pitch (Lee & Lee, 2010; Lee, Lee & Shr, 2011) and those without absolute pitch (Lee & Hung, 2008; Lee, Lekich & Zhang, 2014). However, since none of the English-speaking musicians actually met the criterion for absolute pitch, the null correlations should be considered inconclusive. We will need to identify English-speaking musicians with absolute pitch to further test the association.

More broadly, findings from this series of studies are consistent with evidence showing that musical training facilitates non-tone language users' ability to produce and perceive lexical tones (Alexander, Wong & Bradlow, 2005; Gottfried, 2007; Gottfried & Riester, 2000; Gottfried, Staby & Ziemer, 2001). By comparing the perception of contour and level tones, our studies further contribute to the literature by identifying the source of the musician's advantage. What remains unclear is the association between absolute pitch and lexical tones. Several studies, including our own, showed higher prevalence of absolute pitch in tone language speakers (Deutsch et al., 2006; Deutsch, Dooley, Henthorn & Head, 2009), suggesting a common origin between absolute pitch and the lexical use of pitch. Absolute pitch is also associated with the age of onset of musical training. That is, the earlier musical training commences, the more prevalent absolute pitch is. This developmental course is similar to the acquisition of speech.

On the other hand, there are fundamental differences between the use of pitch in music and the use of pitch in lexical tones. First, the degree to which musical and lexical tone perception relies on pitch may be different. Identifying musical notes relies primarily if not exclusively on pitch perception. Identifying lexical tones, in contrast, involves additional acoustic correlates such as duration and amplitude contours (Liu & Samuel, 2004; Whalen & Xu, 1992). In other words, the internal category structure and the linguistic function that musical pitch and lexical tone serve are quite distinct despite the common use of pitch. In addition, the association between pitch and verbal labels in lexical tones can be acquired by any normally developing speaker of a tone language. The verbal labels for musical pitch, however, have to be taught explicitly. Anecdotal experience also suggests that many tone language speakers cannot identify or produce musical notes reliably, but they have no difficulty in identifying or producing lexical tones. These observations suggest that linguistic and non-linguistic pitch processing may involve distinct processing mechanisms. In summary, musical experience facilitates lexical tone perception. However, whether absolute pitch is responsible for the superior performance by musicians is still inconclusive.

6 Conclusion

In this chapter I reviewed a series of studies on the effects of acoustic variability and listener characteristics on the perception of lexical tones. The studies on native versus non-native tone perception suggest that non-native tone perception is affected disproportionately by most sources of acoustic variability, but speaker variability appears to be an exception. The studies on musicians versus non-musicians in tone perception suggest that musical training is beneficial to lexical tone perception primarily due to its advantage in identifying F0 contour rather than relative F0 height. Taken together, these studies suggest that not all sources of acoustic variability affect lexical tone perception equally, and that listener characteristics play a significant role in tone perception.

References

Abramson, A. S. (1972). Tonal experiments with whispered Thai. In A. Valdman (Ed.), *Papers in Linguistics and Phonetics to the Memory of Pierre Delattre* (pp. 31–44). The Hague: Mouton.

Abramson, A. S. (1978). Static and dynamic acoustics in distinctive tones. *Language and Speech*, 21, 319–325.

Alexander, J., Wong, P. C. M. & Bradlow, A. (2005). Lexical tone perception in musicians and nonmusicians. Proceedings of Interspeech' 2005 – Eurospeech– 9th European Conference on Speech Communication and Technology. Lisbon, Portugal.

Bishop, J. & Keating, P. (2012). Perception of pitch location within a speaker's range: Fundamental frequency, voice quality and speaker sex. *Journal of the Acoustical Society of America*, 132, 1100–1112.

Blicher, D. L., Diehl, R. L. & Cohen, L. B. (1990). Effects of syllable duration on the perception of the Mandarin tone 2/tone 3 distinction: Evidence of auditory enhancement. *Journal of Phonetics*, 18, 37–49.

Bradlow, A. R. & Alexander, J. A. (2007). Semantic and phonetic enhancements for speech-in-noise recognition by native and non-native listeners. *Journal of the Acoustical Society of America*, 121, 2339–2349.

Creelman, C. D. (1957). Case of the unknown talker. *Journal of the Acoustical Society of America*, 29, 655.

Cutler, A., Weber, A., Smits, R. & Cooper, N. (2004). Patterns of English phoneme confusions by native and non-native listeners. *Journal of the Acoustical Society of America*, 116, 3668–3678.

Deutsch, D. (2006). The enigma of absolute pitch. *Acoustics Today*, 2, 11–19.

Deutsch, D., Dooley, K., Henthorn, T. & Head, B. (2009). Absolute pitch among students in an American music conservatory: Association with tone language fluency. *Journal of Acoustical Society of America*, 125, 2398–2403.

Deutsch, D., Henthorn, T. & Dolson, M. (2004). Absolute pitch, speech, and tone language: Some experiments and a proposed framework. *Music Perception*, 21, 339–356.

Deutsch, D., Henthorn, T., Marvin, E. & Xu, H. (2006). Absolute pitch among American and Chinese conservatory students: Prevalence differences, and evidence for a speech-related critical period. *Journal of the Acoustical Society of America*, 119, 719–722.

Dolson, M. (1994). The pitch of speech as a function of linguistic community. *Music Perception*, 11, 321–331.

Gandour, J. (1983). Tone perception in Far Eastern languages. *Journal of Phonetics*, 11, 149–175.

Gandour, J. T. & Harshman, R. A. (1978). Crosslanguage differences in tone perception: A multidimensional scaling investigation. *Language and Speech*, 22, 1–33.

Gårding, E., Kratochvil, P., Svantesson, J.-O. & Zhang, J. (1986). Tone 4 and Tone 3 discrimination in Modern Standard Chinese. *Language and Speech*, 29, 281–293.

Gottfried, T. L. & Riester, D. (2000). Relation of pitch glide perception and Mandarin tone identification. *Journal of the Acoustical Society of America*, 108, 2604.

Gottfried, T. L. & Suiter T. L. (1997). Effects of linguistic experience on the identification of Mandarin Chinese vowels and tones. *Journal of Phonetics*, 25, 207–231.

Gottfried, T. L. (2007). Effects of musical training on learning L2 speech contrasts. In Bohn, O.-S. & Munro, M. J. (Eds.), *Language Experience in Second Language Speech Learning* (pp. 221–237). Amsterdam: John Benjamins Publishing Company.

Gottfried, T. L., Staby, A. M. & Ziemer, C. J. (2001). Musical experience and Mandarin tone discrimination and imitation. *Journal of the Acoustical Society of America*, 115, 2545.

Honorof, D. N. & Whalen, D. H. (2005). Perception of pitch location within a speaker's F0 range. *Journal of the Acoustical Society of America*, 117, 2193–2200.

Howie, J. M. (1976). *Acoustical Studies of Mandarin Vowels and Tones*. Cambridge: Cambridge University Press.

Ladefoged, P. & Broadbent, D. E. (1957). Information conveyed by vowels. *Journal of the Acoustical Society of America*, 29, 98–104.

Laver, J. (1994). *Principles of Phonetics*. Cambridge: Cambridge University Press.

Leather, J. (1983). Speaker normalization in perception of lexical tone. *Journal of Phonetics*, 11, 373–382.

Lee, C.-Y. (2009). Identifying isolated, multispeaker Mandarin tones from brief acoustic input: A perceptual and acoustic study. *Journal of the Acoustical Society of America*, 125, 1125–1137.

Lee, C.-Y. & Hung, T.-H. (2008). Identification of Mandarin tones by English-speaking musicians and nonmusicians. *Journal of the Acoustical Society of America*, 124, 3235–3248.

Lee, C.-Y. & Lee, Y.-F. (2010). Perception of musical pitch and lexical tones by Mandarin-speaking musicians. *Journal of the Acoustical Society of America*, 127, 481–490.

Lee, C.-Y., Dutton, L. & Ram, G. (2010). The role of speaker gender identification in F0 height estimation from multispeaker, brief speech segments. *Journal of the Acoustical Society of America*, 128, 384–388.

Lee, C.-Y., Lee, Y.-F. & Shr, C.-L. (2011). Perception of musical and lexical tones by Taiwanese-speaking musicians. *Journal of the Acoustical Society of America*, 130, 526–535.

Lee, C.-Y., Lekich, A. & Zhang, Y. (2014). Perception of pitch height in lexical and musical tones by English-speaking musicians and nonmusicians. *Journal of the Acoustical Society of America*, 135, 1607–1615, doi: 10.1121/1.4864473

Lee, C.-Y., Tao, L. & Bond, Z. S. (2008). Identification of acoustically modified Mandarin tones by native listeners. *Journal of Phonetics*, 36, 537–563.

Lee, C.-Y., Tao, L. & Bond, Z. S. (2009). Speaker variability and context in the identification of fragmented Mandarin tones by native and non-native listeners. *Journal of Phonetics*, 37, 1–15.

Lee, C.-Y., Tao, L. & Bond, Z. S. (2010a). Identification of acoustically modified Mandarin tones by non-native listeners. *Language and Speech*, 53, 217–243.

Lee, C.-Y., Tao, L. & Bond, Z. S. (2010b). Identification of multi-speaker Mandarin tones in noise by native and non-native listeners. *Speech Communication*, 52, 900–910.

Lee, C.-Y., Tao, L. & Bond, Z. S. (2013). Effects of speaker variability and noise on identifying isolated Mandarin tones by native and non-native listeners. *Speech, Language and Hearing*, 16, 46–54

Lee, C.-Y., Zhang, Y., Li, X., Tao, L. & Bond, Z. S. (2012). Effects of speaker variability and noise on Mandarin fricative identification by native and non-native listeners. *Journal of the Acoustical Society of America*, 132, 1130–1140.

Liu, S. & Samuel, A. G. (2004). Perception of Mandarin lexical tones when F0 information is neutralized. *Language and Speech*, 47, 109–138.

Moore, C. B. & Jongman, A. (1997). Speaker normalization in the perception of Mandarin Chinese tones. *Journal of the Acoustical Society of America*, 102, 1864–1877.

Mullennix, J. W., Pisoni, D. B. & Martin, C. S. (1989). Some effects of talker variability on spoken word recognition. *Journal of the Acoustical Society of America*, 85, 365–378.

Nusbaum, H. C. & Morin, T. M. (1992). Paying attention to differences among talkers. In Tohkura, Y., Sagisaka, Y. & Vatikiotis-Bateson, E. (Eds.), *Speech perception, speech production, and linguistic structure* (pp. 113–134). Tokyo: OHM.

Patel, A. D. (2008). *Music, Language, and the Brain*. New York, NY: Oxford University Press.

Shen, X. S. & Lin, M. (1991). A perceptual study of Mandarin tones 2 and 3. *Language and Speech*, 34, 145–156.

Shen, X. S., Lin, M. & Yan, J. (1993). F0 turning point as an F0 cue to tonal contrast: A case study of Mandarin tones 2 and 3. *Journal of the Acoustical Society of America*, 93, 2241–2243.

Strange, W., Jenkins, J. J. & Johnson, T. L. (1983). Dynamic specification of coarticulated vowels. *Journal of the Acoustical Society of America*, 74, 695–705.

Summerfield, Q. & Haggard, M. P. (1973). Vocal tract normalization as demonstrated by reaction times. In, *Report of speech research in progress*, Vol. 2 (pp. 1–12). Ireland: The Queen's University of Belfast.

Tseng, C. -Y. (1981). *An acoustic phonetic study on tones in Mandarin Chinese*. Ph.D. dissertation, Brown University.

Verbrugge, R. R., Strange, W., Shankweiler, D. P. & Edman, T. R. (1976). What information enables a listener to map a talker's vowel space? *Journal of the Acoustical Society of America*, 60, 198–212.

Whalen, D. H. & Xu, Y. (1992). Information for Mandarin tones in the amplitude contour and in brief segments. *Phonetica*, 49, 25–47.

Wong, P. C. M. & Diehl, R. L. (2003). Perceptual normalization for inter- and intratalker variation in Cantonese level tones. *Journal of Speech, Language, and Hearing Research*, 46, 413–421.

Xu, Y. (1994). Production and perception of coarticulated tones. *Journal of the Acoustical Society of America*, 95, 2240–2253.

Zhou, N., Zhang, W., Lee, C.-Y. & Xu, L. (2008). Lexical tone recognition with an artificial neural network. *Ear and Hearing*, 29, 326–335.

Sara Guediche
Flexible and adaptive processes in speech perception

Abstract: The perception of speech can be flexible, influenced by multiple sources of information, and plastic, tuned over time to cumulative experience. This chapter provides examples of cognitive neuroscience research, presented at a workshop on speech and lexical processing. Section I demonstrates effects of different sources of semantic information on perception and brain activity. Section II presents evidence for the role of internally generated linguistic predictions in guiding adaptive plasticity, and for the potential involvement of a cerebellar-mediated supervised learning mechanism. Finally, Section III examines the relationship between flexibility and adaptive plasticity and underscores the need for considering their underlying neurobiological mechanisms and their interactions with cognitive processes, and other factors that contribute to generalization in order to further elucidate this relationship.

The perception of speech depends on mapping a highly variable and complex acoustic signal onto meaningful sounds and words. However, when the speech signal violates learned regularities due to natural, environmental, or synthetic distortions of the speech signal, accurate perception can be maintained through adjustments in mapping the acoustic signal onto more abstract linguistic information. Such adjustments are facilitated by disambiguating contexts that influence perception of the acoustic signal to be more consistent with the context. They can also accumulate, over brief periods of exposure, and affect perception of later instances of the distorted speech (adaptive plasticity). Current cognitive neuroscience research continues to investigate the underlying mechanisms and neural systems that support these flexible and adaptive properties of speech processing.

The main goal of this chapter is to review findings presented at a workshop on speech and lexical processing, largely from our research group and collaborators, on studies investigating flexible and adaptive processes in speech perception. Section I of this chapter describes behavioral and functional neuroimaging results that provide evidence for interactions across multiple levels of language

Sara Guediche, Department of Cognitive, Linguistic & Psychological Sciences, Brown University; Basque Center on Cognition Brain and Language

and speech processing. The first part of Section II shows that both external sources of disambiguating information and internally-generated predictions, stimulus-driven and based on prior linguistic experience (e. g., lexical information and predictions), contribute to adaptive plasticity. The second part of Section II presents a study that investigates a potential learning mechanism, established in other domains (sensorimotor adaptation) that may mediate adaptive changes in perception. Specifically, the study examines evidence for a cerebellar-mediated supervised learning guided by sensory prediction errors. Finally, Section III summarizes Sections I and II and reviews the potential relationship between flexibility and adaptive plasticity, raising questions for future research. In particular, we highlight unanswered questions about the nature of the underlying neural systems and neurobiological mechanisms that link these two processes. We also discuss potential interactions with cognitive processes and current investigations on the factors that may affect generalization.

1 SECTION I: Flexibility in speech perception: integrating meaning with the acoustic speech signal

How listeners perceive an acoustic speech signal is influenced by the context in which it is presented. Studies have shown effects of context on the perception of ambiguous, distorted, and degraded acoustic input (Ganong, 1980; Schwab, Nusbaum & Pisoni, 1985; Bradlow & Alexander, 2007). For example, a speaker who is pointing at his watch may produce an acoustically ambiguous word that can be perceived as *"dime"* or *"time"*. The overarching idea of contextual influences on perception is that a listener will more likely perceive the uttered word as consistent with the context, and (for this made-up example) perceive "time". Studies have shown that speech perception is sensitive to many different types of contexts including lexical (Ganong, 1980), articulatory (Bertelson, Vroomen & de Gelder, 2003), temporally adjacent nonlinguistic sounds (Holt & Lotto, 2006), and speaker (Theodore & Miller, 2010). In many cases, the context provides supporting information that facilitates perception and improves comprehension of the speech input.

Our understanding of the mechanisms that underlie these effects has been primarily shaped by how context affects behavioral performance on categorization, discrimination, and word recognition tasks. These findings have been pivotal in the development of models of speech perception. Traditionally, models of speech recognition have focused on the processes involved in mapping the acoustic speech signal onto words. Consequently, the computational models that underlie flexibility in effects of context on speech perception have mostly attended to word level (lexical) influences on the perception of ambiguous or degraded sounds (e. g., McClelland & Elman, 1986; Marslen-Wilson, 1987; Gaskell & Marslen-Wilson, 1997; Norris, McQueen & Cutler, 2000).

The "lexical effect" (also known as "Ganong effect") is a well-established effect of context on perception in which an ambiguous sound is more likely to be perceived as a member of a category that forms a word over a nonword (Ganong, 1980). For example, "*kiss*" is a more likely interpretation than "*giss*" if the onset is ambiguous and can be heard as either [g] or [k]. One of the biggest controversies has been whether information at higher levels of abstraction (e. g., lexical information) in a hierarchically organised model, feeds back to directly impact perceptual processing of the acoustic speech input (interactive models such as TRACE and Predictive Coding) (McClelland & Elman, 1986), or whether the effect of context on perception is a result of post-perceptual and decision-making processes (autonomous models such as MERGE) (Norris, McQueen & Cutler, 2000). Thus, interactive and autonomous models have competing views, often difficult to dissociate with behavioral tasks (McClelland, Mirman & Holt, 2006).

Functional neuroimaging methods have been employed to characterize the nature and locus of changes in brain activity associated with effects of context on speech perception. To the extent that different models of speech perception make different predictions about changes in brain activity, functional neuroimaging findings have been used to weigh in on this debate. Models that support feedback of lexical information onto lower levels, for example, predict that activity in auditory cortex (and surrounding speech perceptual areas in the temporal cortex) will be modulated by the lexical effect. Indeed, many studies have supported this hypothesis (see Mattys et al., 2012 for review). A functional magnetic resonance imaging (fMRI) experiment that examined the lexical effect showed that the biasing lexical context does modulate activity in the superior temporal gyrus (STG) (Myers & Blumstein, 2008), an area known to support auditory processing of acoustic speech stimuli (Hickok & Poeppel, 2007).

Results from other functional neuroimaging methods that have higher temporal resolution than fMRI such as Electroencephalography (EEG) and Magnetoencephalography (MEG) (e. g., Gow et al., 2008) converge with the fMRI findings. An EEG study shows effects of lexical information in the superior temporal gyrus (STG) and provides evidence that activity in STG is modulated through interactions with the supramarginal gyrus (SMG) (Gow et al., 2008), an area sensitive to the lexical status of an item (e. g., Prabhakaran et al., 2006). Together, the data support interactions between lexical and pre-lexical sources of information.

Such effects of lexical context on perceptual processing would not be predicted by a strictly feedforward autonomous post-perceptual account of lexical effects

Many contextual sources of information influence the perception of acoustically-manipulated speech including matching priors (e. g., Clos et al., 2012), semantic associates (Golestani, Hervais-Adelman & Scott, 2013), sentence predictability (cloze probability and coherence) (Obleser et al., 2007; Davis et al., 2011). Many of these studies also show contextual modulation of activity in STG that extend beyond word-level influences.

Until now, research on flexible speech perception has mostly focused on the modulatory effects in early auditory cortex (Gagnepain, Henson & Davis, 2012; Kilian-Hutten et al., 2011; Wild, Davis & Johnsrude, 2012). Consequently, models that incorporate the effects of predictive sources of information on early speech perceptual processing have become increasingly popular. They suggest that predictive coding generates feedback signals that suppress activity in lower levels such as in areas involved in early sensory processing. Suppression of activity reflects the modulatory effect due to the expected stimulus such that any change in activity in the corresponding sensory area, in response to the incoming stimulus, would represent the discrepancy between the expected and actual sensory input (Rao & Ballard, 1999; Alink et al., 2010; Friston, 2008; Bastos et al., 2012).

Importantly, in a predictive framework, the processing of the sensory input also feeds forward and contributes to perception; stimulus-driven predictions-based on experience or prior knowledge-are generated even if the sensory signal is degraded (Panichello, Cheung & Bar, 2013; Bastos et al., 2012). This feedforward processing interacts with the feedback provided by the predictive context. Indeed, there is accumulating evidence for interactions between feedback and feedforward signals in perception (Bastos et al., 2012, Panichello Cheung & Bar, 2013) at multiple stages of processing. Similar claims have been made in speech perception, based on findings that effects of contextual and acoustic manipulations permeate multiple levels of processing with effects of context also impacting early perceptual processes and effects of acoustic manipulations propagating to later stages of processing (Aydelott, Dick & Mills, 2006). There is evidence for modulation of activity in perceptual areas (Clos et al., 2012; Sohoglu & Davis, 2012; Wild & Davis, 2012; Blank & Davis, 2016). There is also evidence that interactions between multiple sources of information enhance speech intelligibility (Obleser et al., 2007, 2010; Peelle et al., 2013; Gross et al., 2013).

As in the domain of visual perception, existing neuroanatomical frameworks for spoken language and speech processing are also hierarchically organized into multiple levels (e. g., phonological, lexical, semantic, conceptual). An underlying assumption of these frameworks is that different brain regions are involved in different linguistic processes (Davis and Johnsrude, 2003; Peelle, Johnsrude & Davis, 2010; Scott, 2012; Price, 2012). Thus, one prediction that emerges is that different brain regions may be recruited depending on the source of the predictive context. The other is that the feedback (and its interactions with feedforward processes) should have an effect that modulates activity at multiple stages of processing, as has been proposed in the visual domain. Thus, investigating the nature of the effects of different contexts at different levels of processing may provide insight into the neural architecture that supports flexibility in speech perception.

In this section, we focus on effects of meaning on the perception of acoustically manipulated speech. Meaning can be extracted from multiple levels of processing, derived from a word, a sentence, or a combination of sentences. Meaning can also be accessed from different stimulus input modalities (visual, auditory). We describe functional magnetic resonance imaging studies that examine changes in brain activity associated with effects of meaning on perception, across different levels of abstraction (within a sentence and between two sentences), and across different modalities (visual/written, auditory). Part I describes the details of two studies that investigate sentence context effects on acoustic phonetic perception, within and across modalities. Part II describes a study that shows effects of meaning relationships between two sentences on the perception of acoustically degraded speech.

1.1 Part I: Within-sentence effects of sentence meaning on acoustic phonetic perception

The meaning of a sentence is more abstract than each lexical item that makes up the sentence (Hickok & Poeppel, 2007; Lau, Phillips & Poeppel, 2008). Consequently, in a hierarchically organized speech processing system, sentence meaning is separated by additional level(s) from sound-based pre-lexical representations, and recruits brain regions involved in higher level processes (Davis and Johnsrude, 2003; Peelle, Johnsrude & Davis, 2010; Scott, 2012; Price, 2012). Therefore, the nature of the interactions between meaning and acoustic phonetic properties of speech, and their locus, will elucidate influences of feedback (across multiple levels of processing) on perception.

Prior behavioral work has established that the semantic bias of a sentence context influences acoustic phonetic perception (Connine, 1987; Borsky, Tuller & Shapiro, 1998). For example, Borsky et al. (1998) created a continuum of tokens from 'goat' to 'coat' by varying the voice onset time (VOT) of the onset consonant.

Tokens were presented in different types of sentence contexts that biased the interpretation towards either 'goat' or 'coat'. Results showed significant differences in the perception of the ambiguous stimuli that depended on the semantic bias of the sentence context.

The experiments described below investigated this type of sentence context effect on acoustic phonetic perception using fMRI to examine the nature and locus of changes in brain activity that resulted from each manipulation and their interaction (Guediche, Salvata & Blumstein, 2013). To this end, both the ambiguity of the acoustic phonetic information (ambiguous, unambiguous), and the semantic bias of the sentence context were manipulated by including a neutral condition in the design of the experiment (biased, neutral). Thus, three sentence contexts – goat-biased (e. g., *he fed the*), neutral (e. g., *he drew the*), and coat-biased (e. g., *he buttoned the*) – and three word targets (unambiguous '*goat*', ambiguous '*goat/coat*', unambiguous '*coat*') were used. The ambiguous word, created by manipulating the voice onset time (VOT) of the initial consonant (an acoustic-phonetic parameter), could be perceived as either '*goat*' or '*coat*'. Each of the tokens was presented in each type of sentence context. Interactions between sentence context and acoustic phonetic properties of speech should manifest as 1) a semantic influence on the perception of acoustically ambiguous speech, and 2) interactions between semantic bias and target ambiguity on changes in brain activity.

In the first study (Study 1), auditory presentation was used for both the sentence context and target word, whereas in the second study (Study 2), the sentence context was delivered through orthographic (written) presentation and the target word through auditory presentation. Both studies showed a significant behavioral influence of semantic context on the perception of the ambiguous stimulus (Guediche, Salvata & Blumstein, 2013). In both cases, however, the effect of sentence context was asymmetric; listeners' categorization of the ambiguous target was significantly more likely to be a 'goat' response in the goat-biasing contexts but there was no significant difference in 'coat' responses in coat-biasing sentence contexts. This finding was not surprising; in Guediche, Salvata & Blumstein (2013), we noted that asymmetric effects of context on the perception of ambiguous acoustic phonetic information are common and that they have been reported in a number of studies (Burton & Blumstein, 1995; Myers & Blumstein, 2008; Reinisch & Holt, 2014).

To elucidate the nature of the interaction between semantic and acoustic phonetic information, we were only interested in cases where the semantic bias successfully influenced perception, therefore, the fMRI analyses focused on interactions between the goat-biasing and neutral sentence contexts paired with either the ambiguous or unambiguous 'goat' tokens.

1.1.1 Study 1: Within-modality

The current study investigated the influence of semantic context on acoustic phonetic perception within the auditory modality. This is the first functional neuroimaging study that manipulated both the semantic bias of a sentence context and the ambiguity of the acoustic phonetic properties of a target word, making it possible to examine the effect of their interactions on changes in brain activity.

The fMRI results showed a significant interaction between Sentence Context (goat-biased, neutral) and Target Type (unambiguous 'goat', ambiguous 'coat/goat') in the left middle temporal gyrus extending into parts of the superior temporal gyrus (MTG/STG) (Guediche, Salvata & Blumstein, 2013). The MTG is an important component of neuroanatomical models of speech processing. One of the main functions attributed to the region is lexical processing (Hickok, 2009; Fiez et al., 1996). The interactions showed that Sentence Context (biased, neutral) modulated brain activity in different directions depending on the Target Type (ambiguous, unambiguous); the unambiguous target in the congruent biasing sentence context increased activity, whereas the ambiguous target decreased activity. This crossover interaction was taken as evidence that both sources of information have an interdependent effect that modulates activity in a common area associated with lexical processing, potentially reflecting the integration of information provided by both the semantic context and by acoustic signal.

We also observed main effects for Sentence Context and Target Type. A relative increase in activity for the biasing compared to neutral context (i. e., Sentence Context) emerged in two frontal clusters, whereas the effects of Target Type showed a relative increase in activity in inferior frontal gyrus (IFG), and a relative decrease in activity in STG. Enhanced activity for the biasing context and the ambiguous stimulus in the IFG could result from the effect of the semantic predictions that provided the source for top-down modulation and the resulting propagated error that denotes the differences between the expected and unexpected sensory input, generated in auditory cortex (Davis & Sohoglu, 2016; Blank & Davis, 2016). Enhanced activity for the ambiguous target in the IFG may be due to increased difficulty of category decisions (e. g., Binder et al., 2004; Myers et al., 2009). Of interest, the region that showed a crossover interaction between the semantic bias of the sentence context and the ambiguity of the acoustic input (LMTG) was not sensitive to each manipulation alone and did not emerge in frontal areas. These results suggest that the LMTG/STG region may be an area that integrates both sources of information in such a way that depends on the bias of the semantic context and the ambiguity of the acoustic phonetic properties of the speech signal.

This study extends our knowledge on effects of meaning on speech perception at stages of processing that extend beyond early perceptual processing of the auditory signal but not related to decision-making (also see Toscano, McMurray, Dennhardt & Luck, 2010; Li & Zhao, 2014). The findings provide additional evidence that interactions occur across traditional, hierarchically defined levels of processing during flexible perception (Bastos et al., 2012, Panichello, Cheung & Bar, 2013), and are in favor of more interactive and dynamic models of speech perception.

1.1.2 Study 2: Across-modality

Meaning can be extracted from multiple independent modalities (visual, auditory) or through a combination of several of them. At the neural level, the pathways for reading and spoken language are distinct in the early stages of sensory processing of written and auditory input. However, they engage several common brain areas at later stages, and may converge onto the same amodal semantic representations (Marinkovic & Dhond, 2003). Although a number of studies have examined semantic influences on speech perception, the effect of the presentation modality of semantic information has been largely overlooked. This may be due to an implicit assumption that meaning exerts its contextual influence only after converging onto amodal representations, suggesting its effect on brain activity is unchanged by presentation modality. However, given the potential role of feedforward and feedback interactions such an assumption may be misleading.

The current study investigated the influence of a written semantic context on acoustic phonetic perception, across modalities, to determine 1) if there is a crossmodal effect of a written semantic context on acoustic phonetic perception. As reported above, this was the first study to show an influence of meaning, derived from reading, on the perception of acoustic phonetic properties of speech allowing us to investigate 2) if there is an effect of crossmodal semantic-phonetic interactions on brain activity and 3) the locus of the potential interactions.

The fMRI results showed an interaction between Sentence Context (goat-biased, neutral) and Target Type (ambiguous, unambiguous 'goat') in two clusters in the right hemisphere, MTG extending into parahippocampal gyrus (RMTG), and the anterior temporal gyrus (RATG), and an additional uncorrected cluster in the left anterior temporal gyrus (LATG) (Guediche, Zhu, Minicucci & Blumstein, *submitted*). Importantly, the same pattern of changes in activity that were observed in Study 1 were found in all three of the clusters identified in this study. This finding suggests that the mechanisms underlying semantic-perceptual interactions, across two modalities, may be similar in nature, relying on the same types of computations as those that involve processing of auditory information in the auditory modality alone. The right hemisphere lateralization and more anterior locus of the interactions, in Study 2, is consistent with studies that have shown more right hemisphere activation for reading compared to listening (e. g., Horowitz-Kraus et al., 2015). Thus, despite similar mechanisms, the presentation modality may impact the locus of semantic-phonetic interactions, emerging in crossmodal areas common to reading and auditory speech/language processing.

We also observed each of the main effects of Sentence Context and Target Type in visual areas, confirming the involvement of modality-specific pathways. The main effect of Sentence Context showed greater activity in the angular gyrus for biased compared to neutral sentence context, consistent with a role of this region in semantic processing, and consistent with other reported effects of context (e. g., Golestani et al., 2013). However, less activation was found for the biased compared to neutral sentence context. Even more surprisingly, the main effect of Target Type, which also emerged in a number of temporal areas (anterior and mid-superior middle temporal gyri), showed significantly greater activity for the unambiguous compared to the ambiguous target in visual cortex (middle occipital cortex, MOC).

In summary, Study 2 demonstrates that the semantic bias of an orthographically presented sentence context influences the perception of acoustic-phonetic properties of speech. Semantic-phonetic interactions emerged in regions common to reading and spoken language processing. In addition, the main effects of meaning and target type modulated activity in visual areas, suggesting that the orthographic presentation of the sentence context has an impact on the brain regions that respond to manipulations of sentence meaning and acoustic phonetic ambiguity.

Together, the results of Studies 1 and 2 contribute to our understanding of speech and language processing by characterizing the nature of the interaction between semantic and acoustic phonetic information within and across modalities. Together, they provide compelling evidence against a purely post-perceptual view of context effects on perception. 1) Semantic-perceptual interactions occur in temporal cortex not in post-perceptual decision-making areas. 2) Activity is modulated in different directions depending on the bias of a semantic context and the quality of acoustic phonetic information, providing evidence that they may influence one another. 3) Decision-related changes in activity should not change as a function of presentation modality, yet we observed differences in the *locus* of crossmodal semantic-phonetic interactions, and main effects of semantic context. Thus, perception is influenced by interactions between different sources of information, across different modalities, which may contribute to the recruitment of specific regions.

Importantly, Guediche et al. (submitted) discuss research showing that greater convergence between the neural systems that support reading and speech perception relates to greater reading proficiency (Rueckl et al., 2016; Preston et al., 2016). If reading and speech perception also interact across multiple levels of processing, it begs the following question: Could greater crossmodal semantic-perceptual integration also relate to reading proficiency?

1.2 Part II: Between sentence-effects of conceptual meaning relationships on perception of degraded speech

A re-emerging theme in speech perception research suggests a great deal of interactivity among different sources of information and different brain areas. Such a high degree of interactivity predicts that the factors influencing perception of degraded speech would not be confined to interactions between acoustic speech information and single words, or between words within a single sentence.

To test this hypothesis, in a recent study (Guediche et al., 2016), we examined effects of meaning on perception that extend beyond a single word or sentence by manipulating the overall semantic relationship between two different sentences. Sentences that were related in meaning consisted of different content words. For example, the sentence *"She babysat her niece."* is related in meaning to the sentence *"She took care of her sister's daughter."* Even though each individual word across the sentences, alone, is not necessarily related in meaning. Listeners were presented with pairs of sentences that were either the same, related in meaning, or unrelated in meaning. The pairs consisted of a clear sentence followed by a sentence degraded by background noise (speech babble −5dB) (stimuli created using BLISS) (mertus.org). In the Same condition, the sentences were made up of the same words in both sentences, whereas the in the Related and Unrelated conditions, the sentences were made up of different content words.

Listeners were asked to produce the words they heard in the target sentence (written response). Performance was measured as the proportion of accurately recognized content words (word recognition accuracy) in the degraded target sentence. As expected, when the degraded sentence was preceded by the same sentence, performance (measured as content word recognition accuracy) was higher than for a preceding related or unrelated sentence. Importantly, listeners' performance was also significantly higher for the Related condition than for the Unrelated condition. Hence, in this case, overall sentence meaning seems to mediate perceptual facilitation.

fMRI was used to examine changes in brain activity associated with conceptual meaning effects on degraded speech by comparing differences between the Related and Unrelated sentence conditions. Importantly, the only systematic difference between the two conditions is the conceptual relationship; therefore, any Related compared to Unrelated condition advantage in the perception of the second sentence occurs from successfully integration of the overall related sentence meanings. Thus, differences in brain activity between the two conditions should reflect this advantage, providing insight into the neural systems involved in the conceptual meaning effects degraded speech perception. The effect of Related vs. Unrelated sentence pairs on brain activity enhanced activation of several regions including bilateral middle frontal gyri, the left inferior frontal gyrus, inferior parietal areas (Left angular gyrus (AG), RSMG), and the left middle temporal gyrus (LMTG) (Guediche et al., 2016). This fronto-temporo-parietal network includes areas previously associated with lexical and semantic processing, in addition to a frontal area previously linked to processing semantic relationships (LMFG) (Binder et al., 2009).

The effect of the related sentence on perception of the subsequent degraded sentence requires building meaning from the words within one sentence and integrating this meaning with the meaning of another sentence. This may co-activate multiple areas that potentially correspond to different levels of processing. One possibility is that the areas work together optimizing the simultaneous constraint satisfaction of multiple sources of information. Alternatively, changes in activation in some areas may be due to other factors that are unrelated to improvements in perception. For this reason, we examined the relationship between the observed changes in brain activity and changes in behavior.

In order to be able to assess the association between behavioral performance and brain activity, one half of the fMRI experiment was designed to include a spoken response output, which was collected and analyzed. Overall, performance was lower in the scanner, however, the pattern of results was the same showing a significant advantage for the Related compared to Unrelated condition. In addition, recognition accuracy did not correlate with maximum semantic associations between individual words across the related prime and degraded sentences. Individual behavioral performance (content word recognition accuracy), on the Related condition from this part of the experiment, was positively correlated with individual brain activity in the areas identified above including the MFG, IFG, IPL, and MTG. The LMFG, LIFG, and LMTG. These findings led us to conclude that the two left frontal regions and left middle temporal areas may be involved in integrating conceptual and acoustic information. Indeed, others have pointed to the importance of fronto-temporal coupling during semantic processing (Peelle et al., 2013; Gross et al., 2013; Molinaro et al., 2015). In addition, the angular gyrus may be implicated in modulating predictability gain for degraded speech, based on a recent finding that inactivation through repetitive transcranial magnetic stimulation (rTMS) significantly reduces predictability effects on word comprehension (Hartwigsen, Golombek & Obleser, 2015). Results from a functional connectivity analysis conducted in this study, using the LMFG as a seed region, suggest that the LMFG is part of a fronto-temporo-parietal network that is involved in integrating conceptual meaning across sentences.

We also examined the effect of phonological integration with the degraded signal in an analysis that compared the Related to the Same. The contrast between the Same and Related conditions showed relatively greater activity for the Same condition in the STG, and relatively greater activity for the Related in the IFG. Since the STG is a region involved in early perceptual and phonological processing (Rauschecker and Tian, 2000; Rauschecker and Scott, 2009; Hickok and Poeppel, 2004), the findings suggest that the facilitation effect in the Same sentence condition relies more on perceptual similarity between sentences rather than meaning relationships. This is consistent with the greater performance observed on the Same compared to Related conditions.

The relative contribution of each of these regions to lexical access, lexical selection, semantic processing, and conceptual integration may differ. Semantic facilitation of degraded speech perception, mediated by meaning relationship across two sentences, requires access to multiple levels of linguistic processes.

We proposed at least two possible ways that semantic/conceptual information may facilitate speech perception in a hierarchically organized stream; 1) the fine details of the degraded acoustic input may propagate through different levels and may be integrated at each successive stage of processing or 2) the degraded acoustic input may activate each level in a graded fashion without preserving the fine acoustic details at higher levels of abstraction (Guediche et al., 2016). The findings of this study cannot distinguish between these different possibilities. However, interactions between semantic information and intelligibility observed in previous studies, in parietal (Golestani et al., 2013), and in frontal and temporal areas (Davis et al., 2011; Gow et al., 2008; Guediche, Salvata & Blumstein, 2013; Obleser & Kotz, 2010) suggest the possibility that at least some properties of the details of the acoustic speech signal are retained throughout different levels of processing. The results are consistent with highly interactive models such as those that support mutual constraint satisfaction (e. g., McClelland et al., 2014).

In sum, Section I provides evidence that effects of meaning on perception can involve multiple levels of speech processing and multiple modalities. The involvement of different regions may be dictated by the levels of processing needed to facilitate perception of degraded speech, and thus may depend on the type of information provided by the context.

2 SECTION II: Adaptive plasticity in speech perception

Changes in speech perception are not only momentary but can also accumulate over time, and persist influencing the perception of subsequent speech input. Listeners often encounter atypical speech, such as the accented speech of a non-native speaker, or background noise. These distortions can often lead to poor intelligibility. However, after some experience, listeners' perception of the distorted input can improve and become more intelligible demonstrating successful adaptive changes in perception (adaptive plasticity). How are new relationships between the acoustic signal and sounds/words formed to accommodate atypical distortions to the speech signal?

Whereas Section I described immediate effects of context on perception, Section II focuses on effects of context on changes in perception that are cumulative. In particular, we explore evidence for the potential involvement of a supervised learning mechanism that relies on internally-generated sensory prediction errors to mediate adaptive plasticity (Marr, 1969; Albus, 1971).

Effects of lexical context on adaptive plasticity (a.k.a., perceptual learning) have previously been examined using a paradigm in which listeners are repeatedly exposed to ambiguous sounds in a lexical context that biases the interpretation of the sound towards one category over another (Norris, McQueen & Cutler, 2003). In one study, listeners heard an ambiguous sound in between an /s/ and /ʃ/ that was embedded in either a context that favored the /s/ or a context that favored the /ʃ/ interpretation (e.g., Arkansas) (Kraljic & Samuel, 2005). Each group of listeners subsequently performed a syllable categorization task on a continuum from "a/s/i" to "a/ʃ/i/". Post-test differences between the two groups in acoustic phonetic perception of ambiguous phonemes depended on the contextual bias they experienced during training. Therefore, the effect of the lexical context that provided the disambiguating information and influenced perception, during training, persisted after training-affecting perception of subsequent speech in the absence of any disambiguating context.

The traditional interactive and autonomous models of speech perception, discussed earlier in the chapter, have each been modified from their original instantiation in order to account for adaptive plasticity; although they differ in their implementation of context effects, both suggest that interactions between lexical and phonological processing support adaptive changes in perception. Myers and Mesite (2014) specifically examined lexically-mediated perceptual adjustments in category boundary judgments, and showed LIFG involvement associated with decision making, and increased sensitivity of LSTG (extending into middle temporal gyrus) – associated with increasing differences between boundary and non-boundary over time. These findings provide evidence that changes in phonological processing that are mediated by lexical information are linked to changes in activity in areas involved in speech perceptual processing, STG.

In many common listening situations, an entire word (not just one sound) is acoustically degraded. Thus, listeners cannot merely disambiguate the sound based on one possible lexical context, rather they may rely on (stimulus-driven) internal predictions that are generated based on existing linguistic (e. g., lexical) knowledge. If a supervised learning mechanism (that relies on prediction accuracy) supports adaptive changes in the absence of external information, then the accuracy of internally-generated predictions will affect the degree of adaptive plasticity.

In the current section, we describe studies that examine whether internally-generated lexical predictions contribute to adaptive changes in perception. Part I presents a set of behavioral experiments that manipulated these two potential contributing factors during exposure to distorted stimuli: 1) the presence of external information and 2) the accuracy of internally-generated lexical predictions on adaptive plasticity. Part II describes an fMRI experiment that investigated evidence for the involvement of the cerebellum in adaptive plasticity in speech perception, a key structure implicated in supervised learning mechanism that relies on internally-generated sensory predictions, in domains outside of speech perception (e. g., sensorimotor adaptation).

2.1 Part I: Effects of internally generated linguistic predictions

In some cases, perception of degraded speech can improve after a very brief period of exposure, however, in other cases, exposure alone is not sufficient and improvements in perception only occur if there is some external source of information that disambiguates the speech signal during exposure. In the absence of any other disambiguating source of information, Guediche, Fiez & Holt (2016) suggested that internally-generated linguistic predictions (e. g. lexical predictions) may mediate adaptive plasticity. To examine this hypothesis, a distortion manipulation that systematically affects intelligibility was employed (Shannon et al., 1995; Fu & Galvin, 2003) impacting the accuracy of internally-generated predictions. The prediction was that more intelligible speech leads to more accurate internal predictions compared to unintelligible speech and should improve adaptive plasticity. When speech is unintelligible, external information can facilitate access to lexical information that can be used to generate predictions and mediate adaptive plasticity. For this reason, we predicted that the effect of external information would be greater in the Severe compared to the Incremental conditions.

Listeners' performance on the most severe distortion was assessed before (Pretest-50 trials) and after (Posttest-50 trials) a period of exposure (250 trials). During exposure, two factors were manipulated: the presence of external disambiguating information (Present, Absent), and the acoustic distortion (Severe, Incremental). The external information provided was a post-response written version of the stimulus paired with the distorted auditory stimulus. The presentation of the distortion was either abrupt, consisting of only the most severely distorted stimuli (Severe), or was initially mild, and gradually incremented in 10 trial intervals until it reached the most severe distortion.

The incremental manipulation was used as a way to increase the probability of successful predictions. Mild distortions increase the probability of successful mapping between the acoustic input and existing linguistic knowledge. With gradual increases in the distortion, adjustments in this mapping extended to the more severe (less intelligible) distortions, through progressive alignment, until reaching the most severe distortion used in the posttest (for discussion, see Guediche, Fiez & Holt 2016). Listeners in the Severe condition, only heard the severe distortion which was less intelligible, and accurate predictions about the stimulus were less likely.

Improvements in perception (adaptive plasticity) were measured as the difference in word recognition accuracy on the Posttest compared to the Pretest. The results showed that, in the Severe condition, external information significantly increased improvements in perception. In contrast, there was no effect of external information in the Incremental condition. Thus, accurate predictions contribute to adaptive changes in perception. A correlation analysis between word recognition performance during training and improvements from Pretest to Posttest showed significant positive correlations providing additional evidence for the role of internally-generated predictions in adaptive plasticity. Based on the interaction between external information and distortion severity, and on the correlation results, we concluded that both internal and external sources of information that facilitate accurate predictions about the speech signal contribute to adaptive plasticity.

Such adaptive changes to distorted sensory input are not unique to speech perception. Understanding the mechanisms involved in other types of adaptation may inform the mechanisms that support adaptive plasticity in speech perception. We turned to the case of sensorimotor short-term adaptation, which is also presumed to rely on internally-generated predictions, and to occur over a similarly short timecourse of adaptation (Vroomen et al., 2007; Vroomen & Baart, 2012).

In sensorimotor tasks, such as visually-guided reaching, a distorted sensory input initially leads to incorrect/unintended motor output. For example, a visual distortion can be introduced with prism goggles that shift the visual field towards one direction. Such distorted visual input impairs reaching accuracy toward a desired target. However, over the course of multiple reaches, incremental adjustments in motor output correct for the distorted visual input enabling more accurate reaches to the desired target (Redding, 2006).

In sensorimotor adaptation, extensive research suggests that internally-generated predictions about the sensory consequences of a motor plan serve as a basis for determining discrepancies between expected and actual sensory input, and are used to derive an internal sensory prediction error signal that guides the adaptation through supervised learning; the cerebellum appears to be a key component involved in this supervised learning mechanism (Kawato, 1999; Wolpert, Miall & Kawato, 1998; Golfinopoulos et al., 2011). A growing literature shows cerebellar involvement in nonmotor functions (Desmond & Fiez, 1998; Petacchi et al., 2005; Stoodley & Schmahmann, 2009; Stoodley, Valera & Schmahmann, 2012; Rothermich & Kotz, 2013; Roth, Synofzik & Lindner, 2013). The possibility that other cerebellar functions, including supervised learning, extend beyond the motor domain continues to build (for recent reviews discussing the plausibility of nonmotor cerebellar function, see Argyropoulos 2015 and Moberget & Ivry 2016).

2.2 Part II: Is there evidence for cerebellar-dependent supervised learning in speech perception?

Part I of this section presented evidence that internally-generated predictions from prior linguistic knowledge (e. g., lexical information) contribute adaptive plasticity (Guediche, Fiez & Holt, 2016). One suggested mechanism is that the predictions are used to compute predictions error signals and used to guide supervised learning. If the supervised learning mechanism that mediates adaptation in other domains (e. g., sensorimotor adaptation), contributes to adaptive plasticity in speech perception, the cerebellum may play a role (Guediche et al., 2014). The fMRI study described below examines the involvement of the cerebellum in adaptive changes in speech perception by comparing differences in cerebellar activity before and after adaptation to acoustically manipulated speech.

Participants listened to severely distorted words during a Pretest (30 trials). They were then exposed to another set of less severely distorted words during Exposure (60 trials). The Posttest, consisted of yet another set of severely distorted words (30 trials). The severe distortion level of the same distortion manipulation used in the study discussed in Part I was used for the Pretest and Posttest. An intermediate level of the distortion was used for the Exposure phase. There was no explicit information provided about the stimuli (no feedback) and therefore, predictions about the speech were based solely on internally (stimulus-driven) generated sources of information (e. g., lexical information). On some of the trials, participants passively listened, whereas on other trials, participants were asked to provide a written response of what they thought they heard. This response manipulation (Response, No-Response) was included to assess motor-related changes in activity and determine whether cerebellar areas identified in the Pretest vs. Posttest were sensitive to motor processing.

Several regions in the cerebellum showed differences between the Pretest and Posttest (Guediche et al., 2015). Three of the regions were sensitive to the response condition, showing greater changes in brain activity for Written compared to the No-Response condition. However, one sub region that has been implicated in nonmotor tasks, including language functions (right Crus I), was not sensitive to the response condition. In this area, activity during the exposure phase correlated with improvements in performance from Pretest to Posttest (Guediche et al., 2015). Therefore, we concluded that this region might contribute to the learning mechanisms that mediate adaptive plasticity in speech perception.

In order to examine the functional connectivity of Crus I during adaptive plasticity, a simple correlation analysis was conducted for the exposure phase using this subregion of the cerebellum as a seed region (Guediche et al., 2015). Changes in activity in right Crus I were significantly correlated with activity in inferior parietal lobe, and a region that encompassed portions of auditory cortex during the exposure phase. For comparison, the same analysis was conducted with the other subregions of the cerebellum (sensitive to the motor response) that were identified. In contrast to Crus I, the other regions showed significant correlations with motor cortex.[1] Indeed, a growing number of neuroanatomical and functional neuroimaging studies confirm differences in connectivity between different subregions of the cerebellum cerebral cortex. Thus, nonmotor subregions of the cerebellum may also contribute to adaptive plasticity in speech perception through interactions with cerebral cortical areas involved in speech processing. This conclusion is consistent with a number of other studies that examined adaptation to degraded speech input and show changes in STG (Leech et al., 2009;

---

[1] We were specifically interested in the functional correlations that present during exposure/learning. We note that these functional correlations are assessed during the entire exposure phase (and include task-related correlations), thus they do not reflect intrinsic patterns of connectivity but *see* Allen et al., 2005; and Buckner, Krienen, Castellanos, and Yeo, 2011 for resting state connectivity patterns).

Adank and Devlin, 2010; Kilian-Hutten et al., 2011; Kilian-Hutten, Vroomen & Formisano, 2011; Myers & Mesite, 2014), and parietal areas (Eisner, et al., 2010)

Callan, Callan & Jones (2014) showed that changes in speech perception, after perceptual training on a non-native phonetic category also drive changes in cerebellar activity. Based on their findings, they concluded that the cerebellum is involved in remapping the signal onto articulatory-based representations, consistent with cerebellar involvement in motor processing (see Callan et al., 2014 and Gambi et al., 2015 for discussion). The Guediche et al. (2015) findings suggest that articulatory processes are not necessarily involved in generating the predictions needed for cerebellar-mediated supervised learning. Of course, associations between phonological and articulatory processes activate motor cortex during speech perception (Wilson et al., 2004; Watkins et al., 2003), and the potential involvement of intermediate articulatory processes in lexically-mediated adaptive plasticity cannot be completely ruled out. Nonetheless, the evidence that distinct subregions of the cerebellum are 1) involved in cognitive functions (Desmond & Fiez, 1998; Stoodley & Schmahmann, 2009; Stoodley et al., 2016), 2) anatomically connected to distinct cerebral cortical structures (Kelly and Strick, 2003), and 3) functionally connected to nonmotor areas – including the superior temporal cortex (Sokolov et al., 2014) together, offer the possibility that predictions generated (and the corresponding errors computed) could be derived from multiple sources of motor and nonmotor information. For within the context of the dual stream framework of speech processing, Hickok (2012) highlighted the importance of the predictions generated by ventral stream (word recognition) over the dorsal (motor) stream for influencing speech recognition. Others have also emphasized the need for generative models that incorporate predictions from both motor and nonmotor sources of information, to account for multiple cue integration in speech perception (for discussion see Jaeger & Ferreira, 2013; Farmer et al., 2013).

Here, we considered the possibility that a cerebellar-mediated supervised learning mechanism, previously established in the sensorimotor adaptation, may be domain-general for its role in timing-related speech processes (see Schwartze & Kotz, 2015; Lametti et al., 2016). In Guediche et al. (2014), we likened the proposal that cerebellar involvement in speech perception contributes to a domain-general supervised learning mechanism to the proposal that basal ganglia involvement in speech perception contributes to a domain-general reinforcement learning mechanism; just as sensory prediction errors mediate supervised learning, reward prediction errors mediate reinforcement learning (Doya, 2000). Indeed, previous studies confirm the involvement of the basal ganglia in reinforcement learning during speech perception (Tricomi et al., 2006; Lim, Fiez & Holt, 2014). However, more research that considers the role of subcortical structures (also see Erb et al., 2013) in speech perception and bridges established learning mechanisms in other domains with adaptive processes in speech perception is needed.

3 Section III. *Conclusions*

In this section, we point to the potential relationship between flexibility and adaptive plasticity. Unanswered questions, specifically related to mechanism, are raised. In addition, the importance of research on interactions between flexibility/adaptive plasticity and other cognitive processes is discussed. The section ends by turning to generalization in adaptive perception as an avenue of research that may inform additional details about the relevant acoustic properties of speech and how they contribute to flexibility and adaptive plasticity. Together, the different sections emphasize the need for linking findings across areas of speech perception research to further elucidate the underlying systems and mechanisms involved.

3.1 Part I: Relationship between flexibility and plasticity in speech perception

Together, Sections I and II suggest a potential relationship between flexibility and adaptive plasticity, in speech perception, that highlight the importance of interactions between *disambiguating contexts and acoustic input*.

The studies presented in Section I shift the focus of effects of context from their influence on the dynamics of early perceptual/auditory areas to the interactions between context and acoustic information-the different sources of information (and predictions that can be generated from them) – across multiple levels – and show that the *effect of a disambiguating context on perception depended on the ambiguity of the acoustic-phonetic input*. Moreover, across studies, the effects emerged in brain areas that extend beyond regions associated with early auditory and speech perception processing.

The studies presented in Section II provide evidence that training conditions that provide external source of information (disambiguating context) and those that promote accurate internally-generated predictions (related to intelligibility), have an interactive effect *on adaptive plasticity. Specifically, the effect of external information depends on the intelligibility of the acoustic input effect*. Thus, changes in perception that occur over time are also modulated by interactions between context and the quality of the acoustic signal. Importantly, the effects generalize and transfer to new instances of speech, absent any disambiguating context, and therefore suggest that changes in the feedforward processing (or mapping) of the acoustic input must take place.

The link between Sections I and II is consistent with overarching frameworks that allow for predictions, from multiple sources, to influence perception and guide learning (Mumford, 1992; Rao & Ballard, 1999; Friston, 2008; Friston, 2010; Alink et al., 2010). A recent computational model of speech perception by Kleinschmidt & Jaeger (2015) applies a Bayesian approach to cue integration that weights different sources of information, according to their reliability, and uses recent experience to update predictions about the incoming acoustic speech signal. Although this model focuses on visual and acoustic cue integration, the general principle leads to a straightforward hypothesis, namely that any contextual sources of information that influences perception (e. g., effects of sentence meaning) may also lead to adaptive changes in perception. Models such as these can be used to generate and test predictions about the potential influence of multiple factors on adaptive speech perception.

With respect to the underlying neural computations that support adaptation, there is still debate. The traditional models of speech perception (TRACE and MERGE) were modified from their original instantiation to implement adaptive changes in perception. A Hebbian learning mechanism was incorporated in TRACE (Hebb-TRACE) (Mirman, McClelland & Holt, 2006), and interactions between different levels that are dedicated for learning and guide adaptive plasticity (the learning mechanism is not specified) were incorporated in MERGE (Norris, McQueen & Cutler, 2003). However, these traditional models do not extend beyond the lexical level and are not implemented in such a way that captures the rapid timecourse of adaptation.

Models from other perceptual domains can continue to provide insight for models of speech perception. For example, the reverse hierarchy model of visual perceptual learning (e. g., Ahissar, 2004) suggests that different sources of predictive information originate from different brain regions and that learning influences activity in a reverse hierarchy affecting intermediate levels of processing. Alternatively, there may be other non-hierarchical functional structures that offer other plausible solutions.

Current computational models that link flexibility and plasticity have also incorporated some neuro-anatomical constraints such as Adaptive Resonance Theory and Predictive Coding (Grossberg et al., 2013; Sohoglu & Davis, 2016). The hierarchical Bayesian predictive coding computational model by Sohoglu & Davis (2016) consists of two layers – frontal cortex and superior temporal cortex (STG). Importantly, they relate the model's predictions to changes in brain activity. Specifically, they used EEG to examine the effect of context (matching vs. mismatching orthographic prime) on different levels of a degraded speech signal; they showed decreases in activity in perceptual areas (STG in their model) for both effects of predictive context and perceptual learning. The model accounts for both flexible and adaptive processes with a common computation that minimizes the prediction error (also see more recent paper by Blank & Davis, 2016).

Clearly the two processes are related; both Davis and Sohoglu (2016) and Guediche, Fiez & Holt (2016) showed significant correlations between individual performance on word recognition during exposure to degraded speech stimuli, and measures of perceptual learning. However, even if a common mathematical computation can account for the two phenomena (e. g., Sohoglu & Davis, 2016; Blank & Davis, 2016), the underlying neural and biological mechanisms that support flexible vs. adaptive processes may differ. We proposed that the cerebellum contributes to adaptive changes in perception by using prediction errors, potentially at multiple levels of processing to guide learning (for alternative cerebellar role, see Lametti et al., 2016).

3.2.1 Mechanism?

Studies at the cellular level suggest that experience-dependent plasticity may invoke additional neurobiological changes that alter subsequent feedforward processing of sensory input. For example, in other domains, supervised learning is thought to result from long-term depression of parallel fiber-purkinje cell synapses (and long-term potentiation of parallel fiber and interneuron synapses) in the cerebellum (De Zeeuw et al., 1998; Ito, 2002; Jorntell, 2016; Hirano, Yamazaki & Nakamura, 2016), implicating γ-aminobutyric acid (GABA-ergic) dependent plasticity (e. g., Lee et al., 2015). Phosphorylation mechanisms that are dependent on sustained protein kinase activation may regulate AMPA receptor internalization and long-term depression in the cerebellum, as suggested recent neurobiological computational (Gallimore et al., 2016). If these mechanisms apply to other domains, including speech perception, adapting perception to distorted sensory input, may involve neurobiological changes that occur over time and thus do not contribute to immediate effects of context on flexibility in perception.

Ultimately, the challenge for future research on speech perception will be to develop models that incorporate additional known and newly discovered neuro-anatomical and neurobiological constraints. Clark (2013) revisited the possibility that the processing of predictions and the processing of incoming sensory input may occur in the same brain areas, but in distinct cortical layers. However, little is known about how neurons in different cortical layers contribute to flexible and adaptive perception. There is at least one study in barrel cortex sensory processing that showed changes in neural responses to different types of sensory stimuli differ for layers 4–6 compared to layers 1–3 (Ramirez et al., 2014). Indeed, more research at the meso-scale is needed (Badre, Frank & Moore, 2015) to bridge the gap between our understanding at a cellular and the systems level mechanisms involved in flexible and adaptive changes in behavior. Doing so may lead to an eventual unifying framework that accounts for both flexibility and adaptive short-term plasticity in speech perception with detailed neurobiological mechanisms.

3.2.2 Interaction with cognitive factors

Flexibility and adaptive plasticity interact with other cognitive processes. The relationship between verbal working memory and context effects has been examined (Zekveld et al., 2011; Zekveld et al., 2012), showing correlations between verbal working memory measures and semantic facilitation of perception (and with activation in frontal areas involved in verbal working memory). Mattys & Wiget (2011) showed that the lexical effect is modulated by cognitive load. Specifically, increased cognitive load led to increased reliance on the lexical context. Recent work provides compelling evidence that lexically-mediated adaptive plasticity also requires attention (Samuel, 2016). Interactions between perception and cognitive processes also extend to recognition memory. Theodore, Blumstein & Luthra (2015) showed that attention to specific features modulates word recognition accuracy; attention to speaker during encoding showed a talker specific word recognition advantage, whereas attention to lexical information instead did not facilitate talker specific word recognition. Thus, it is important to keep in mind that perceptual processing is heavily intertwined with many cognitive processes. Talsma & Durk (2015) went so far as to suggest that attentional accounts may provide a unifying framework for Predictive coding and integration mechanisms.

Cognitive processes also impact adaptive plasticity. In an fMRI study, Eisner et al. (2010) showed that activity in prefrontal cortex was correlated with both individual phonological working memory and intelligibility scores for spectrally shifted speech. Other cognitive factors such as attention also play a role as in the case of phoneme restoration (Samuel & Ressler, 1986), or in perception of speech in noise (Moradi et al., 2014). Kraljic, Samuel & Brennan (2008) even showed that adaptive changes in perception that normally occur in response to a speaker's unusual pronunciations can be abolished when listeners are provided with information that the source of the distortion is not caused by the speaker (e. g., a pen in a speaker's mouth). These types of interactions will have to be investigated further and incorporated in subsequent models of speech perception (Mattys et al., 2012).

3.2.3 Generalization

All of the previous sections point to a highly dynamic, flexible, and adaptive speech perception system. Yet, speech perception is not always flexible nor is it always plastic. Rather, the adaptive properties of speech perception operate within a highly stable system. An interesting area of research on the generalizability of the flexibility and plasticity of speech perception points to potential contributing factors that affect this equilibrium. Adaptive changes in perception sometimes generalize across different categories, speakers, and languages, and sometimes do not (Kraljic & Samuel, 2006; Sumner, 2011; Reinisch & Holt, 2014; Reinisch, Weber & Mitterer, 2013; Dahan, Drucker & Scarborough, 2008). One study showed that exposure to multiple speakers rather than one speaker promoted generalization across different speakers (e. g., Banai & Lavner, 2012). Furthermore, changes in perception have been shown for some acoustic distortions but not for others. Exposure to changes in the dimensional relationship between two properties of speech leads to changes in perception (dimension-based statistical learning) but only if the manipulation did not violate typical learned long-term relationship regularity between the two dimensions (e. g., Idemaru & Holt, 2011). Recent examples show that changes in perception are sensitive to specific languages (Schertz, 2014), individual biases (Schertz, Lotto & Warner, 2015), and to linguistic experience (Cooper, 2016). What is the basis for these differences?

Many open questions still remain. If multiple equally reliable sources of information provide conflicting predictions about the speech signal, will the weighting of different sources of information always be probabilistic? How do flexible and adaptive processes in speech perception contend with a bilingual system with multiple co-existing consistent or conflicting maps (e. g., acoustic-phonological, pre-lexical-lexical, etc.)? Answers to some of these questions may depend, in part, on the nature of representations of speech categories.

Therefore, characterizing the acoustic parameters that contribute to different sound categories (*for discussion see* Blumstein and Jongman & McMurray in this volume) and understanding the level of specification (Eulitz & Lahiri, 2004) is crucial to this work. New developments in functional neuroimaging methods that establish the underlying relationship between properties of the acoustic speech signal and brain activity, (e. g., Lutti et al., 2014; Leonard & Chang, 2014; Leonard et al., 2016), and reveal the nature of contextual linguistic influences at a individual neuron level (Cibelli et al., 2015) will provide further constrain models of speech perception. In sum, cognitive neuroscience research on speech perception has the potential to help advance our knowledge of linguistic processes and the mechanisms that allow stability, flexibility, and adaptive plasticity by making links across topics and methodologies. Together, the synthesis of different areas of research will help to elucidate the underlying mechanisms that maintain equilibrium between stability and plasticity in speech perception.

Acknolwedgments: This research would not have been possible without the support of Dr. Fiez, Holt, Blumstein, and their respective labs. The experiments discussed in Section 1 of this chapter were funded by RO1 DC 006220 to Blumstein and a 2T32MH09118-19 NIH postdoctoral training grant. The experiments discussed in Section 2 of this chapter were funded by RO1 DC 004674 to Holt, RO1MH59256 and NSF 1125719 to Fiez and a Kenneth P. Dietrich School of Arts and Sciences, and Andrew Mellon Predoctoral Fellowship.

References

Adank, P. & Devlin, J. T. (2010). On-line plasticity in spoken sentence comprehension: Adapting to time-compressed speech. *Neuroimage 49*(1). 1124–1132.
Adank, P. & Janse, E. (2009). Perceptual learning of time-compressed and natural fast speech. *Journal of the Acoustical Society of America 126*(5). 2649–2659.
Ahissar, M. & Shaul, H. (2004). The reverse hierarchy theory of visual perceptual learning. *Trends in cognitive sciences 8*(10). 457–464.
Albus, J. S. (1971). "A theory of cerebellar function." *Mathematical Biosciences 10*(1). 25–61.
Alink, A., Schwiedrzik, C. M., Kohler, A., Singer, W. & Muckli, L. (2010). Stimulus predictability reduces responses in primary visual cortex. *Journal of Neuroscience 30*(8). 2960–2966.
Allen, G., McColl, R., Barnard, H., Ringe, W. K., Fleckenstein, J. & Cullum, C. M. (2005). Magnetic resonance imaging of cerebellar–prefrontal and cerebellar–parietal functional connectivity. *Neuroimage 28*(1). 39–48.
Argyropoulos, G. P. D. (2015). "The cerebellum, internal models and prediction in 'non-motor' aspects of language: A critical review." *Brain and language*.
Aydelott, J., Dick, F. & Mills, D. L. (2006). "Effects of acoustic distortion and semantic context on event-related potentials to spoken words." *Psychophysiology 43*(5). 454–464.
Badre, D., Frank, M. J. & Moore, C. I. (2015). "Interactionist Neuroscience." *Neuron 88*(5). 855–860.
Banai, K. & Lavner, Y. (2012). Perceptual learning of time-compressed speech: More than rapid adaptation. *PLoS One 7*(10). e47099.
Bastos, A. M., Usrey, W. M., Adams, R. A., Mangun, G. R., Fries, P. & Friston, K. J. (2012). Canonical microcircuits for predictive coding. *Neuron 76*(4). 695–711.
Bertelson, P., Vroomen, J. & de Gelder, B. (2003). Visual recalibration of auditory speech identification: A McGurk aftereffect. *Psychological Science 14*(6). 592–597.

Binder, J. R., Liebenthal, E., Possing, E. T., Medler, D. A. & Ward, D. B. (2004). Neural correlates of sensory and decision processes in auditory object identification. *Nature Neuroscience* 7(3). 295–301.

Binder, J. R., Desai, R. H., Graves, W. W. & Conant, L. L. (2009). "Where is the semantic system? A critical review and meta-analysis of 120 functional neuroimaging studies." *Cerebral Cortex* 19(12). 2767–2796.

Blank, H. & Davis, M. H. (2016). "Prediction Errors but Not Sharpened Signals Simulate Multi-voxel fMRI Patterns during Speech Perception." *PLoS Biology* 14(11). e1002577.

Borsky, S., Tuller, B. & Shapiro, L. P. (1998). "How to milk a coat:" The effects of semantic and acoustic information on phoneme categorization. *Journal of the Acoustical Society of America 103*. 2670–2676.

Bradlow, A. R. & Bent, T. (2008). Perceptual adaptation to non-native speech. *Cognition* (106). 2.

Bradlow, A. R. & Alexander, J. A. (2007). Semantic and phonetic enhancements for speech-in-noise recognition by native and non-native listeners. *Journal of the Acoustical Society of America 121*(4). 2339–2349.

Buckner, R. L., Krienan, F. M., Castellanos, A., Diaz, J. C. & Yeo, B. T. T. (2011). "The organization of the human striatum estimated by intrinsic functional connectivity." *Journal of Neurophysiology 106*(5). 2322–2345.

Burton, M. & Blumstein, S. E. (1995). Lexical effects on phonetic categorization: The role of stimulus naturalness and stimulus quality. *Journal of Experiment Psychology: Human Perception and Performance 21*. 1230–1235.

Callan, D., Callan, A. & Jones, J. A. (2014). Speech motor brain regions are differentially recruited during perception of native and foreign-accented phonemes for first and second language listeners. *Frontiers in neuroscience 8*.

Cibelli, E. S., Leonard, M. K., Johnson, K. & Chang, E. F. (2015). "The influence of lexical statistics on temporal lobe cortical dynamics during spoken word listening." *Brain and language. 147*, 66–75.

Clark, A. (2013). "Whatever next? Predictive brains, situated agents, and the future of cognitive science." *Behavioral and Brain Sciences 36*(3). 181–204.

Clos, M., Langner, R., Meyer, M., Oechslin, M. S., Zilles, K. & Eickhoff, S. B. (2012). Effects of prior information decoding degraded speech: An fmri study. *Human Brain Mapping 35*(1). 61–74.

Connine, C. M. (1987). Constraints on interactive processes in auditory word recognition: The role of sentence context. *Journal of Memory and language*. 527–538.

Cooper, A. (2016). *Perceptual Learning of Accented Speech by First and Second Language Listeners* (Doctoral dissertation, Northwestern University).

Dahan, D., Drucker, S. J. & Scarborough, R. A. (2008). Talker adaptation in speech perception: Adjusting the signal or the representation?.". *Cognition 108*(3). 710–718.

Davis, M. H., Ford, M. A., Kherif, F. & Johnsrude, I. S. (2011). Does semantic context benefit speech understanding through "top-down" processes? Evidence from time-resolved sparse fmri. *Journal of Cognitive Neuroscience 23*(12). 3914–3932.

Davis, M. H. & Johnsrude, I. S. (2003). Hierarchical processing in spoken language comprehension. *Journal of Neuroscience 23*(8). 3423–3431.

Desmond, J. E. & Fiez, J. A. (1998). Neuroimaging studies of the cerebellum: Language, learning and memory. *Trends in Cognitive Sciences 2*(9). 355–358.

De Zeeuw, C. I., Hansel, C., Bian, F., Koekkoek, S. K. E., Van Alphen, A. M., Linden, D. J. & Oberdick, J. (1998). "Expression of a protein kinase C inhibitor in Purkinje cells blocks cerebellar LTD and adaptation of the vestibulo-ocular reflex." *Neuron 20*(3). 495–508.

Doya, K. (2000). Complementary roles of basal ganglia and cerebellum in learning and motor control. *Current Opinion in Neurobiology 10*. 732–739.

Eisner, F., McGettigan, C., Faulkner, A., Rosen, S. & Scott, S. K. (2010). Inferior frontal gyrus activation predicts individual differences in perceptual learning of cochlear-implant simulations. *Journal of Neuroscience 30*(21). 7179–7186.

Erb, J., Henry, M. J., Eisner, F. & Obleser, J. (2013). The brain dynamics of rapid perceptual adaptation to adverse listening conditions. *Journal of Neuroscience 33*(26). 10688–10697.

Eulitz, C. & Lahiri, A. (2004). Neurobiological evidence for abstract phonological representations in the mental lexical during speech recognition. *Journal of Cognitive Neuroscience 16*(5). 577–583.

Farmer, T. A., Brown, M. & Tanenhaus, M. K. (2013). "Prediction, explanation, and the role of generative models in language processing." *Behavioral and Brain Sciences 36*(03). 211–212.

Fiez, J. A., Raichle, M. E., Balota, D. A., Tallal, P. & Petersen, S. E. (1996). "PET activation of posterior temporal regions during auditory word presentation and verb generation." *Cerebral cortex 6*(1). 1–10.

Friston, K. (2008). Hierarchical models in the brain. *PLos Computational Biology 4*(11). e1000211.

Friston, K. (2010). The free-energy principle: A unified brain theory? *Nature Neuroscience Reviews 11*(2). 127–138.

Fu, Q.-J. & Galvin III, J. J. (2003). The effects of short-term training for spectrally mismatched noise-band speech. *Journal of the Acoustical Society of America 113*(2). 1065–1072.

Gagnepain, P., Henson, R. N. & Davis, M. H. (2012). Temporal predictive codes for spoken words in auditory cortex. *Current Biology 22*. 615–621.

Gallimore, A. R., Aricescu, A. R., Yuzaki, M. & Calinescu, R. (2016). "A Computational Model for the AMPA Receptor Phosphorylation Master Switch Regulating Cerebellar Long-Term Depression." *PLoS Computational Biology 12*(1). e1004664.

Gambi, C., Cop, U. & Pickering, M. J. (2015). "How do speakers coordinate? Evidence for prediction in a joint word-replacement task." *Cortex 68*. 111–128.

Ganong, W. F. (1980). Phonetic categorization in auditory word perception. *Journal of Experimental Psychology: Human Perception and Performance 6*(1). 110–125.

Gaskell, M. G. & Marslen-Wilson, W. D. (1997). Integrating form and meaning: A distributed model of speech perception. *Language and cognitive Processes 12*(5–6) 613–656.

Golestani, N., Hervais-Adelman, A., Obleser, J. & Scott, S. K. (2013). Semantic versus perceptual interactions in neural processing of speech-in-noise. *Neuroimage 79*. 52–61.

Golfinopoulos, E., Tourville, J. A., Bohland, J. W., Ghosh, S. S., Nieto-Castanon, A. & Guenther, F. H. (2011). FMRI investigation of unexpected somatosensory feedback perturbation during speech. *Neuroimage 55*(3). 1324–1338.

Gow, D. W., Segawa, J. A., Ahlfors, S. P. & Lin, F.-H. (2008). Lexical influences on speech perception: A granger causality analysis of MEG and EEG source estimates. *Neuroimage 43*(3). 614–623.

Gross, J., Hoogenboom, N., Thut, G., Schyns, P., Panzeri, S., Belin, P. & Garrod, S. (2013). "Speech rhythms and multiplexed oscillatory sensory coding in the human brain." *PLoS Biol 11*(12). e1001752.

Grossberg, S. (2013). Adaptive Resonance Theory: How a brain learns to consciously attend, learn, and recognize a changing world. *Neural Networks 37*. 1–47.

Guediche, S., Blumstein, S. E., Fiez, J. A. & Holt, L. L. (2014). Speech perception under adverse conditions: Insights from behavioral, computational, and neuroscience research. *Frontiers in Systems Neuroscience 7*. 126.

Guediche, S., Fiez, J. A. & Holt, L. L. (2016). Incremental exposure to a speech distortion facilitates adaptive plasticity in the absence of external information, *Journal of Experimental Psychology: Human Perception and Performance 42*(7), 1048–59.

Guediche, S., Yuli Zhu, Y., Minicucci, M. & Blumstein, S. E. Written sentence context effects on acoustic phonetic perception: fMRI reveals cross-modal semantic/acoustic-phonetic interactions, *submitted*.

Guediche, S., Holt, L. L., Laurent, P., Lim, S.-J. & Fiez, J. A. (2015). Evidence for cerebellar contributions to adaptive plasticity in speech perception. *Cerebral Cortex 7*(25). 1867–1877.

Guediche, S., Reilly, M., Santiago, C., Laurent, P. & Blumstein, S. E. (2016). An fMRI study investigating effects of conceptually related sentences on the perception of degraded speech, *Cortex 79*. 57–74.

Guediche, S., Salvata, C. & Blumstein, S. E. (2013). Temporal cortex reflects effects of sentence context on phonetic processing. *Journal of Cognitive Neuroscience 25*(5). 706–718.

Hartwigsen, G., Golombek, T. & Obleser, J. (2015). Repetitive transcranial magnetic stimulation over left angular gyrus modulates the predictability gain in degraded speech comprehension. *Cortex 68*. 100–110.

Hickok, G. (2012). The cortical organization fo speech processing: Feedback control and predictive coding the context of a dual-stream model. *Journal of Communication Science Disorders 45*(6). 393–402.

Hickok, G. (2009). The functional neuroanatomy of language. *Physics of Life Reviews 6*(3). 121–143.

Hickok, G. & Poeppel, D. (2007). The cortical organization of speech processing. *Nature Reviews Neuroscience 8*(5). 393–402.

Hickok, G. & Poeppel, D. (2004). Dorsal and ventral streams: A framework for understanding aspects of the functional anatomy of language. *Cognition 92*. 67–99.

Hirano, T., Yamazaki, Y. & Nakamura, Y. (2016). "LTD, RP, and motor learning." *The Cerebellum*. 1–3.

Horowitz-Kraus, T., Grainger, M., DiFrancesco, M., Vannest, J., Holland, S. K. & CMIND Authorship Consortium. Right is not always wrong: DTI and fMRI evidence for the reliance of reading comprehension on language-comprehension networks in the right hemisphere. *Brain imaging and behavior 9*(1). 19–31.

Holt, L. L. & Lotto, A. J. (2006). Cue weighting in auditory categorization: Implications for first and second language acquisition. *Journal of Acoustical Society of America 119*(5 Pt 1). 3059–3071.

Idemaru, K. & Holt, L. L. (2011). Word recognition reflects dimension-based statistical learning. *Journal of Experiment Psychology: Human Perception and Performance 37*. 1939–1956.

Ito, M. (2002). "The molecular organization of cerebellar long-term depression." *Nature Reviews Neuroscience 3*(11). 896–902.

Jaeger, T. F. & Victor, F. (2013). Seeking predictions from a predictive framework. *Behavioral and Brain Sciences 36*(4). 359–360.

Jörntell, H. (2016). "Cerebellar synaptic plasticity and the credit assignment problem." *The Cerebellum 15*(2): 104–111 1–8.

Kawato, M. (1999). Internal models for motor control and trajectory planning. *Current Opinion in Neurobiology 9*. 718–727.

Kelly, R. M. & Strick, P. L. (2003). Cerebellar loops with motor cortex and prefrontal cortex of a nonhuman primate. *The Journal of Neuroscience 23*(23). 8432–8444.

Kilian-Hutten, N., Valente, G., Vroomen, J. & Formisano, E. (2011). Auditory cortex encodes the perceptual interpretation of ambiguous sound. *The Journal of Neuroscience 31*(5). 1715–1720.

Kilian-Hutten, N., Vroomen, J. & Formisano, E. (2011). Brain activation during audiovisual exposure anticipates future perception of ambiguous speech. *Neuroimage 57*(4). 1601–1607.

Kleinschmidt, D. F. & Jaeger, T. F. (2015). Robust speech perception: Recognize the familiar, generalize to the similar, and adapt to the novel. *Psychological Review 122*(2).148.

Kraljic, T. & Samuel, A. G. (2006). Generalization in perceptual learning for speech. *Psychonomic Bulletin and Review 13*(2). 262–268.

Kraljic, T. & Samuel, A. G. (2005). Perceptual learning for speech: Is there a return to normal? *Cognitive Psychology 51*(2). 141–178.

Kraljic, T., Samuel, A. G. & Brennan, S. E. (2008). First impressions and last resorts how listeners adjust to speaker variability. *Psychological Science 19*(4). 332–338.

Lametti, D. R., Oostwoud Wijdenes, L., Bonaiuto, J., Bestmann, S. & Rothwell, J. C. (2016). "Cerebellar tDCS dissociates the timing of perceptual decisions from perceptual change in speech." *Journal of Neurophysiology 116*(5). 2023–2032.

Lau, E. F., Phillips, C. & Poeppel, D. (2008). A cortical network for semantics: (de)constructing the N400. *Nature Reviews Neuroscience 9*(12). 920–933.

Leech, R., Holt, L. L., Devlin, J. T. & Dick, F. (2009). Expertise with artificial nonspeech sounds recruits speech-sensitive cortical regions. *The Journal of Neuroscience 29*(16). 5234–5239.

Lee, K. Y., Kim, Y. I., Kim, S. H., Park, H. S., Park, Y. J., Ha, M. S., Jin, Y. & Kim, D. K. (2015). "Propofol effects on cerebellar long-term depression." *Neuroscience letters 609*. 18–22.

Leonard, M. K. & Chang, E. F. (2014). Dynamic speech representations in the human temporal lobe. *Trends in Cognitive Sciences 18*(9). 472–479.

Li, X., Lu, Y. & Zhao, H. (2014). "How and when predictability interacts with accentuation in temporally selective attention during speech comprehension." *Neuropsychologia 64*. 71–84.

Lim, S.-J., Fiez, J. A. & Holt, L. L. (2014). How may the basal ganglia contribute to auditory categorization and speech perception? *Frontiers in neuroscience 8*.

Lutti, A., Dick, F., Sereno, M. I. & Weiskopf, N. (2014). Using high-resolution quantitative mapping of r1 as an index of cortical myelination. *Neuroimage 93*. 176–188.

Marinkovic, K., Dhond, R. P., Dale, A. M., Glessner, M., Carr, V. & Halgren, E. (2003). Spatiotemporal dynamics of modality-specific and supramodal word processing. *Neuron 38*(3). 487–497.

Marr, D. (1969). A theory of cerebellar cortex. *Journal of Physiology 202*. 437–470.

Marslen-Wilson, W. D. (1987). Functional parallelism in spoken word-recognition. *Cognition 25*(1). 71–102.

Mattys, S. L., Davis, M. H., Bradlow, A. R. & Scott, S. K. (2012). Speech recognition in adverse conditions: A review. *Language and Cognitive Processes 277*(8). 953–978.

Mattys, S. L. & Wiget, L. (2011). Effects of cognitive load on speech recognition. *Journal of Memory & Language 65*(2). 145–160.

McClelland, J. L., Mirman, D., Bolger, B. D. J. & Khaitan, P. (2014). Interactive activation and mutual constraint satisfaction in perception and cognition. *Cognitive Science 38*(6). 1139–1189.

McClelland, J. L. & Elman, J. L. (1986). The trace model of speech perception. *Cognitive Psychology 18*(1). 1–86.

McClelland, J. L., Mirman, D. & Holt, L. L. (2006). Are there interactive processes in speech perception? *Trends in Cognitive Sciences 10*(8). 363–369.

Mirman, D., McClelland, J. L. & Holt, L. L. (2006). An interactive hebbian account of lexically guided tuning of speech perception. *Psychonomic Bulletin & Review 13*(6). 958–965.

Moradi, S., Lidestam, B., Saremi, A. & Ronnberg, J. (2014). Gated auditory speech perception: Effects of listening conditions and cognitive capacity. *Frontiers in Psychology 5.*

Moberget, T. & Ivry, R. B. (2016). Cerebellar contributions to motor control and language comprehension: searching for common computational principles. *Annals of the New York Academy of Sciences*, *1369*(1), 154–171.

Molinaro, N., Paz-Alonso, P. M., Duñabeitia, J. A. & Carreiras, M. (2015). "Combinatorial semantics strengthens angular-anterior temporal coupling." *Cortex 65*. 113–127.

Mumford, D. (1992). On the computational architecture of the neocortex. II. The role of corticocortical loops. *Biological Cybernetics 66*(3). 241–51. [arAC, TE, KF]

Myers, E. B. & Blumstein, S. E. (2008). The neural bases of the lexical effect: An fmri investigation. *Cerebral Cortex 18*(2). 278–288.

Myers, E. B. & Mesite, L. M. (2014). Neural systems underlying perceptual adjustment to nonstandard speech tokens. *Journal of memory and language 76*. 80–93.

Myers, E. B., Blumstein, S. E., Walsh, E. & Eliassen, J. (2009). Inferior frontal regions underlie the perception of phonetic category invariance. *Psychological Science 20*(7). 895–903.

Norris, D., McQueen, J. M. & Cutler, A. (2000). Merging information in speech recognition: Feedback is never necessary. *Behavioral and Brain Sciences 23*(3). 299–325.

Norris, D., McQueen, J. M. & Cutler, A. (2003). Perceptual learning in speech. *Cognitive Psychology 47*. 204–238.

Obleser, J., Wise, R. J. S., Dresner, M. A. & Scott, S. K. (2007). Functional integration across brain regions improves speech perception under adverse listening conditions. *Journal of Neuroscience 27*(9). 2283–2289.

Obleser, J. & Kotz, S. A. (2011). Multiple brain signatures of integration in the comprehension of degraded speech. *Neuroimage 55*. 713–723.

Obleser, J. & Kotz, S. A. (2010). Expectancy constraints in degraded speech modulate the language comprehension network. *Cerebral Cortex 20*(3). 633–640.

Panichello, M. F., Cheung, O. S. & Bar, M. (2013). Predictive feedback and conscious visual experience. *Frontiers in Psychology 3*. 620.

Peelle, J. E., Johnsrude, I. S. & Davis, M. H. (2010). Hierarchical processing for speech in human auditory cortex and beyond. *Frontiers in Human Neuroscience 4*. 1–3.

Peelle, J. E. (2013). Cortical responses to degraded speech are modulated by linguistic predictions. In *Proceedings of Meetings on Acoustics 19*(1). 060108. Acoustical Society of America.

Peelle, J. E., Gross, J. & Davis, M. H. (2013). "Phase-locked responses to speech in human auditory cortex are enhanced during comprehension." *Cerebral Cortex 23*(6). 1378–1387.

Petacchi, A., Laird, A. R., Fox, P. T. & Bower, J. M. (2005). Cerebellum and auditory function: An ALE meta-analysis of functional neuroimaging studies. *Human Brain Mapping 25*(1). 118–128.

Prabhakaran, R., Blumstein, S. E., Myers, E. B., Hutchison, E. & Britton, B. (2006). An event-related fmri investigation of phonological-lexical competition. *Neuropsychologia* 44(12). 2209–2221.
Preston, J. L., Molfese, P. J., Frost, S. J., Mencl, W. E., Fulbright, R. K., Hoeft, F., ... & Pugh, K. R. (2016). Print-Speech Convergence Predicts Future Reading Outcomes in Early Readers. *Psychological science* 27(1), 75–84.
Price, C. J. (2012). A review and synthesis of the first 20 years of PET and fMRI studies of heard speech, spoken language and reading. *Neuroimage*.
Ramirez, A., Pnevmatikakis, E. A., Merel, J., Paninski, L., Miller, K. D. & Bruno, R. M. (2014). "Spatiotemporal receptive fields of barrel cortex revealed by reverse correlation of synaptic input." *Nature neuroscience* 17(6). 866–875.
Rao, R. P. N. & Ballard, D. H. (1999). Predictive coding in the visual cortex: A functional interpretation of some extra-classical receptive-field effects. *Nature Neuroscience* 2(1). 79–87.
Rauschecker, J. P. (2012). Ventral and dorsal streams in the evolution of speech and language. *Frontiers in Evolutionary Neuroscience* 4(7).
Rauschecker, J. P. & Scott, S. K. (2009). Maps and streams in the auditory cortex: Nonhuman primates illuminate human speech processing. *Nature Neuroscience* 12(6). 718–724.
Rauschecker, J. P. & Tian, B. (2000). Mechanisms and streams for processing of "what" and "where" in auditory cortex. *Proceedings of the National Academy of Sciences* 97(22). 11800–11806.
Redding, G. M. (2006). Generalization of prism adaptation. *Journal of Experimental Psychology: Human Perception and Performance* 32(4). 1006–1022.
Reinisch, E. & Holt, L. L. (2014). Lexically-guided phonetic returning of foreign-accented speech and its generalization. *Journal of Experimental Psychology: Human Perception and Performance* 40(2). 539–555.
Reinisch, E., Weber, A. & Mitterer, H. (2013). Listeners retune phoneme categories across languages. *Journal of Experiment Psychology: Human Perception and Performance* 39. 75–86.
Roth, M. J., Synofzik, M. & Lindner, A. (2013). The cerebellum optimizes perceptual predictions about external sensory events. *Current Biology* 23. 930–935.
Rothermich, K. & Kotz, S. A. (2013). Predictions in speech comprehension: FMRI evidence on the meter-semantic interace. *Neuroimage* 70. 89–100.
Rueckl, J. G., Paz-Alonso, P. M., Molfese, P. J., Kuo, W. J., Bick, A., Frost, S. J., ... & Samuel, A. G. (2016). Lexical representations are malleable for about one second: Evidence for the non-automaticity of perceptual recalibration." *Cognitive Psychology* 88: 88–114.
Samuel, A. G. & Ressler, W. H. (1986). Attention within auditory word perception: Insights from the phonemic restoration illusion. *Journal of Experimental Psychology: Human Perception and Performance* 12(1). 70.
Schertz, J. L. (2014). The structure and plasticity of phonetic categories across languages and modalities.
Schertz, J., Cho, T., Lotto, A. & Warner, N. (2015). "Individual differences in phonetic cue use in production and perception of a non-native sound contrast." *Journal of phonetics* 52. 183–204.
Schwab, E. C., Nusbaum, H. C. & Pisoni, D. B. (1985). Some effects of training on the perception of synthetic speech. *Human Factors* 27(4). 395–408.
Schwartze, M. & Kotz, S. A. "Contributions of cerebellar event-based temporal processing and preparatory function to speech perception." *Brain and language* (2015).

Scott, S. K. (2012). The neurobiology of speech perception and production-can functional imaging tell us anything we did not already know? *Journal of Communication Science Disorders* 45(6). 419–425.

Shannon, R. V., Zeng, F.-G., Kamath, V., Wygonski, J. & Ekelid, M. (1995). Speech recognition with primarily temporal cues. *Science* 270(5234). 303–304.

Sokolov, A., Erb, M., Grodd, W. & Pavlova, M. (2014). Structural loop between the cerebellum and STS: Evidence from diffusion tensor imaging. *Cerebral Cortex* 24(3). 626–632.

Spratling, M. W. (2008). Reconciling predictive coding and biased competition models of cortical function. *Frontiers in Computational Neuroscience* 2: 4.

Sohoglu, E. & Davis, M. H. (2016). Perceptual learning of degraded speech by minimizing prediction error. *Proceedings of the National Academy of Sciences*, 113(12). E1747–E1756.

Stoodley, C. J. & Schmahmann, J. D. (2009). Functional topogaphy in the human cerebellum: A meta-analysis of neuroimaging studies. *Neuroimage* 44(2). 489–501.

Stoodley, C. J., Valera, E. M. & Schmahmann, J. D. (2012). Functional topography of the cerebellum for motor and cognitive tasks: An FMRI study. *Neuroimage* 59. 1560–1570.

Stoodley, C. J., MacMore, J. P., Makris, N., Sherman, J. C. & Schmahmann, J. D. (2016). "Location of lesion determines motor vs. cognitive consequences in patients with cerebellar stroke." *NeuroImage: Clinical* 12. 765–775.

Sumner, M. (2011). "The role of variation in the perception of accented speech." *Cognition* 119(1). 131–136.

Talsma, D. (2015). "Predictive coding and multisensory integration: an attentional account of the multisensory mind." *Frontiers in integrative neuroscience* 9.

Theodore, R. M., Blumstein, S. E. & Luthra, S. (2015). Attention modulates specificity effects in spoken word recognition: Challenges to the time-course hypothesis. *Attention, Perception & Psychophysics*. 1–11.

Theodore, R. M. & Miller, J. L. (2010). Characteristics of listener sensitivity to talker-specific phonetic detail. *The Journal of the Acoustical Society of AmericaI* 128(4). 2090–2099.

Toscano, J. C., McMurray, B., Dennhardt, J. & Luck, S. J. (2010). "Continuous perception and graded categorization electrophysiological evidence for a linear relationship between the acoustic signal and perceptual encoding of speech." *Psychological Science* 21(10). 1532–1540.

Tricomi, E., Delgado, M. R., McCandliss, B. D., McClelland, J. L. & Fiez, J. A. (2006). Performance feedback drives caudate activation in a phonological learning task. *Journal of Cognitive Neuroscience* 18(6). 1029–1043.

Vroomen, J. & Baart, M. (2012). Phonetic recalibration in audiovisual speech. Micah M. Murray and Mark T. Wallace (eds.), *The neural bases of multisensory processes*. Chap. 19. Boca Raton (FL): CRC Press.

Vroomen, J., van Linden, S., deGelder, B. & Bertelson, P. (2007). Visual recalibration and selective adaptation in auditory-visual speech perception: Contrasting build-up courses. *Neuropsychologia* 45(3). 572–577.

Watkins, K. E., Strafella, A. P. & Paus, T. (2003). "Seeing and hearing speech excites the motor system involved in speech production." *Neuropsychologia* 41(8). 989–994.

Wild, C. J., Davis, M. H. & Johnsrude, I. S. (2012). Human auditory cortex is sensitive to the perceived clarity of speech. *Neuroimage* 60. 1490–1502.

Wilson, S. M., Saygin, A. P., Sereno, M. I. & Iacoboni, M. (2004). "Listening to speech activates motor areas involved in speech production." *Nature Neuroscience* 7(7). 701–702.

Wolpert, D. M., Miall, R. C. & Kawato, M. (1998). Internal models in the cerebellum. *Trends in Cognitive Sciences 2*(9). 338–346.

Zekveld, A. A., Rudner, M., Johnsrude, I. S., Heslenfeld, D. J. & Ronnberg, J. (2012). Behavioral and fmri evidence that cognitive ability modulates the effect of semantic context on speech intelligibility. *Brain and Language 122*(2). 103–113.

Zekveld, A. A., Rudner, M., Johnsrude, I. S., Festen, J. M., Van Beek, J. H. M. & Rönnberg, J. (2011). The influence of semantically related and unrelated text cues on the intelligibility of sentences in noise. *32*(6). e16–e25.

Jack Ryalls and Rosalie Perkins
Foreign accent syndrome: Phonology or phonetics?

Abstract: This chapter considers at what stage of planning Foreign Accent Syndrome (FAS) takes its toll in speech production. Consideration of the scientific literature leads to the conclusion that FAS is a post-phonological process that has an effect at the stage of phonetic outputting in the speech production planning.

Foreign Accent Syndrome (FAS) is defined as a foreign sounding accent, acquired on the basis of a neurological disorder. Strictly speaking, the person has never learned a foreign language, has not visited the foreign country in question, and does not have a family history of association with that foreign country. Typically, the area of neurological damage is known, usually involving the left hemisphere in or near to speech or language areas or subcortical areas near known speech and language areas.

In 2013, we published a rather comprehensive review of the literature on FAS (Perkins & Ryalls, 2013). Miller (2015) offers a full history of FAS since its first mention in medical reports. Thus here we shall first review newer relevant references. Then we shall turn our attention to the question of whether FAS is more a reflection of impairment at the phonological or phonetic levels.

Recent studies compare the speech of FAS to more commonplace motor speech disorders such as dysarthria and apraxia of speech (AOS). Kanjee, Watter, Sévigny & Humphries (2010) examined the speech of a female patient from Southern Ontario, Canada whose accent was perceived as Atlantic Canadian following a left hemispheric stroke. Acoustic-phonetic analyses showed changes in both phonetic and prosodic speech features when compared to those of native Southern Ontario control speakers. The nature of these changes contributed to the perception of foreign rather than disordered speech. However, certain anomalies, particularly inconsistency in consonant distortions (i. e., alveolar stopping of dental fricatives), variability in vowel production, and reduced pitch variability in sentence production, led the researchers to conclude that FAS may be considered a milder form of AOS.

Jack Ryalls, Department of Communication Sciences and Disorders, University of Central Florida
Rosalie Perkins, Department of Communication Sciences and Disorders, University of Central Florida

Roy, Macoir, Martel-Sauvageau & Boudrealt (2012) consider FAS a subtype of AOS as well. They report acoustic-phonetic analyses on two French Canadians with FAS speech. Both patients were originally from Quebec but were perceived differently as Acadian French and German, respectively. Measures of vowel duration, formant frequencies, and VOT derived from phrase readings were taken. In addition, recordings of paragraph readings and spontaneous speech were used to assess suprasegmentals. When compared to matched control speakers, intonation contours and fundamental frequency ranges were relatively unremarkable. However, both patients with FAS demonstrated slowed speaking rate, simplified rhythm comprised of frequent, inappropriate pauses, and certain sound distortions (such as stopping of affricates) that likely correlate with difficulty controlling speech gestures. These problems in particular tend to fall in line with those seen in AOS. Because symptoms mimic foreign speech and are milder than those found in AOS, the authors hold the position that FAS should be considered a "mild form" or even "subtype of AOS" (p. 943).

Kuschmann, Lowit, Miller & Mennen, (2012) report one of the first detailed analyses on the intonation system of four English patients with FAS. The study aimed to differentiate between core impairments and the use of compensatory strategies to account for deviations in intonation patterns. Speech rate, pitch range and variation, and three maximum performance tests (maximum phonation duration to assess respiratory support, a loudness glide for volume control, and a pitch glide for pitch modulation, respectively) were examined during various connected speech tasks (reading passage, picture description, and monologue) and compared to those of age-, gender-, and dialect-matched controls. Results from MPTs showed that speakers with FAS had reduced breath support which contributed to a division of their utterances into shorter phrases. This also correlates with a greater number of observed pitch accents than the healthy controls.

The authors concluded that FAS speakers were not solely affected by an underlying disturbance of prosody, as suggested by some earlier studies. Rather, the patients were aware of intonational rules but were confined by physiological constraints such as breath support, coordination, and articulatory effort. Intonation changes, therefore, were viewed as compensatory mechanisms to deal with these primary speech deficits.

Sakurai, Itoh, Sai, Lee, Terao & Manen (2014) examined changes in prosody and laryngeal control in relation to underlying neurological damage of a 42 year old Japanese woman. The patient reportedly sounded Chinese or Korean following an infarct in the left motor and premotor cortices, per MRI results. An acoustic analysis involving measurements of VOT (/p, t, k/ and /b, d, g/), formant frequencies (F1 and F2 of /i, e, a, o, u/), pitch, intensity, and glottal pulsing were conducted at both 3 weeks post-onset and one year post-onset and compared to those of normal speakers. Like many published FAS cases, this patient's acoustic analyses showed both segmental and suprasegmental speech impairments. In general, there was little difference overall between VOT for voiced and voiceless stop consonants. Voiced consonants (/b, d, g/), usually produced with a negative VOT in Japanese, were in the positive range in both the acute (3 weeks post) and chronic phases (1 year post). Pitch and intensity variances were lower 3 weeks post onset and, while improved one year later, never matched that of a normal speaker. Glottal pulsing, measured on the vowel of syllables /pa, ta, ka/, were significantly reduced in the acute phase but relatively recovered after one year. Collectively, reduced pitch and intensity variability and reduced glottal pulsing suggest inconsistency in intrinsic laryngeal muscle functioning that is likely associated with damage to the patient's precentral motor cortex (Area 6), and is often observed in cases of laryngeal apraxia.

Another avenue of inquiry into FAS involves that of neuroimaging. The first functional Magnetic Resonance Imaging (fMRI) of FAS is that of Frikrikson, Ryalls, Rorden, Morgen, George & Baylis (2005). Initially this rather young gentleman demonstrated Broca-like aphasic symptoms and bucco-facial apraxia which quickly resolved. Functional Magnetic Resonance Imaging revealed that this male participant was apparently recruiting larger areas of the left cortical areas to a significantly greater degree than 14 neurologically healthy control participants in the same object-naming task. This leads us to speculate that what we see in FAS is a 'stage of recovery'. While the popular media has put the emphasis on the sudden emergence of FAS, many cases only are heard as having a foreign accent after a period of time after more obvious aphasia symptoms. These results are certainly congruent with current aphasia recovery findings that the 'best' recovery from aphasia occurs among individuals who eventually learn to 'shift' from the apparently less efficient right hemisphere activation patents to recruit undamaged areas of the left hemisphere. In this view FAS may represent a stage of recovery from a more impaired to a more or less complete recovery.

A factor that should also be considered in this recovery perspective is the preponderance of female FAS patients. Out of the 27 contributors with FAS, for Ryalls & Miller (2015), there was only a single male. Now this could be due to a very intriguing gender-based neurological difference; or it could be due to the much more neurologically mundane behavior difference that males are simply less willing to share experiences in which they could be viewed as 'vulnerable.' In any case, better understanding of the factors that predict this recovery pattern obviously holds great potential for neuro-rehabilitation in general.

In a more recent fMRI imaging study of FAS, Katz, Garst, Briggs, Cheskov, Ringe, Gopinath, Goyal & Allen (2012) partially replicated Fridriksson et al.'s orginal fMRI study of a patient with FAS (2005). These authors also found evidence of a similar 'brain reorganization for speech motor control', suggesting a compensatory effect. However, the Katz et al. study found some degree of bilateral participation of subcortical structures including the thalamus. One summary interpretation of these results is that while increased cortical activation can compensate for damaged subcortical structures (Fridriksson et al., 2005); increased subcortical activation can apparently compensate for abnormal cortical activation (Katz et al., 2012).

Tomasino, Marin, Maieron, Ius, Budai, Fabbo & Skrap (2013) have also employed fMRI in an attempt better understand FAS. Similar to Fridriksson and colleagues (2005), they also found increased cortical activation which they also interpret as a compensatory mechanism. Furthermore, they advance the hypothesis that the particular pattern of results in their patient should be viewed as a disorder of the 'feed foward' control commands thought to be important in fine motor control of speech production which they attribute to activation changes in the caudo-ventral portion of the precentral gryus.

Such studies remind us that the brain is ultimately an integrated and self-regulating network that seeks to compensate for the effects of neural structures through increased activation of others. More studies investigating neural activation after FAS promise not only to shed light on FAS specifically, but are promising in the better understanding of brain compensation and rehabilitation in general.

FAS: phonology or phonetics?

In our view, FAS represents a deficit after phonemic selection has occurred and therefore clearly a phonetic level impairment. Although from time to time there are reports of FAS which has apparently affected phoneme selection (i. e., a language level impairment) these cases may reflect the mixing of FAS impairments with more aphasic symptoms. Thus, we believe that FAS is similar to a 'pure' apraxia of speech. Indeed, many studies have viewed FAS being similar to an apraxia of speech.

Whiteside & Varley (1998) have advanced a hypothesis to characterize the particular level of processing that FAS takes its toll. But it remains to be seen whether the empirical data across a variety of languages will support this hypothesis.

Moreno-Toreres & colleagues (2013) have recently considered FAS in terms of planning (phonological) and execution (phonetics) in a detailed case study of FAS, and, based on detailed arguments, have come down squarely on the side of execution or a phonetic level impairment. They have added to the avenues of treatment for FAS and even suggested that one previously unexplored avenue of rehabilitation may involve the exploration of "enhancing cholinergic activitiy with drugs (e. g. donepezil)" (p. 512).

Gilbers, Jonkers, van der Scheer & Feiken (2013) have attempted to account for FAS changes in terms of "a larger amount of fortition (force of articulation) put in the speech of the FAS speaker". However, it appears that there are a fair amount of counter examples to this force of articulation hypothesis.

Another view commonly found in the literature is that FAS is a linguistic prosodic disturbance, not necessarily a form of apraxia (Blumstein et al., 1987; Blumstein & Kurowski, 2006). However, in other reported cases, prosody appears intact, with segmental errors contributing to the perception of foreignness (Kurowski et al., 1996; Verhoeven & Mariën, 2010). In Verhoeven and Mariën (2010), a Belgian Dutch woman had a stroke in the fronto temporal parietal region of the brain resulting in a brief period of anarthria followed by FAS and verbal apraxia. Samples of pre-recorded speech prior to the stroke were compared to recordings of conversational speech following the stroke. Acoustic analyses revealed problems mainly at the segmental level with regard to voicing, articulation, and coordination of speech. Voice quality was characterized by a creaky voice, quantified as such by jitter and shimmer measures of vowels. Many of these reported changes in voicing, place and manner of articulation contributed to the perception of a French accent, and correlated with a tense articulatory setting, including (1) devoicing of fricative sounds which could not be explained by coarticulatory effects; (2) articulatory overshoot (i. e., fricative /h/ produced as a glottal stop); (3) aleveolar /r/ produced as uvular /r/; and (4) a smaller vowel space with poor differentiation between [i] and [ɪ] compared to Dutch speaking controls. Suprasegmental errors included a slower speech rate with prolonged vowels and consonants and a more syllable-timed speech rhythm. However, compared to previous research which asserts that FAS is a prosodic disturbance (Blumstein & Kurowski, 2006), the prosodic processing of this patient, namely pitch contours, was relatively normal. Of note, in the intonation analysis, the patient did demonstrate over-usage of a "continuation contour" common in Dutch, but this was interpreted by the researchers as an adaptation of a slow speaker to indicate that her speaking turn is not over.

Another attempt to characterize the underlying pattern in the speech of those with FAS comes from studies which have compared the speech of individuals with FAS with speech patterns after the speaker has regained their former speech patterns (Perkins & Ryalls, 2013). In three such cases there was a clear and consistent pattern of backing of posterior vowels, and compression of vowel height. A preliminary explanation of this observation is that there are less touch receptors at the back at the tongue than at the tongue tip. Consequently, it appears that FAS interrupts the proprioceptive processes for the back of the tongue to a greater degree than for the tip of the tongue. Admittedly this casts FAS as more of a motor-speech disorder than the linguistically based disorder of typical interpretations. In other words, in this view FAS may be closer to a dysarthria or an apraxia of speech than an aphasia. This observation again fits in with a view that FAS is more a phonetic level impairment and not phonological in nature.

References

Blumstein, S. E., Alexander, M. P., Ryalls, J. H., Katz, W. & Dworetzky, B. (1987). On the nature of the foreign accent syndrome: A case study. *Brain and Language*, *31*, 215–244.
Blumstein, S. E., Kurowski, K. (2006). The Foreign Accent Syndrome: A perspective. *Journal of Neurolinguistics*, *19*(5), 346–355.
Fridriksson, J., Ryalls, J., Rorden, C., Morgan, P., George, M. & Baylis, G. (2005). Brain damage and cortical compensation in Foreign Accent Syndrome, *Neurocase*, *11*, 1–6.
Gilbers, D., Jonkers, R., van des Scheer, F. & Feiken, J. (2013). On the force of articulation in foreign accent syndrome. *Phonetics in Europe*, 11–33.
Katz, W., Garst, D., Briggs, R., Cheshkov, S., Ringe, W., Gopinath K., Goyal, A. & Allen, G. (2012). Neural bases of the foreign accent syndrome: A functional magnetic resonance imaging case study. *Neurocase*, *18* (3), 199–211.
Kanjee, R., Watter, S., Sévigny, A. & Humphreys, K. R. (2010). A case of foreign accent syndrome: Acoustic analyses and an empirical test of accent perception. *Journal of Neurolinguistics*, *23*(6), 580–598.
Kurowski, K. M., Blumstein, S. E. & Alexander, M. (1996). The Foreign Accent Syndrome: A reconsideration. *Brain and Language*, *54*, 1–25.
Kuschmann, A., Lowit, A., Miller, N. & Mennen, I. (2012). Intonation in neurogenic foreign accent syndrome. *Journal of Communication Disorders*,*45*(1), 1–11.
Millller, N. (2015). All about Foreign Accent Syndrome. In J. Ryalls & N. Miller (Eds). *Foreign Accent Syndromes: The Stories People Have to Tell*, Psychology Press, London, U.K.
Moreno-Torres, I., Berthier, M., del Mar Cid, M., Green, C., Guttierez, A., Garcia- Casares, N., Walsh, S. Anarozidiz, A., Sidorova, J., Davila, G. & Carnero-Pardo, C. (2013). Foreign accent syndrome: A multimodel evaluation in the search of neuroscience-driven trreatments. Neuropsychologia, *51*: 520–537.
Perkins, R. & Ryalls, J. Vowels. (2013). In Foreign Accent Syndrome. In M. Ball & F. Gibbons (Eds.) *Handbook of Vowels and Vowel Disorders* Routledge Press. New York, N.Y. and London, U.K.
Roy, J. P., Macoir, J., Martel-Sauvageau, V. & Boudreault, C. A. (2012). Two French- speaking cases of foreign accent syndrome: an acoustic-phonetic analysis. *Clinical Linguistics & Phonetics*, *26*(11–12), 934–945.
Ryalls, J. & Miller, N. (2015) (Eds.) *Foreign Accent Syndromes: The Stories People Have to Tell*, Psychology Press, London, U.K.
Sakurai, Y., Itoh, K., Sai, K., Lee, S., Abe, S., Terao, Y. & Mannen, T. (2014). Impaired laryngeal voice production in a patient with foreign accent syndrome. *Neurocase*, 1–10.
Tomasino, B., Marin, D., Maieron, M, Ius, T., Budai, R, Fabbro, F. & Skrap, M. (2013). Foreign accent syndrome: A multimodal mapping study. *Cortex*, *49*(1), 18–39.
Verhoeven, J. & Mariën, P. (2010). Neurogenic foreign accent syndrome: Articulatory setting, segments and prosody in a Dutch speaker. *Journal of Neurolinguistics*, *23*(6), 599–614.
Whiteside, S. & Varley, R. (1998). A reconceptualization of apraxia of speech: Asynthesis of evidence. *Cortex*, *34*, 221–231.

Joan A. Sereno
How category learning occurs in adults and children

Abstract: A central issue in the field of speech perception involves phonetic category formation. The present chapter examines speech category learning in order to understand how linguistic categories develop. One productive approach has been to examine how second language categories are learned, with recent research showing that the adult perceptual system is more plastic than previously thought. The present chapter extends this research on the learning of second language contrasts by investigating *how* this learning occurs. Little is known about the acquisition pattern itself, that is, the time course of learning. Is the learning of a new language contrast a slow gradual process or does learning exhibit spurts of rapid growth punctuated by periods of little change? This proposed chapter also examines age differences in the acquisition patterns, addressing whether acquisition is faster and/or qualitatively different in adults as compared to children. The present chapter thus provides a view of the acquisition of novel language contrasts by adults and children, contributing to understanding how listeners are able to learn new phonetic categories and clarifying the temporal constraints in learning these new phonetic contrasts.

1 Introduction

The formation of linguistic categories is a necessary step in language learning. Recent research has shown that the adult perceptual system may be more plastic than previously thought in acquiring new linguistic contrasts. The present chapter extends this research on the learning of language contrasts by examining age differences to determine whether learning of second language contrasts differs for adults versus children. Are there significant age differences in the acquisition of novel second language contrasts? In addition, most of the second language learning research has not scrutinized the time course of the learning process. By observing the learning that occurs during the process of acquisition, a clearer image of precise behavioral consequences of learning is possible, understanding not only what is learned but also how it is learned. What is the shape

---

Joan A. Sereno, Department of Linguistics, University of Kansas

DOI 10.1515/9783110422658-010

of the learning curve for the novel linguistic contrasts? The aim of this chapter therefore is to investigate how novel second language categories develop, comparing adults and children.

2 Adult language learning

While children's learning abilities are often unquestioned, adults are also capable of learning throughout their lifetime. Studies indicate that cortical representations may be continuously shaped throughout life (Van Turennout, Ellmore & Martin, 2000). For language, research has concentrated on expanding adult second language learners' ability to perceive and produce non-native contrasts at any age (Strange, 1995; Flege, 1999). These studies are based on the assumption that the perceptual system of adults can be modified, with the goal of helping listeners create new phonetic categories that are usable in various phonetic contexts and can be retained in long-term memory.

Language training studies

The notion that modification of perceptual representations is possible formed the basis for the early auditory training studies that attempted to alter or create phonetic categories. The initial focus of these experiments was the nature of the training itself: what types of stimuli were presented to the learners, who produced these stimuli, and what was the linguistic context of the presented utterances? The goal of these initial experiments was to identify the training procedures that were necessary to modify learners' perceptual representations.

An early attempt was made to train American listeners, accustomed to distinguishing only voiced and voiceless aspirated stops, to recognize a three-way (voiced, voiceless unaspirated, voiceless aspirated) voice onset time (VOT) distinction (Pisoni, Aslin, Perey & Hennessy, 1982; McClaskey, Pisoni & Carrell, 1983). These studies were closely followed by training studies examining two other phonetic contrasts. Jamieson and Morosan (1986, 1989) trained French listeners to identify the English /θ/-/ð/ contrast and Strange and Dittmann (1984) trained Japanese listeners to identify the English /ɪ/-/l/ contrast. Most of the recent training studies concentrate on the /ɪ/-/l/ distinction (Logan, Lively & Pisoni, 1991; Logan, Lively & Pisoni, 1993; Lively, Pisoni, Yamada, Tohkura & Yamada, 1994; Bradlow, Pisoni, Yamada & Tohkura, 1997). The major question addressed by these studies was how compliant learning is to perceptual training.

Interestingly, the early studies showed little, if any, improvement in perceptual accuracy. Strange and Dittmann employed discrimination training (three week duration) using synthetic stimuli in one phonetic environment. They reported no significant effect of training. Later studies, however, did show an effect of training using a similar training time frame. Jamieson and Morosan (1986), for example, reported that French trainees' identification of natural stimuli (containing /θ/ or /ð/) improved from pretest (68 % correct) to posttest (79 % correct) by 11 %. Studies of Japanese listeners' identification of English /ɹ/ and /l/ showed significant increases of 8 %, from pretest (78 %) to posttest (86 %) (Logan et al., 1991). Similarly, there was a 16 % increase (from 65 % to 81 %) in Japanese trainees' /ɹ-l/ identification accuracy in Bradlow et al. (1997). More recently, similar gains have been reported for the identification of Spanish /ɾ/ and /r/ by American learners of Spanish (Herd, Jongman & Sereno, 2013).

These later studies concluded that specific types of training can instill formation of a robust phonemic category. Logan et al. (1991) demonstrated clearly that a high-variability training paradigm encouraged the long-term modification of listeners' phonetic perception. High-variability in the training paradigm meant that natural stimuli were produced by various speakers in various contexts. Studies have shown this type of auditory training to be quite effective in the identification of non-native segmental contrasts.

Mandarin tone training

Our research (Wang, Spence, Jongman & Sereno, 1999; Wang, Jongman & Sereno, 2001) has examined auditory training at the suprasegmental level. In a series of experiments, we investigated how well American listeners could be trained to identify Mandarin tones. Mandarin phonemically distinguishes 4 tones: a high level pitch (Tone 1); a high rising pitch (Tone 2); a low dipping pitch (Tone 3); and a high falling pitch (Tone 4) (Chao, 1948). These tones differ in fundamental frequency and duration (see Figure 1).

Wang, Spence, Jongman & Sereno (1999) used a high-variability training paradigm to train American listeners to identify Mandarin tones. Eight American learners of Mandarin were trained over two weeks to identify the four Mandarin tones produced by 2 male and 2 female native speakers in a variety of phonetic contexts (natural words). Performance was assessed by comparing pre-test and post-test scores. The results revealed a significant 21 % improvement in tone identification for trainees compared to a matched, untrained control group. This improvement, importantly, generalized to new stimuli and to new speakers. In addition, the improvement in tone identification was retained six months after training. Non-native learners' identification of suprasegmental linguistic contrasts can also be substantially improved with brief perceptual training.

These changes in perceptual identification ability reflecting increases in language proficiency are accompanied by modifications at the cortical level as well. Wang, Sereno, Jongman and Hirsch (2003) employed functional magnetic resonance imaging (fMRI) to investigate the cortical effects of this second language training. Although cortical activation was consistently observed at pre-test and at post-test, following training there was greater activation in Wernicke's area in Brodmann's Area 22 and an expansion of activation in Brodmann's Area 42 in the left hemisphere superior temporal gyrus. These imaging data document cortical changes, specifically an enlargement of cortical representations and recruitment of additional brain regions, concomitant with language learning.

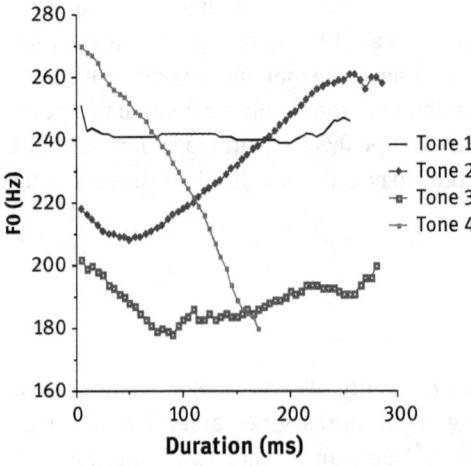

Figure 1: F0 contours for each of the four Mandarin Chinese tones for the segmental context *ma* spoken in isolation by a female speaker.

In addition, using the high variability training procedure, knowledge gained during perceptual learning of novel linguistic contrasts has also been shown to transfer to the production domain, resulting in not only more precise acoustic targets for the non-native productions (Wang, Jongman & Sereno, 2003) but also more accurate native speaker judgments of these utterances (Bradlow, Pisoni, Yamada & Tohkura, 1997; Wang, Jongman & Sereno, 2003).

These high variability training experiments clearly demonstrate that within a two-to-four week period (most of the training studies use this time frame), there is significant improvement in both perceptual and production accuracy for novel second language sounds as well as a concomitant modification of cortical representations. New phonetic categories can be learned by adults.

3 Age and learning

In considering language learning processes, arguments about the existence of a critical period often arise (Birdsong, 1999). The critical period hypothesis states that cerebral lateralization, completed by puberty, is accompanied by the loss of neurological plasticity, resulting in a reduction in language learning abilities (Lenneberg, 1967). Much of the evidence for the critical period hypothesis has come from research in first language acquisition, often examining language learning abilities following neurological damage.

Some research in second language (L2) acquisition also supports the critical period hypothesis, with adults often being inferior to children in the ability to perceive and produce foreign speech sounds. This diminution of speech learning ability at puberty predicts a concrete relationship between a learner's age and the potential for success in second language acquisition. For proponents of the critical period, the perceptual system of adults may be modified but learning is qualitatively different than that which occurs in children.

One of the most-cited studies that address the age issue in second language acquisition is a study by Snow and Hoefnagel-Höhle (1978). This report investigated naturalistic acquisition of Dutch by English speakers. Three groups were contrasted: 8–10 year old children, 12–15 year old adolescents, and adults. Over a ten-month period, learners' proficiency was measured. In most of the pronunciation, morphology and syntax measures, adults actually outperformed children initially. However, differences between adults and children at the end of the ten-month period were minimal, with children showing gains over time. Krashen, Long, and Scarcella (1979) reviewed much of the research addressing the age issue. They concluded that adult learners have an initial advantage where rate of learning is concerned. However, they will eventually be overtaken by child learners, who are more likely to reach higher levels of attainment.

While many studies have shown that individuals who learn a second language at an early age usually outperform their older counterparts, a significant difference between these groups is their prior linguistic background, with older learners more likely to have a fully developed linguistic system in place. This topic has been systematically studied with regard to the prominence of an "accent" in second language learning and explained on phonological grounds (e.g., Flege, 1992, 1995; Best, 1994, 1995). This alternative account to the critical period hypothesis argues that age effects can result from the interaction of two phonetic systems. In contrast to children, adults perceive and produce second language sounds with reference to linguistic categories of a highly entrenched native language system. The influence of the adult's first language system is largely responsible for the foreign accent. Interestingly, under this phonological claim, an adult's ability to master second language sounds depends on the degree of similarity of such sounds to familiar first language sounds. Unlike the critical period hypothesis, the phonological hypothesis does not posit a diminution of speech learning ability across the board. Research supporting a phonological account suggests that, given sufficient exposure, second language learners exhibit differential behavior. Sounds judged to have no first language (L1) counterparts are learned more readily, while similar sounds present considerably difficulty (e.g., Flege, 1987).

Critical period or phonological explanations of second language learning can be explored by directly comparing adults to children. However, it is difficult, if not impossible, to directly compare children and adults as second language learners. Young learners have more opportunities to hear and use the language, more time to devote to language learning, less social pressure to speak fluently and, generally, a more informal language learning environment. Older learners are often faced with a situation which demands much more complex language use and they also must contend with a sense of inadequacy and frustration in their lack of mastery of the language. For these reasons, it is often problematic to directly compare these groups under normal language learning situations.

The high variability training paradigm described above, however, provides an opportunity to compare adults and children with a methodology that minimizes these extraneous variables. Although adults and children differ along a number of exposure-related and motivational variables, the structured nature of the training paradigm may be able to generate data that minimize the influence of these factors in order to compare the language learning abilities of adults and children. Wang and Kuhl (2003) used the high-variability tone training paradigm developed by Wang et al. (1999) to successfully train English-speaking children aged 6, 10, and 14 years as well as adults. All groups showed comparable gains after training, ranging from 6–9 %.

While including both adults and children spanning a range of ages as training groups affords important insight into the extent to which age may affect acquisition, the comparison of adult versus child learning must also address the time course of the learning. Very little is known about the nature of the second language acquisition process. Neither the early work on segmental contrasts nor our research on suprasegmentals document the time course of the learning process. Rather, these studies usually examine the end product of training. By examining the learning that occurs during the process of acquisition, a more systematic comparison of adult versus child learning can be achieved. The main objective of the present paper was to determine whether learning of new linguistic contrasts occurs in a slow, gradual manner or whether learning is characterized by abrupt changes.

Early training studies with adults clearly showed that, although initially counterintuitive, phonetic variability in the training stimuli (in terms of contexts and speakers) was advantageous, with more variability turning out to be better for learning. This finding has significantly changed our notion of category formation. The present chapter extends this line of investigation to delineate the process of acquiring new language contrasts. Two specific issues are addressed. First, a direct comparison of adult learners versus child learners is presented. The training process itself is key to understanding the learning process. The training procedures allow for a direct comparison of adult and child learning, by controlling the nature and quality of the input. Second, the nature of the learning over time is also examined by obtaining not only pretest and posttest scores, similar to previous research, but also evaluation scores throughout training. Gains in accuracy throughout the training procedure will provide data to precisely track the time course of learning. The present chapter will thus systematically compare adult learners to child learners and assess the learning at different stages in the training regime.

4 Experiment 1: Adult second language learning

Both our research examining suprasegmental contrasts and previous research examining segmental contrasts have shown that modification of listeners' perception is possible using a high-variability training paradigm. Learners show, with a short 2–3 week training program, sizeable gains (approximately 10 %-20 %) in identification accuracy. While all these training studies show overall gains (posttest compared to pretest) in accuracy, none document the rate of acquisition. This experiment used the suprasegmental tonal contrast (4 Mandarin tones) that has been used productively in our past research. The goal was to obtain not only pretest and posttest scores, similar to previous research, but also evaluation scores throughout training. The present experiment was conducted to determine the daily gains in accuracy throughout the training procedure.

Participants

Nine adult native speakers of American English participated. All were undergraduate students at the University of Kansas who had no experience with a tone language.

Stimuli

The stimuli were all real monosyllabic Mandarin words presented in isolation. Five different talkers of Mandarin (3 male, 2 female) recorded the stimuli, one talker for the test stimuli (Pretest and Posttests) and 4 talkers for the Training stimuli.

Procedure

All testing was done in the Kansas University Phonetics and Psycholinguistics Laboratory. The procedure consisted of a Pretest, 6 Training sessions, and 6 Posttests. Stimuli were presented over headphones and listeners were instructed to indicate which of the four Mandarin tones they heard by pressing one of 4 buttons in front of them.

The Pretest consisted of 100 randomized stimuli (25 for each tone) from one talker. Participants were to respond to each stimulus. No feedback was given. Immediately after Pretest, participants undertook a training program, during which they were trained auditorily with the stimuli. Training consisted of 6 sessions using stimuli from 4 different talkers. For each session, 96 stimuli were presented, including all 4 tones and all 4 different speakers. Subjects' task was four-alternative forced-choice identification. Immediately after each response, feedback was given both visually (smiley/non-smiley face) and auditorily (voice identifying the correct tone and then repeating the stimulus). Immediately after each of the 6 Training sessions, a Posttest was given. The Posttests were identical to the Pretest, except that the stimuli were re-randomized. No feedback was given for the Posttests. Overall, then, participants took one Pretest and 6 Posttests.

The procedures used in this experiment were slightly modified from those used in the original tone training study (Wang, Spence, Jongman & Sereno, 1999), with fewer tokens during training, fewer training sessions, and more explicit feedback (auditorily and visually). The simpler procedures were developed so that the training program could also be used with children (see Experiment 2 below).

Results

The results of 9 adult participants are shown below in Figure 2. Scores represent percent correct identification of the 4 Mandarin tones for Pretest and the 6 Posttests. Overall, adult trainees improved by 17% from Pretest (57%) to the final

Posttest (74 %). The 17 % increase in accuracy scores is very similar to our earlier results showing an overall 21 % improvement (Wang, Spence, Jongman & Sereno, 1999).

The more interesting aspect here is revealed by a detailed look at the individual subjects and their scores across Posttests. We will start by comparing two participant groups. Both sets of subjects show comparable improvement, with the first group (3 participants) showing an average improvement of 25 % and the second (late) group (4 participants) showing an improvement of 21 %. The remaining participants did not show any improvement over the course of the training sessions, with 57 % accuracy at Pretest and 56 % accuracy at Posttest. A detailed look at the subjects who showed improvement during the course of the experiment reveals very different learning over time (See Figure 3).

The first group (early) shows significant improvement after the first training session (Post1), with an initial 20 % improvement. After that initial session, these participants' scores do not change very much, with the next five training sessions showing very little additional improvement (83 % to 88 %). These trainees show initial improvement and then very little change after that.

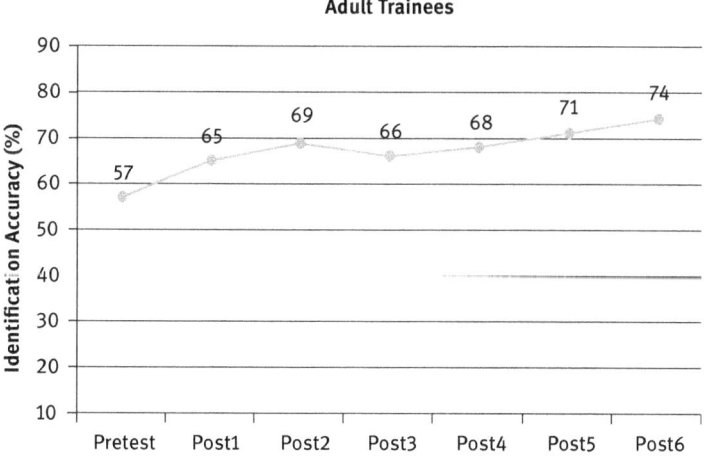

Figure 2: Adult trainees' correct identification accuracy (percent) of the four Mandarin tones for Pretest and the six Posttests.

While the second group (late) shows similar overall improvement to the first group, they show a very different pattern of learning over time. These participants show gradual improvement throughout the training regime, with larger gains in later sessions. Initial levels of accuracy (52 %) show small increases each training session, with gains averaging around 3% each session. In the final training sessions, gains average around 5% each session. For this late group, learning seems to gradually increase with increasing training, a noticeably different pattern from the early group.

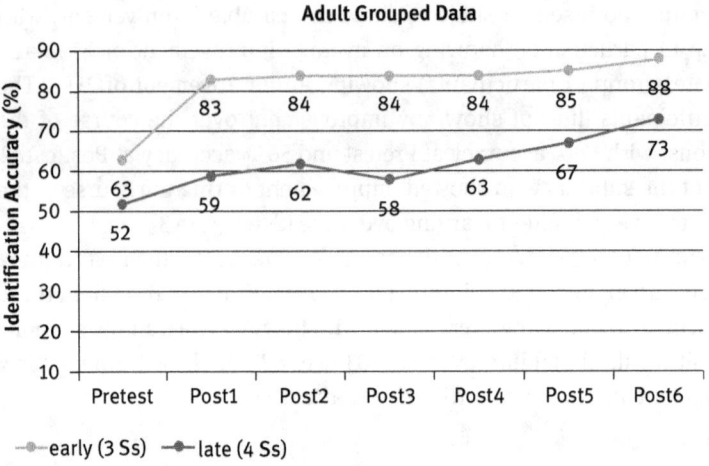

Figure 3: Grouped data for the adult trainees (early learning group, late learning group) for four Mandarin tones for Pretest and the six Posttests.

These adult training data reveal distinct patterns of learning. For some trainees, learning takes place in an initial abrupt cycle, punctuated by a period of relative stability. The learning process exhibits a fast burst of incremental growth followed by a plateau, where little change occurs. However, for some trainees, learning occurs gradually over time in which there is a fairly uniform rate of change. The acquisition process seems to be slower and reveal a gradual accumulation of information over time. Small improvements are evident at each stage of the learning process.

5 Experiment 2: Child second language learning

A second training experiment was conducted to examine learning in children. Similar to the earlier pilot study examining training in adults, not only overall learning was examined but also data related to the nature of the learning throughout the training paradigm were collected.

Participants

Ten children who were native speakers of American English participated in the experiment. All were elementary students at the Century Elementary School in Lawrence, Kansas. None had any experience with a tone language. The children ranged in age from 6 to 11 years of age. Five children were 6–8 years old and the other five children were 9–11 years of age. Different ages were selected in order to sample the critical period range and to see if the task was doable at different ages.

Stimuli

The Mandarin stimuli were identical to those used for the adults.

Procedure

All testing was done at Century School. All other procedures were identical to those used for the adults, with a schedule consisting of Pretest, Training, and Posttest in a two-week time frame.

Results

The results of the 10 child participants are shown in Figure 4. Scores represent percent correct identification of the four Mandarin tones for Pretest and the 6 Posttests. Overall, children showed significant improvement (11%) over the 6 training sessions, with average scores at Pretest of 26% correct and at Posttest of 37% correct. These scores were lower than our earlier adult improvement scores of 17%, using identical stimuli and procedures. The children were quite capable of doing the task. However, overall accuracy rates were below those of the adults, with the children only achieving a final 37% correct identification rate while the adults averaged 74% correct identification after all training sessions.

Similar to the adults, the child participants also displayed distinct patterns across Posttests. Two distinct groups were evident. Both sets of subjects show improvement, with the first group (3 participants) showing an average improvement of 21% and the second (late) group (3 participants) showing an improvement of 12%. The remaining participants (4 participants) did not show any improvement over the course of the training sessions, with 33% accuracy at Pretest and 34% accuracy at Posttest. A detailed look at the children who showed improvement during the course of the experiment reveals very different learning over time (See Figure 5).

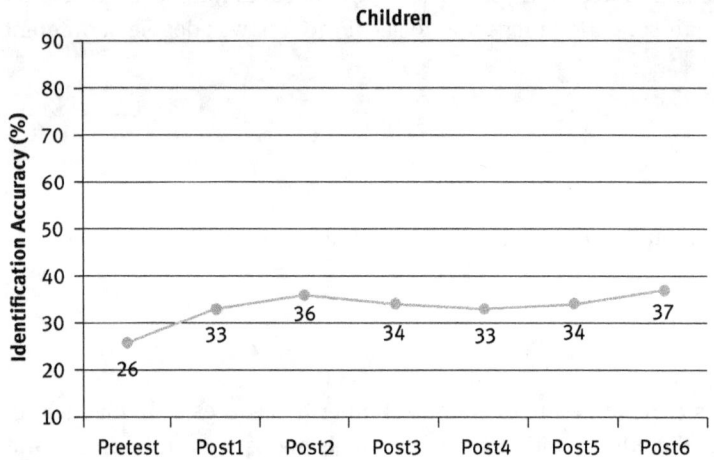

Figure 4: Child trainees' correct identification accuracy (percent) of the four Mandarin tones for Pretest and the six Posttests.

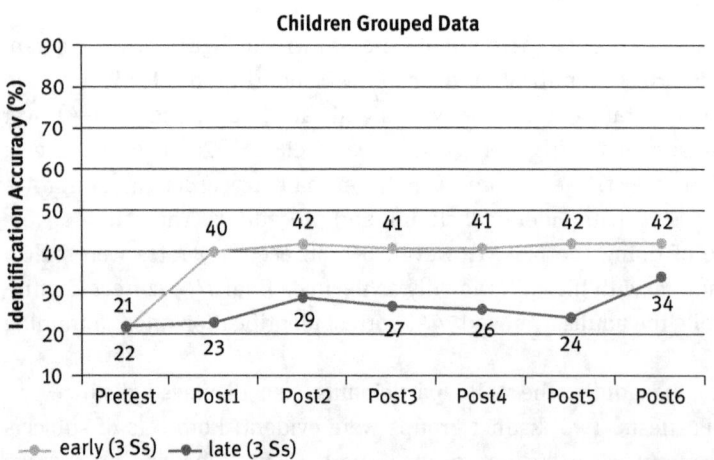

Figure 5: Grouped data for the child trainees (early learning group, late learning group) for the four Mandarin tones for Pretest and the six Posttests.

The first group (early) shows significant improvement after the first training session (Post1), with an initial 19% improvement. After that initial session, these participants' scores do not change very much, with the next five training sessions showing very little additional improvement (40% to 42%). These trainees show initial improvement and then very little change after that.

The second group (late) shows a very different pattern of learning over time. The initial training sessions don't seem to affect accuracy. These participants show improvement only at the end of the training regime. Initial levels of accuracy (22%) show little increase after 5 training sessions, from 22% to 24%. It is not until the final training session that these participants show an increase in accuracy to 34%. For this late group, learning seems to take time, with a number of training sessions necessary for an increase in accuracy, a noticeably different pattern from the early group. This second (late) group also shows less overall improvement compared to the first (early) group, 12% versus 21%, respectively.

6 Discussion

The present chapter presents two experiments examining second language learning, comparing adults and children. Both experiments exploit the high variability training paradigm using a variety of speakers and phonetic contexts to examine learning a novel second language tonal contrast. Unlike previous experiments, the present experiments systematically assess learning at different stages in the training regime. To accomplish this goal, learning in both adults and children was assessed at different stages in the training regime, examining the step-by-step acquisition of a non-native language contrast. For both the adult trainees (Experiment 1) and the child trainees (Experiment 2), the time course of learning a language contrast was examined.

Overall, adult trainees (Experiment 1) improved by 17% from Pretest (57%) to the final Posttest (74%). The 17% increase in accuracy scores is very similar to our earlier results showing an overall 21% improvement (Wang, Spence, Jongman & Sereno, 1999). Using identical methods and assessment, children were also trained on the same novel tonal contrast. Overall, children (Experiment 2) also showed improvement (11%) over the 6 training sessions, with average scores at Pretest of 26% correct and at Posttest of 37% correct.

While the children were capable of doing the task, overall accuracy rates were well below those of the adults, with the children only achieving a final 37% correct identification rate while the adults averaged 74% correct identification after all training sessions. In addition, the gain for the children (11% increase) was significantly smaller than for the adults (17% increase). The adult trainees did show both more substantial improvement in learning as well as more accurate perception. Instead of children outperforming adults on this task, the adults showed greater improvement and also started and ended at higher accuracy levels than the children.

For the child trainees, two age ranges of children were included, a younger (6–8 years old) group (5 children) and an older (9–11 years old) group (5 children). The groups did show different levels of improvement over training sessions, with the younger group improving very little (5%) and, as a group, not reaching above chance levels of accuracy in the final sessions (26%) (See Figure 6).

The older group, however, showed much higher correct identification rates, with initial accuracy levels at 31% and final posttest accuracy reaching 47%, a 16% improvement in identification with training. Interestingly, although overall accuracy was lower for these older children as compared to the adults, the gains in identification accuracy were comparable to the adults. The older children patterned very similarly to the adults. While Wang & Kuhl (2003) reported similar training benefits across all age groups, they did find that participants' pre-training scores consistently increased with age (6-year olds: 55%, 10-year olds: 67%, 14-year olds 74%, and adults 86%). We also observed the latter effect (6–8 year olds: 21%, 9–11 year-olds: 31%; adults: 57%). In addition, the present study also shows increased post-training gains with age (6–8 year olds: 5%, 9–11 year-olds: 16%; adults: 17%).

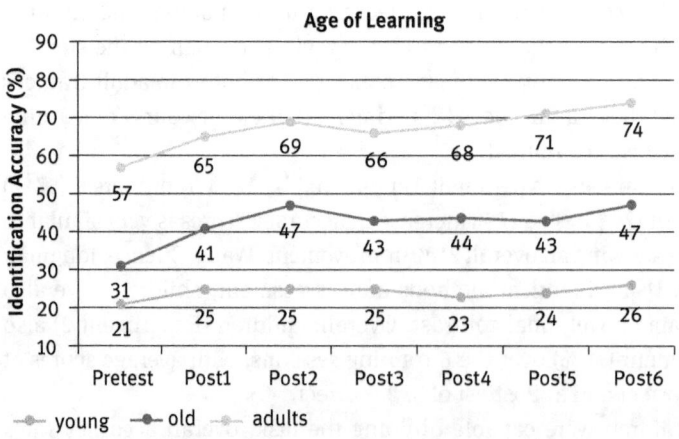

Figure 6: Adult and child (young, old) trainees' correct identification accuracy (percent) of the four Mandarin tones for Pretest and the six Posttests.

The present research also examined not only what is learned but also how it is learned. The present data provide information about the mechanisms responsible for learning by examining the step-by-step acquisition process. Both the adult training data and the child training data reveal distinct patterns of learning. For some trainees, learning takes place early in training. The learning process exhibits an immediate burst of incremental growth followed by little improvement. However, for some trainees, learning seems to take longer to appear. The acquisition process is slower and reveals learning only later in the training sessions. These distinct patterns are observed for both the adult and the child participants. The relevant issue that is raised by these data is whether different learning strategies produce different types of learning.

While new phonetic categories can be learned by adults, the present data show that individual differences in learning do exist. Some individuals show fast acquisition followed by very little change and others show a slower, more gradual, acquisition process. Few studies systematically examine performance of individual participants. The variables that influence both initial accuracy levels as well as overall improvement in both adults and children is key. A larger number of participants and a more detailed documentation of their abilities may help bring us closer to maximizing learning.

An additional variable that may influence learning is the nature of the contrast itself that is to be learned. Within second language research, many studies have observed that individuals who learn a second language at a later age often exhibit an "accent". This topic has been explained on phonological grounds (e.g., Flege, 1992, 1995; Best, 1994, 1995). Older learners are more likely to have a fully developed linguistic system already in place. This phonological account argues that age effects result from the interaction of two phonological systems. In contrast to children, adults perceive and produce second language sounds with reference to linguistic categories of a highly entrenched native language system. Under this phonological claim, an adult's ability to master second language sounds depends on the degree of similarity of such second language sounds to familiar first language sounds. A number of these studies have drawn the distinction between second language sounds that are relatively similar to sounds in the first language as opposed to second language sounds that are more dissimilar or novel. This research has provided some evidence that second language sounds not found in the first language inventory (new or novel L2 sounds) may eventually be produced more accurately than are second language sounds with a counterpart in the first language inventory. These data suggest that all language contrasts may not be equally potent in the learning process.

Research suggests that the benefits of high-variability training do depend on the contrast that is to be acquired. For example, in their study of Spanish learners of English, Wade, Jongman & Sereno (2004) showed that high-variability training was helpful for less-confusable vowel distinctions but actually hurt the acquisition of more confusable vowel pairs. In addition, individual aptitude has also been shown to influence the success of high-variability training. Perrachione et al. (2011) reported that high-aptitude perceivers (participants who scored above 70 % on a pitch-contour perception pre-test) benefitted from high-variability training when learning pseudowords that differed in terms of their pitch contour. However, low-aptitude perceivers did worse on high-variability as compared to low-variability training. Sadakata & McQueen (2014) showed a similar pattern of results for Dutch learners of Mandarin. An examination of additional language contrasts is needed.

The present experiments investigated the perceptual training of non-native adult and child listeners, revealing that tone perception accuracy can be improved with minimal exposure in both adults and children. However, learning in adults and children was not the same. Overall, accuracy rates for adults were significantly greater than those of children. In addition, while adults and older children (age 9–11 years old) showed sizeable improvements in identification accuracy of novel second language contrasts, younger children (ages 6–8 years old) did not. Finally, the rate of learning in both adults and children was distinct, with some learners showing early improvements in accuracy and others requiring a number of training sessions before the contrast was learned. Future research will assess the role of individual aptitude and its interaction with the degree of variability during training in the acquisition of second language phonetic categories.

References

Best, C. (1994). The emergence of native-language phonological influences in infants: A perceptual assimilation model. In J. Goodman and H. Nusbaum (eds.), *The Development of Speech Perception: The Transition from Speech Sounds to Spoken Words*, Cambridge: MIT Press, pp. 167–224.

Best, C. (1995). A direct realist view of cross-language speech perception. In W. Strange (ed.), *Speech Perception and Linguistic Experience: Issues in Cross-Language Research*, York: Timonium, pp. 174–204.

Birdsong, D. (1999). *Second Language Acquisition and the Critical Period Hypothesis*. Mahwah, NJ: Lawrence Erlbaum.

Bradlow, A. R., Pisoni, D. B., Yamada, R. A. & Tohkura, Y. (1997). Training Japanese listeners to identify English /r/ and /l/ IV: Some effects of perceptual learning on speech production. *Journal of the Acoustical Society of America*, 101, 2299–2310.

Chao, Y. R. (1948). *Mandarin Primer*. Cambridge: Harvard University Press.

Flege, J. (1987). The production of "new" and "similar" phones in a foreign language: Evidence for the effect of equivalence classification. *Journal of Phonetics*, 15, 47–65.

Flege, J. (1992). Speech learning in a second language. In C. Ferguson, L. Menn, and C. Stoel-Gammon (eds.), *Phonological Development: Models, Research, and Applications*, York: Timonium, pp. 565–604.

Flege, J. (1995). Second language speech learning: Theories, findings and problems. In W. Strange (ed.), *Speech Perception and Linguistic Experience: Issues in Cross-Language Research*, York: Timonium, pp. 233–277.

Flege, J. (1999). Age of learning and-second language speech. In D. Birdsong (Ed.) *Second Language Acquisition and the Critical Period Hypothesis*. Hillsdale, NJ: Lawrence Erlbaum. pp. 101–131.

Herd, W., Jongman, A. & Sereno, J. (2013). Perceptual and production training of intervocalic /d, r, r/ in American English learners of Spanish. *Journal of the Acoustical Society of America*, 133 (6), 4274 – 4255.

Jamieson, D. G. & Morosan, D. E. (1986). Training non-native speech contrasts in adults: Acquisition of the English /θ/-/ð/ contrast by francophones. *Perception and Psychophysics* 40, 205–215.

Jamieson, D. G. & Morosan, D. E. (1989). Training new, nonnative speech contrasts: A comparison of the prototype and perceptual fading techniques. *Canadian Journal of Psychology* 43, 88–96.

Krashen, S., Long, M. & Scarcella, R. (1979). Age, rate and eventual attainment in second language acquisition. *TESOL Quarterly*, 13(4), 573–582.

Lenneberg, E. (1967). *Biological Foundations of Language*, New York: Wiley.

Lively, S. E., Pisoni, D. B., Yamada, R. A., Tohkura, Y. & Yamada, T. (1994). Training Japanese listeners to identify English /r/ and /l/ III: Long-term retention of new phonetic categories. *Journal of the Acoustical Society of America*, 96, 2076–2087.

Logan, J. S., Lively, S. E. & Pisoni, D. B. (1991). Training Japanese listeners to identify English /r/ and /l/: A first report. *Journal of the Acoustical Society of America*, 89, 874–886.

Logan, J. S., Lively, S. E. & Pisoni, D. B. (1993). Training listeners to perceive novel phonetic categories: How do we know what is learned? *Journal of the Acoustical Society of America*, 94, 1148–1151.

McClaskey, C. L., Pisoni, D. B. & Carrell, T. D. (1983). Transfer of training of a new linguistic contrast in voicing. *Perception and Psychophysics*, 34, 323–330.

Perrachione, T. K., Lee, J., Ha, L. Y. Y. & Wong, P. C. (2011). Learning a novel phonological contrast depends on interaction between individual differences and training paradigm design. *Journal of the Acoustical Society of America*, 130, 461–472.

Pisoni, D. B., Aslin, R. N., Perey, A. J. & Hennessy, B. L. (1982). Some effects of laboratory training on identification and discrimination of voicing contrasts in stop consonants. *Journal of Experimental Psychology: Human Perception and Performance*, 8, 297–314.

Sadakata, M. & McQueen, J. M. (2014). Individual aptitude in Mandarin lexical tone perception predicts effectiveness of high-variability training. Frontiers in Psychology, 5. DOI=10.3389/fpsyg.2014.01318

Snow, C. & Hoefnagel-Höhle, M. (1978). The critical period for language acquisition: Evidence from second language learning. *Child Development*, 49(4), 1114–1128.

Strange, W. (1995). *Speech Perception and Linguistic Experience: Theoretical and Methodological Issues in Cross-Language Speech Research*. Timonium, MD.: York Press Inc.

Strange, W. & Dittman, S. (1984) Effects of discrimination training on the perception of /r-l/ by Japanese adults learning English. *Perception and Psychophysics*, 36, 131–145.

Van Turennout, M., Ellmore, T. & Martin, A. (2000). Long-lasting cortical plasticity in the object naming system. *Nature Neuroscience*, 3, 1329–1334.

Wade, T., Jongman, A. & Sereno, J. A. (2004). Effects of acoustic variability in the perceptual learning of non-native accented speech sounds. *Phonetica*, 64, 122–144.

Wang, Y., Jongman, A. & Sereno, J. A. (2001). Dichotic perception of Mandarin tones by Chinese and American listeners. *Brain and Language*, 73(3), 332–348.

Wang, Y., Jongman, A. & Sereno, J. A. (2003). Acoustic and perceptual evaluation of Mandarin tone productions before and after perceptual training. *Journal of the Acoustical Society of America*, 113(2), 1033–1043.

Wang, Y. & Kuhl, P. K. (2003). Evaluating the "critical period" hypothesis: Perceptual learning of Mandarin tones in American adults and American children at 6, 10, and 14 years of age. *Proceedings of the 15th International Congress of Phonetic Sciences*, 1537–1540.

Wang, Y., Sereno, J. A., Jongman, A. & Hirsch, J. (2003). fMRI evidence for cortical modification during learning of Mandarin lexical tone. *Journal of Cognitive Neuroscience*, 15(7), 1019–1027.

Wang, Y., Spence, M. M., Jongman, A. & Sereno, J. A. (1999). Training American listeners to perceive Mandarin tones. *Journal of the Acoustical Society of America*, 106, 3649–3658.

Vipul Arora and Henning Reetz
Automatic speech recognition: What phonology can offer

Abstract: This chapter presents phonological features as the underlying representation of speech for the purpose of automatic speech recognition (ASR), instead of phones (or phonemes), which are typically used for this purpose. Phonological features offer a number of advantages. Firstly, they can efficiently handle the pronunciation variability found in languages. Secondly, these features form natural classes to represent speech universally, hence they are capable of providing better ways to transfer various models, involved in ASR, across different languages and dialects. Moreover, the ubiquity of the perceptual properties of phonological features is supported by various neuro-linguistic experiments and language studies for different languages of the world. Thus, phonological features can provide a principled way of ASR, thereby reducing the amount of training data and computational resources required.

The main challenge is to develop mathematical models to reliably detect these features from the speech signal, and to incorporate them into ASR systems. Towards this end, we describe here some of our implementations. Firstly, we present a digit recognition system that includes detecting the features with the help of neural networks and a rule-based feature-to-phoneme mapping. Secondly, we describe a deep neural networks based method to extract the features from speech signals. This method improves the detection accuracy by using deep learning. Thirdly, we present a deep neural network based ASR system which detects features and maps them to phonemes using statistical models. This system performs at par with state-of-the-art ASR systems for the task of phoneme recognition.

1 Introduction

Human faculty of speech has allured philosophers, linguists and engineers of all times. The modern devices of recording and reproducing sound trace their roots back to phonograph invented by Edison in 1877. From there, the technology

---

Vipul Arora, Faculty of Linguistics, Philology and Phonetics, University of Oxford
Henning Reetz, Institut für Phonetik, Goethe University Frankfurt

DOI 10.1515/9783110422658-011

evolved and gave rise to interest in audio processing, leading further to speech analysis and recognition. Spectral analysis (Koenig et al., 1946) and linear predictive coding (Markel & Gray, 1976) laid much of the foundations of visualising and representing the acoustics of speech. Around this time the phoneticians and phonologists developed insights into speech acoustics, and came up with ways of characterising sound units for prospectively all spoken languages (Chiba & Kajiyama, 1941; Jakobson et al., 1951; Fant, 1960).

The Advanced Research Projects Agency (ARPA) of the Department of Defense financed in the 1970s the ARPA Speech Understanding Project to boost the development of Automatic Speech Understanding (ASU) technology. The goal was to convert spoken text input into an appropriate computer reaction. Note that Automatic Speech Understanding is different from Automatic Speech Recognition (ASR). The later transcribes an acoustic speech signal into a written text, whereas the first gives an appropriate reaction by a machine, for example, to retrieve a document from a database. Klatt noted in his report (Klatt, 1977: 1353) that the best performing Harpy[1] system's phonetic transcription performance was worse than the other systems in the competition. This is not surprising, since Harpy used only acoustic spectrum matching techniques without a phonetic or phonemic inventory. This was possible since it did not try to 'transcribe' what was said into phonetic labels but used a stochastical Markov chain to match spectral patterns with its internal network of patterns. Its success was mostly based on the restricted syntax of its application, which was decoded in an internal network of possible phrases, and an efficient beam-search method. That is, the system did not try to transcribe every word that was uttered but rather found matching parts in its network to generate an appropriate reaction by the system. Another reason for its good performance was due to its avoidance of early 'hard' decisions on sounds or words. Additionally, the central processing unit was a network of essentially simple nodes, who all have the same structure, and did not need any proprietary rules for each sound. The success of this system over the 'classical' phonetic-based systems, which try to transcribe speech first and find then words in a lexicon, paved the way for nowadays ASR systems and the usage of (stochastical) Hidden-Markov Models in ASR systems. And since there was no need to understand phonetics, phonology, or another linguistic's discipline, the HMM systems could be constructed by programmers. Essentially, this lead to an

---

[1] Harpy is a combination of the Hearsay and Dragon system (Lowerre, 1976). The name, a mythological figure of a bird with a woman's head, was probably chosen to give Dragon, "an entirely different kind of beast from the AI systems being considered in the rest of the speech effort" (Newell, 1978: 1) wings.

end of phonetic/linguistic related speech recognition or speech understanding approaches. Klatt noted further (Klatt 1977: 1345) that the ARPA project was specifically funding technical groups, rather than supporting phonetic or linguistic approaches.

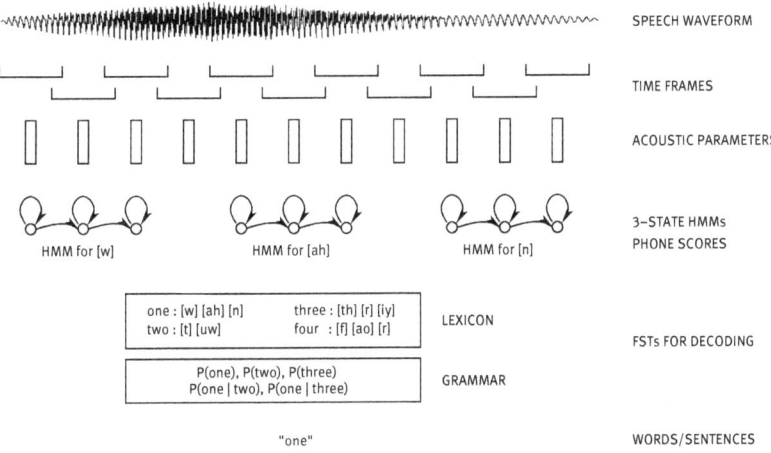

Figure 1: A typical HMM based ASR system

This chapter describes the present approach to automatic speech recognition, the further challenges in speech recognition research and the solutions that phonology can offer. Section 2 of this chapter outlines the typical components of modern ASR systems, followed by various problems faced by them. Section 3 presents the concepts from phonology, systematised in the form of Featurally Underspecified Lexicon (FUL) model, that can be helpful in providing solutions to many of those problems. Our attempts to implement FUL model for building full-fledged ASR system are presented subsequently. Section 4 describes a digit recognition system using shallow neural networks for detection of features from speech spectra, followed by a rule-based ternary matching scheme to map the features onto phonemes, which are then decoded into words. An improved feature detection system, using deep neural networks (DNNs), is detailed in Section 5. Section 6 presents a phoneme recognition system, which uses DNNs for detecting features and mapping them onto phonetic states of HMM. This system achieves accuracy at par with modern state-of-the-art systems.

2 Modern ASR Systems

Modern ASR systems are based on statistical models, which have their parameters trained[2] over speech audio data. The typical steps involved in an ASR system are illustrated in Figure 1. They can be explained as follows:

1. The speech waveform is a continuous signal evolving in time. It is divided into short time frames, with the assumption that the relevant statistical properties of the signal are constant over one frame. To prevent any loss of information, the frame advance length is kept smaller than the frame length, resulting in overlapping frames. In addition, these frames are multiplied by a smoothing window so as to avoid effects of abrupt cut-off at end points.
2. Acoustic parameters o_t are extracted from each frame t for further analysis. These parameters could be spectra, band energies, mel-frequency cepstral coefficients (MFCCs), perceptual linear prediction (PLP) coefficients, or others. In general, these parameters try to represent acoustic properties that are relevant to recognise speech and reduce the amount of data that has to be processed in subsequent steps. Since the human hearing system ignores essentially the phase relations of spectral components in an audio signal when it comes to speech understanding, the power spectrum removes them. Since the frequency resolution of our hearing system is worse for higher frequencies and seems only to evaluate certain frequency bands, band spectra model this behaviour. Furthermore, speech recognition focusses on information about the vocal tract, the MFCCs provide a dataset that claims to represent the auditory system of humans and concentrate of parameter that model the vocal tract. Classical linear prediction coding (LPC) model a simplified speaking apparatus under idealised conditions that is prone to deliver wrong data for e. g. nasals and fails under the presence of background noise. PLP claim to represent more the perceptual side. All these methods deliver some data reduction and represent in a simplified way the acoustic information that is used by human listeners and are equally appropriate for the task.
3. The acoustic parameters are mapped on to some form of representation, which is similar to a sub-phonetic[3] unit. Since a phoneme changes its acoustic properties in time, it is typically modelled with three successive states, corresponding to beginning, middle and end. A statistical model maps the

---

[2] 'Training' and 'learning' means in this context that a system can cluster similar datasets together and treat them as one unit.
[3] ASR literature generally uses the term *phone* to denote the unit which we call as *phoneme*, throughout this chapter.

acoustic parameters $\mathbf{o}_t$ of each successive frame to one of these states q_t. Typical statistical models used are Gaussian mixture models (GMMs), artificial neural networks (ANNs), next to others. A GMM is an efficient clustering method to assign observed data to cluster by assuming they stem from a (multi-dimensional) mixture of normal (Gaussian) distributions. ANNs do not make an assumption about the distribution of some data but try to assign them directly to internal nodes of their network. Essentially, these methods are used to map the datasets of the three-frames onto a sub-phonetic units. For robustness, these models assign each frame t with a probabilistic score $b(\mathbf{o}_t|q_t = i)$ with which it belongs to one of the states i.

4. The sub-phonetic state probabilities along successive frames have to be traced over time so as to obtain phones, words and sentences. For this purpose, hidden markov models (HMMs) are used in conjunction with finite state transducers (FSTs). HMMs have two kinds of parameters – $b(\mathbf{o}_t|q_t = i)$, i. e., probability of observing the given acoustic parameters $\mathbf{o}_t$ from a particular state q_t, and $a(q_t = i|q_{t-1} = j)$ the probability of a particular state i following another state j. FSTs also model probability of one state following another but at a higher level, i. e., the states here are phones or words instead of sub-phonetic states. The best path over these states is the one with maximum overall probability and is obtained by Viterbi algorithm. This step is called *decoding*.

The Viterbi algorithm involves probabilistic parameters $b(\mathbf{o}_t|q_t = i)$, $a(q_t - i|q_{t-1} - j)$, etc., which have to be trained beforehand over speech audio data along with its phonetic transcription. ASR systems based on this scheme have been quite successful in achieving high accuracy speech to text transcription. Recently, a major breakthrough was seen by introducing DNNs to learn the mapping from acoustic to linguistic representation (step 3 above). DNNs are a succession of ANNs, which are supposed to 'learn' patterns on different levels with increasing complexity.

Still, the accuracy of state of the art ASR systems is much below human performance. Moreover, these systems have enormously large number of parameters, which require large amounts of training data and intensive computational resources.

We consider the root of the problem to be overly strong reliance on statistical models while using crude linguistic representations. Present efforts are mostly directed towards higher level modelling, while there is still much room at the bottom, i. e. at acoustic level (O'Shaughnessy, 2013). The next section throws light on some of such principles that have the potential to provide efficient modelling leading to enhanced accuracy.

3 Alternative Feature-based Approaches

All present commercial ASR systems use stochastical models on all levels, converting the audio signal into a sequence of states (a network of quasi-phonetic representation with usually three states representing the left, center and right context of a soneme), which are connected to a higher level of a network of word candidates. All 'linguistic' knowledge is represented by the transition probabilities between theses states, which are based on the training data. There is usually no 'external' linguistic knowledge used to construct these networks, neither is there a interpretation of the states. For example, the acoustic data is often represented by MFCCs, which cannot be easily interpreted as Spectrograms or LPC spectra, where higher energy peaks are associated with formant frequencies of the vocal tract. However, if the underlying representation is made more general and flexible, not only will it enhance the efficiency of systems, but will also enable the models to be transferred easily across different accents as well as languages. There have been some attempts to use some form of linguistic categories articulatory, phonological, etc. for making the ASR systems more robust and efficient.

Various mid-level features (e.g., phonological, articulatory) have been used as input to the conventional HMM framework to improve performance. Scanlon et al. (2007) proposed classification of speech into broad classes (vowel, diphthong, semi-vowel, fricative, stop, nasal, silence), and further into phones by classifiers specific to that class. Mitra et al. (2014) used articulatory characteristics (lip aperture and protrusion, tongue tip and body constriction location and degree, velum and glottal involvement), which they computed on a variety of acoustic measures.

Table 1: Phonological features for some of the phones (TIMIT notation)

	voc	cons	cont	obstr	str	voice	son	stop	low	high	lab	cor	dor	rtr	nas	lat	rho	rad
/aa/	1	-1	0	-1	-1	0	1	-1	1	-1	-1	-1	1	0	0	0	-1	-1
/ae/	1	-1	0	-1	-1	0	1	-1	1	-1	0	1	0	0	0	0	-1	-1
/iy/	1	-1	0	-1	-1	0	1	-1	-1	1	0	1	0	-1	0	0	-1	-1
/uw/	1	-1	0	-1	-1	0	1	-1	-1	1	1	-1	1	-1	0	0	-1	-1
/t/	-1	1	-1	1	1	-1	-1	1	0	0	0	1	0	0	-1	-1	-1	-1
/d/	-1	1	-1	1	-1	1	0	1	0	0	0	1	0	0	-1	-1	-1	-1

Another approach is to *detect* the presence of certain landmarks, originally proposed by Stevens (2002), followed by higher level processing for decoding these landmarks into words or sentences (Jansen & Niyogi, 2009).

3.1 Phonological Features

Each phoneme is characterised by a group of phonological features based on the manner and place of articulation along with their acoustic correlates. Thus, a single feature can characterise a set of phones. The phones here are denoted in TIMIT (Garofalo et al., 1990) notation.

We define our features based on featurally underspecified lexicon model (FUL) (Lahiri & Reetz, 2010). Within FUL, an interesting property of phonological features is that they are not necessarily all specified in the mental lexicon. For instance, the place feature is specified as labial for the phoneme /m/, but is unspecified for /n/. This allows /n/ to easily change to /m/ or /ng/ in running speech, but leaves /m/ unchanged. For example, "green-bag" is often pronounced as "greem-bag" but /m/ in "cream-desk" does not change to /n/. This property of the feature space makes the distance metric asymmetric. We have proposed a ternary-value representation to express the phonological feature vectors. Under this, each phoneme is characterised by a set of phonological features, each of which can take three values, viz., +1, 0 or –1. The value +1 denotes presence, –1 denotes absence and 0 leaves the feature unspecified. E. g., for /m/, the feature LAB (labial) takes value +1, while for /n/, LAB has the value 0 because /n/ is underspecified. The significance of an unspecified value is that the detection or not-detection of that feature does not affect the decoding of the corresponding phone.

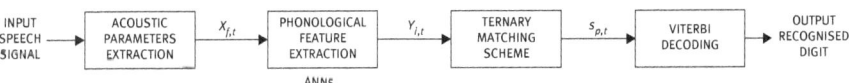

Figure 2: Block schematic of ASR system with rule-based feature-to-phoneme mapping

For this research, we use a set of 18 such features to characterise different phonemes in English. The features used here (Lahiri & Reetz, 2010) include vocalic (VOC) for vowels and consonantal (CONS) for consonants. Pitched phones have the feature sonorant (SON). Features low (LOW) and high (HIGH) correspond to the tongue height, both for vowels and consonants, while features coronal (COR) and dorsal (DOR) pertain to tongue's frontness or backness; and labial (LAB) indicates the involvement of lips. Short vowels (e. g. /ih/, /ax/) have the retracted tongue root (RTR) feature. Feature continuant (CONT) marks the consonants continuing in time (e. g. /f/, /s/) while feature stop (STOP) denotes the stop consonants (e. g. /b/, /t/). A consonant (e. g. /g/) carries voicing feature (VOICE) to distinguish from its unvoiced counterpart (e. g. /k/). Any consonant involving obstruction of the vocal track is associated with the feature obstruent (OBS), with consonants (e. g. /s/, /z/) that involve turbulent streaming of air having the feature strident (STR). Nasal sounds (e. g. /n/, /m/) carry the feature nasal (NAS). Features like rhotic (RHO), lateral (LAT) and radical (RAD) denote certain kinds of consonants, namely /r/, /l/ and /hh/, respectively.

As we have seen, certain features, like those referring to tongue position and height correspond to both vowels as well as consonants. Table 1 shows some examples of phones with the corresponding phonological features. To recapitulate, +1 denotes not only the presence of a feature, and –1 the absence, but also 0 signifies an underspecified condition. For example, /p/ is listed as –1 for COR, and 1 for LAB because COR extracted from the signal (e. g. /t d n/ etc.) mismatches with it. On the other hand, /t/ is listed as 1 for COR and 0 for LAB because the LAB extracted from the signal (e. g. /p b m/ etc.) does not mismatch and is tolerated.

4 ASR with ANN-Based Feature Extraction and Rule-Based Feature-to-Phoneme Mapping

Using these principles, we have attempted to implement a limited-vocabulary ASR system for recognising English digits. The different stages that make up this system are depicted in Figure 2. Acoustic parameters are extracted from the input speech waveform and are used to detect phonological features with a statistical learning system. A rule-based ternary matching scheme, based on the FUL model, is used to map the features to phoneme sequences, which subsequently are decoded into words. The goal of the system is to estimate single isolated digits, from a set of 11 digits with phonetic transcriptions given in Table 2.

The different stages of the ASR system are described in the following subsections.

Table 2: Digits with phonetic transcription

1	w ah n	5	f ay v	9	n ay n
2	t uw	6	s ih k s	z	z iy r ow
3	th r iy	7	s eh v ah n	o	ow
4	f ao r	8	ey t		

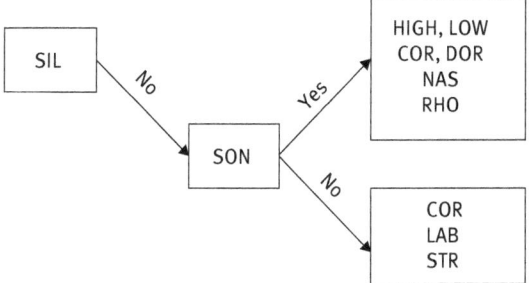

Figure 3: Block schematic for the different stages of phonological feature extraction

4.1 Acoustic Parameters Extraction

The speech signal is transformed to the spectral domain with a 1024-point Fourier transform using a 10 ms Hanning window and 10 ms hop size. Discarding the phase information, each spectrum is converted to dB scale with 60 dB dynamic range (the origin is shifted to make all magnitude values positive), and is normalised to unit norm. This spectral energy distribution, $X_{f,t}$, is used as the input to the ANN, which estimates $Y_{i,t}$, the phonological features, as the output. Before feeding in to the ANN, each tuple of the input vector is also normalised to zero mean and unit variance, for efficient learning.

4.2 Phonological Feature Extraction

Since, digits need only a limited number of phonemes, we construct the set of minimal number of phonological features required to distinguish them. The features used here include:
- sonorant (SON);
- sonorant phonemes are further categorised with the features high (HIGH), low (LOW), coronal (COR), dorsal (DOR), nasal (NAS) and rhotic (RHO);
- non-sonorant or obstruent phonemes are characterised by the features coronal (COR), labial (LAB) and strident (STR).

The label SIL stands for pause or silence. In this implementation, we do not deal with noise, and hence, SIL is simply extracted using the total energy in each time frame. The SON feature directly corresponds to the signal periodicity, i. e., if the frame has got a pitch period, then it is marked as SON.

Most of the above features are usually analysed and characterised in terms of the formant frequencies and formant trajectories. However, formant estimation is highly susceptible to parameters like number of formants, window size, etc. Also, formant extraction becomes quite inconsistent for the formants higher than F2. Instead, we rely on the relative energy distribution over short-time spectrum as the relevant acoustic properties of the speech signal from which we extract the phonological features for sonorant phonemes using a non-linear classifier, i. e. an artificial neural network (ANN). This network takes spectral energy distribution as input and output a score between 0 to 1 for each phonological feature.

However, the nature of these phonological features differ for the sonorant and non-sonorant sounds, hence, separate ANN classifiers have been trained for these two categories. The block-schematic of the scheme is shown in Figure 3. First, the silent frames are separated simply by putting threshold on the total energy. This simple approach is adopted because the input sounds have no noise and at present, we do not handle noisy signals. Then, the son feature, which corresponds to periodicity, is detected with the help of PRAAT pitch estimator (Boersma & Weenink, 2001). The spectral energy distribution of the sonorant frames is used to estimate the phonological features, $Y_{i,t}^{SON}$, and that of the non-sonorant frames is used to estimate $Y_{i,t}^{nonSON}$, with the help of two separate ANNs: NN^{SON} and NN^{nonSON}, respectively. Each ANN has one hidden layer – NN^{SON} has 100 hidden neurons, while NN^{nonSON} has 40 hidden neurons. These ANNs are trained beforehand with desired phonological features using adaptive back-propagation learning (Behera & Kar, 2010).

4.3 Ternary Matching Scheme for Phoneme Estimation

A very important element of our approach is the incorporation of phonological knowledge in the form of the FUL model described as follows.

As we mentioned, FUL provides a scheme for matching phonological features to phonemes. According to this model, the human speech perception system analyses the acoustic signal to extract phonological features, which are subsequently mapped to the lexical representation. The lexicon contains the phonological features determined for each phoneme; let us represent them as $L_{i,p,t}$. Here, i stands for the feature, p for the phoneme and t for the time index. On the other hand, there are features extracted from the speech signal, represented as $Y_{i,t} \in \{0,1\}$. For a phoneme,

Table 3: Digit recognition accuracy, in %

Category	Accuracy
boy	65.2
girl	63.1
man	55.0
woman	65.5
All	62.2

- a 'match' occurs when a feature extracted with high score from the signal is the one expected by the lexicon. It raises the score for that phoneme to be present there in the speech.
- a 'mismatch' occurs when a feature extracted with high score from the signal is the one blocked by the lexicon. It diminishes the score for that phoneme.
- a 'no-mismatch' occurs when a feature extracted with high score from the signal is the one neither expected nor blocked by the lexicon. It can also occur if a feature expected by the lexicon is not detected in the signal. A 'no-mismatch' does not severely diminish the score of the phoneme.

In order to implement these conditions mathematically, the score function for each phoneme is designed as

$$S_{p,t} = \frac{\sum_i L_{i,p,t} Y_{i,t}}{\left(\sum_{i:L_{i,p,t}>0} L_{i,p,t}\right)^{0.7}} \qquad (1)$$

For the phoneme p, $L_{i,p,t}$ takes the values 1, –1 and 0 to incorporate the 'match', 'mismatch' and 'no-mismatch' conditions, respectively. By this formulation, the matched features contribute positively, mismatched features contribute negatively and the no-mismatched features do not contribute to the score function numerator. The denominator aims to normalise the score for phonemes with different number of expected features.

4.4 Experiments

The performance of the proposed ASR system has been evaluated on isolated digit recognition task. The test dataset consists of single digit utterances from the TIDIGITS database (Leonard & Doddington, 1993). The TIDIGITS database has speakers marked with gender and age – *boy, girl, man, woman* – along with their dialect region in USA.

The ANNs have been trained to estimate the phonological features from the normalised spectral energy vectors. This training is carried out using the required phonemes extracted from 2000 speech files randomly selected from the TIMIT database. The TIMIT database has voices from adult male and female speakers, labelled with their gender as well as dialect region in USA. While training, the differences in terms of gender or dialect region have not been considered.

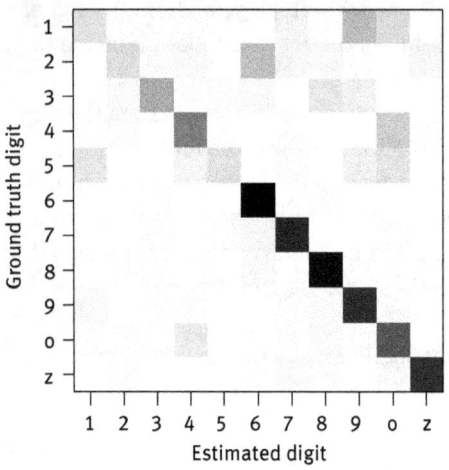

Figure 4: Confusion Matrix showing estimated digit labels with respect to the ground truth digit labels, over all the speakers. The intensity shows the recognition accuracy, normalised along each row. 'z' stands for 'zero'.

The evaluations are performed based on correct isolated digit identification. The digit recognition accuracy is calculated as the number of sound files labelled with correct digit divided by the total number of sound files tested.

Randomly 1000 test files from each category of speakers have been selected and tested. Table 3 shows the recognition accuracy for these tests. To analyse the performance for individual digit, the results of all these files for the four categories are amalgamated and depicted as a confusion matrix in Figure. 4.

As seen in Table 3, the system performance varies over gender and age. Among the adults, women perform better than men, while among the children, boys perform better than girls. We belive that this difference can largely be attributed to the difference in pitch (F0) among these categories, owing to the observation that the formant frequencies vary with F0 (Johnson, 2005). Males have lower F0 than females, while adults have lower F0 than children. According to these factors, boys and women have intermediate F0s. Notably, the feature detector ANNs have been trained on men (low F0) and women (high F0) voices from the TIMIT database. Thus, it is reasonable that the feature detection system works better for the speakers with intermediate range of F0s. The feature detection performance could not be evaluated separately because there is no phonetic or syllabic segmentation in the TIDIGITS database.

The confusion matrix in Figure 4 gives more insights on the general performance over individual digits. As we can see, the system performs very well in identifying the digits '6', '7', '8', '9', 'o' and 'z' (zero), while performing poorly over the digits '1', '2', '3', '4' and '5'. If we perform these tests with the digits '6', '7', '8', '9', 'o' and 'z' as input (output can be one of all the 11 digits), the recognition accuracy reaches 92.4 %.

Although the ternary matching scheme to certain extent takes care of errors originating at the feature detection stage, errors finally appear if the sequence of phonemes in certain digits are very close in the metric space formed by the phonological features. Following is a detailed analysis of these errors on the basis of phonological principles.

Clearly, digits beginning with consonants having the feature STR ('6', '7') perform better than the acoustically weaker fricatives ('3', '4', '5') and the STOP ('2'). The digit '1' is mostly misidentified as '9' or 'o'. The prominent difference is the presence of nasality in the beginning of the digit '1' which spreads regressively from the nasal consonant at its end. Nasality on the onset of '1' is mistaken for '9'. Furthermore, since in our feature metric, '1' and 'o' have very similar initial phonological features, the matching scheme does not effectively correct the errors in feature detection. Thus, if the nasality is detected all over, the '1' is misidentified as '9', and as 'o' if no nasality is detected at all. The digits '2', '3', '4' and '5' are misidentified mainly because of the failure of the system to distinguish the features associated with /t/ (as in '2'), /th/ (as in '3') and /f/ (as in '4', '5') from those associated with /s/. As mentioned above, STR or strident of 's' is identified more easily. However, the aspiration in 't' is also mistaken as the feature strident. This observation is in line with the one made by Jongman (1989), who says that the identification of these phonemes depends much on the duration and becomes worse if the duration is short. At present, our ASR system uses a simple model for silence detection and hence is not yet able to detect /f/ which has weak frication. This accounts for most of the errors in estimating '4' and '5'.

These observations clearly suggest the need to improve the mapping from acoustic signal to specific phonological features. For instance, the non-strident fricatives and plosives need to be distinguished better. Recall, that in the present implementation, we use only a minimal set of phonological features, as required to classify the phonemes of the digits. For full fledged ASR system, some more phonological features need to be put added. Nevertheless, the present system illustrates well the basic value of phonological principles. The next section focuses on using improved statistical learning system, based on deep neural networks, for robust extraction of various phonological features.

5 Detection of Phonological Features

In order to improved the detection of phonological features, we propose in this section a statistical learning system with deep neural networks. This section focuses only on the detection of phonological features and evaluates the performance of the proposed detection system for the detection of each feature.

5.1 Acoustic Parameters

In this work, we use 13 dimensional mel frequency cepstral coefficients (MFCCs), without energy component, as the acoustic parameters for detecting all the features. These MFCCs are calculated for each time frame of 25 ms with a hop size of 10 ms. Many of the above features are associated with time duration. Hence, we use a long context window with 3 frames on each side. Thus, the total number of acoustic parameters to characterise each frame is 13×7.

5.2 Feature Detection

For feature detection we use artificial neural networks with variable number of hidden layers, and with sigmoid function as non-linearity at the output layer. The hidden layers have rectified linear unit function as non-linearity.

The output of the neural network at time frame t is denoted by $y_i(t)$, where i indexes the phonological features. Since $y_i(t)$ is the output of a sigmoid function, it can take values $\in \{0, 1\}$, with 0 denoting the absence and 1 the presence of feature. To incorporate the underspecified features, we allow them to take any value $\in \{0, 1\}$.

5.2.1 Ground truth

The training data is labelled for time intervals of phonemes and not features. The ground truth for training the feature detectors is generated from the ternary feature values illustrated in Table 1. Let $f_i(t)$ denote the ternary feature value associated with feature i at time frame t. The feedback error for training the neural network is given by

$$E(t) = \frac{1}{2} \sum_i (y_i^d(t) - y_i(t))^2 \qquad (2)$$

where $y_i^d(t)$ the desired output at time t. The ternary feature values require the error to be zero for underspecified features. Hence, we define the desired output as

$$y_i^d(t) = \begin{cases} 1 & \text{if } f_i(t) = 1; \\ 0 & \text{if } f_i(t) = -1; \\ y_i(t) & \text{if } f_i(t) = 0. \end{cases} \qquad (3)$$

This ensures that no error is back propagated for $y_i(t)$ when the feature i is underspecified for phoneme at t.

5.2.2 Training of Detectors

The purpose of the detector is to detect the presence of a feature at *any* time point within the time interval of the corresponding phoneme, and not to associate *each* time frame, within that interval, with the particular feature. Hence, it is not wise to use the entire interval of a phoneme to train the corresponding features. Also, many features like stops occur locally in time, and the task of the detector is to search for good acoustic parameters in the local region and learn from them so as to detect the corresponding features.

Let t_p denote the set of all time points (frames) in the pth time interval in phonetic transcription. The weights of the neural network are initialised randomly and are trained for a few epochs from the entire interval of each phoneme. However, after a fixed number of epochs (10 here), the predicted outputs are used to find salient time points $t_{i,p}$ where good acoustic parameters are found for a feature i within the time interval t_p. Since, the purpose of training is to maximise correct detections as well as to minimise false alarms, we define $t_{i,p}$ as

$$t_{i,p} = \begin{cases} \arg\min_{t \in t_p} (y_i^d(t) - y_i(t))^2 & \text{if } f_i(t) = \pm 1; \\ \phi & \text{if } f_i(t) = 0. \end{cases} \qquad (4)$$

where ϕ denotes no time point.

In the subsequent epochs, the training is performed only over these salient time points. The salient time points are re-estimated after every fixed number of epochs (10 here).

The network is trained in order to minimise the mean square error defined in Eq. 2 with back-propagation algorithm. Mini-batches are used to update the weights, with the size of mini-batches increasing linearly from 2048 to 8096, with number of epochs. The learning rate linearly falls from 0.2 to 0.01. The total number of epochs has been set to 500 here.

5.2.3 Detection Process

After the neural networks have been trained, they are used to detect phonological features from the unseen data. The acoustic parameters are extracted from the speech signal and fed into the neural network for detection of the features. The output $y_i(t)$ at each time t is compared with a fixed threshold to register a detection of feature i at that time point. These thresholds are learnt from the training data so as to maximise the detection accuracy.

5.3 Experiments

The proposed algorithm has been tested over TIMIT database, as it provides transcription of the sequence of phonemes. A standard GMM-HMM is used for getting precise time alignments of the phonemes, so as to prepare ground truths for training as well as evaluating test results. For training as well as testing, the audio files in the dataset are corrupted with an additive white gaussian noise of 20 dB SNR. We have used 3696 audio files from the 'train' set of TIMIT for training, while 192 files from the 'test' set for testing.

Since we do not have a standard feature detector available, we have used a monophone GMM-HMM system (Povey et al., 2011), which models each phoneme with three states and estimates for each time frame the state probabilities. Since each state is uniquely associated with a phoneme, we take probability of most probable state as the phoneme probability. The probability of the most probable phoneme at each time frame, is assigned as the probabilities of the associated features (with $f_i = 1$). It is to be noted that the HMM setup (i. e. transition probabilities) is used only while aligning and training the GMMs, and not while testing. During testing, only the GMMs are used to get phoneme probabilities at each time frame. Notably, we cannot use triphone GMM-HMM system as it ties together many states across different phonemes, thereby making the estimation of phoneme probabilities difficult.

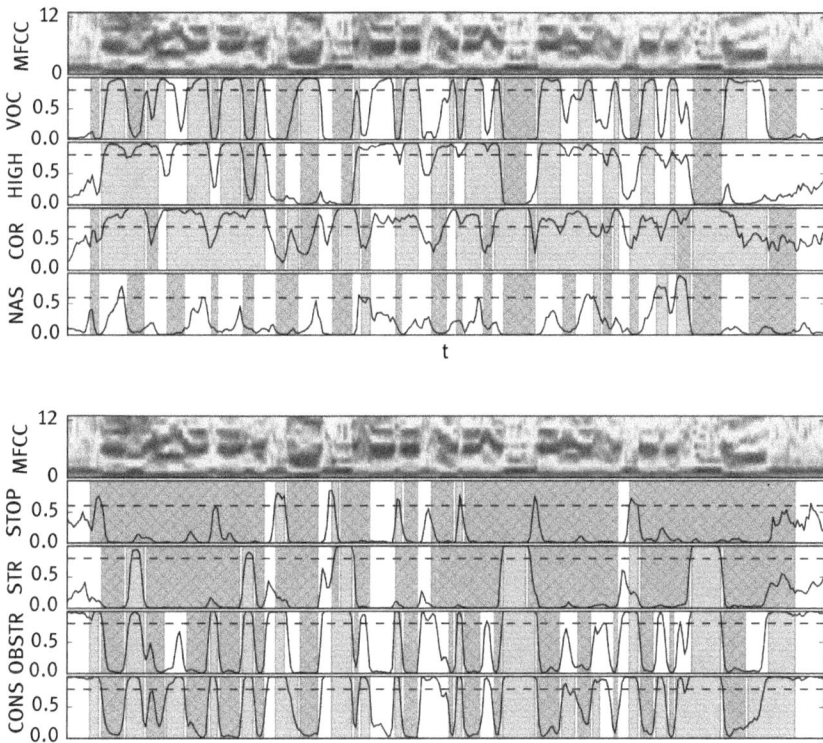

Figure 5: Detection of various features over a test file FDHC0_SI1559 (3.4 seconds long) from TIMIT database, using the proposed method with single hidden layer of 500 units. See text for description.

The detector produces a set of time points t_i corresponding to each detected feature i. At the phoneme interval $\mathbf{t}_p$, a feature i is detected if $\exists\, t_i \in \mathbf{t}_i$ such that $t_i \in \mathbf{t}_p$; in other words, if $\mathbf{t}_i \cap \mathbf{t}_p \neq \phi$. This detection is said to be a correct detection if the phoneme at pth interval has $f_i = 1$, and a false alarm if p has $f_i = -1$; while the result is ignored if $f_i = 0$. However, if phoneme at p has $f_i = 1$ but there is no $t_i \in \mathbf{t}_i$ such that $t_i \in \mathbf{t}_p$, then it is called a miss. The accuracy is determined as the total number of correct detections divided by the sum of correct detections, false alarms and misses.

The proposed system has been tested with different architectures of neural networks – ranging from shallow to deep. We present results for three architectures. Architecture I has single hidden layer with 500 units. Architecture II has two hidden layer with 500 and 200 units, respectively; it is denoted as (500–200). Likewise, architecture III has three hidden layers as (500–500–200).

Table 4: Detection accuracy (in %) for each phonological feature obtained using the baseline and proposed detectors, with neural network architectures mentioned in the header

	Baseline	Proposed		
		(500)	(500–200)	(500–500–200)
VOC	72.2	78.1	81.3	82.4
CONS	73.9	81.7	84.2	84.8
CONT	68.2	79.5	83.1	83.7
OBSTR	77.2	89.4	90.1	91.4
STR	60.1	70.5	73.6	75.2
VOICE	49.4	63.7	67.2	68.4
SON	87.2	92.1	93.5	93.7
STOP	41.7	57.2	62.3	63.5
LOW	72.1	76.3	81.5	83.3
HIGH	72.0	81.5	83.8	85.1
LAB	34.4	45.2	50.4	53.0
COR	72.2	75.1	76.8	79.5
DOR	33.4	42.0	48.9	52.2
RTR	76.5	81.7	84.0	85.5
NAS	59.4	63.8	71.2	72.4
LAT	49.1	54.6	62.6	64.7
RHO	42.9	46.2	50.4	54.5
RAD	13.0	9.1	14.6	17.2

Figure 5 depicts an example of detection over a test file. The topmost plot shows the MFCCs and the subsequent ones are different features. Light gray background with horizontal lines and dark gray background with a cross-hatch pattern mark the intervals having phonemes with $f_i = 1$ and $f_i = -1$, respectively, for the corresponding feature i. Regions with white background correspond to phonemes with $f_i = 0$. The black continuous curve is the output of the detector $y_i(t)$ and the black dashed horizontal line shows the threshold for the corresponding feature detection. The x-axis carries time. The y-axis of MFCC plots has the index, and that of the feature detection plots, the output value for detected features. Ideally, black continuous curve should *at least once* go above the threshold where the background is light gray, and should always stay below the threshold where the background is dark gray. However, it can be anywhere in the regions of white background.

The test results for all the features detected using the baseline as well as the proposed system are presented in Table 4. We can note that the proposed system performs better than the baseline for all the features and the performance improves as the architecture of neural network becomes deeper. While several features are very well detected, some of them are detected poorly in general. RAD performs poorly because the acoustics of /hh/ are statistically very similar to white noise and they have low energy, that makes it difficult to detect it in noisy speech. The poor performance of RHO (/r/) and LAT (/l/) clearly indicates that these features cannot be successfully detected from local acoustics over short time intervals, but are spread over a larger context. The feature LAB and DOR are used in phonology in highly variable acoustic conditions – ranging from vowels to consonants. These results indicate that these features have to be dealt with more carefully, by incorporating larger context and with heavier models (i. e. with more weights) as compare to the other features.

6 ASR with DNN-Based Feature Extraction and Feature-to-Phoneme Mapping

6.1 DNNs for Feature Extraction

The input to the DNN are the acoustic parameters (APs) extracted from the speech signal. Short-time FFT power spectra are calculated with 25ms window and 10ms hop size. They are binned with 23 Mel-scaled filters, whose log scaled outputs form the APs for each time frame. Mean and variance normalisation is applied to these APs, to be used as input to DNN with a context of ±5 frames.

For feature extraction, the DNN consists of three hidden layers, with 500, 500 and 200 neurons, respectively, each with ReLU (rectified linear unit) non-linearity. The output layer corresponds to 19 phonological features, with sigmoid activation function at each neuron.

The target values of feature extraction DNNs are determined by canonical representation of the phonemes in terms of their phonological features. Phonetic state level segmentation is obtained by forced alignment of training data with tri-state GMM-HMM based phoneme recogniser using 13 MFCCs with delta and delta-delta appended. Although the onset and offset times of phonological features do not synchronise exactly with those of phonemes, a practical justification for the above implementation can be found in (King & Taylor, 2000). The target values are set to binary {0,1} values denoting the absence and presence of the corresponding features at a particular time frame.

Training is performed to minimise the squared-error objective function. Network weights are updated using minibatch based stochastic gradient descent algorithm with Nesterov momentum. The learning rate decays linearly from 10^{-2} to 10^{-5}, and the minibatch size increases linearly from 256 to 1024, with each epoch. DNNs are implemented using Lasagne library (github.com/Lasagne).

6.2 Phoneme Recognition System

The phoneme recognition system is based on DNN-HMM framework (Yu & Deng, 2014). For mapping from feature space to phonemes, the neural network consists of single hidden layer with 500 neurons and ReLU activation function. The features are fed directly into this network, without any transformation or stacking.

Output neurons correspond to the conditional state posterior probabilities of monophoneme states of HMM, numbering 3 per phoneme. Monophone models are used here, instead of triphone ones, as some of our preliminary experiments have indicated that they have better portability than triphone models. However, we leave the detailed exploration in this direction for future work.

The target values are obtained using the forced alignment explained in Section 6.1. The output layer has softmax non-linearity. Training is performed to minimise categorical cross-entropy objective function. The weight update scheme is the same as those for feature extraction DNNs (cf. 6.1). The network outputs represent posterior probability of states. These are converted into likelihoods, by dividing with prior probabilities, to be used by HMM. The transition probabilities come from the original GMM-HMM system used for alignment. Bigram language model is trained over phoneme sequences in training data and is used for decoding. The decoding system is implemented using the Kaldi toolkit (Povey et al., 2011).

6.3 Datasets

As before, for training and evaluation, we have used the TIMIT speech database. It consists of clean speech audio files recorded in studio settings. However, we have corrupted them with additive white Gaussian noise with 20dB SNR. All the speech files are phonetically labelled. We use the transcription to get only the sequence of phonemes, without the time-alignment information, which we generate using forced alignment.

TIMIT transcriptions are based on 61 phonemes. Phonemes associated with each phonological feature are shown in Table 5. Diphthongs exhibit change of features over time, and are not considered for training. In TIMIT, phonemes /ay, aw, ey, ix, ow, oy/ are diphthong vowels.

Experiments involve two stages – training and testing. Hence, the corpus is divided into two sets. The training set comes from 3608 files from the TIMIT corpus. Total duration of these files is 2 hours 50 minutes. The test set consists of 192 files with a total duration of 10 minutes. The speaker sets of the above two datasets are mutually non-overlapping.

Table 5: Features associated with phonemes of English (TIMIT)

Feature	Phonemes
VOC	ah axr ax ax-h aa ae eh ih ix iy ao uh ux uw er
CONS	b ch d dh dx el em en eng f g hh hv jh k l m n ng nx p r s sh t th v z zh
CONT	dh el f hh hv l s sh th v z zh
OBSTR	b ch d dh dx f g hh hv jh k p s sh t th v z zh
STR	ch s sh t th z zh
VOICE	b d dh dx g jh v z zh
SON	ah axr ax ax-h aa ae eh el em en eng ih ix hv iy ao l m n ng nx ao r w y uh ux uw er
STOP	b ch d dx g jh k p t
LOW	aa ae
HIGH	ch ih ix iy jh sh w y zh uh ux uw
LAB	b em f ao m p v w uh ux uw
COR	ae eh ch d dh dx eh el en ih ix iy jh l n nx r s sh t th y z zh
DOR	aa eng g ao k ng w uh ux uw
RTR	ah axr ax ax-h eh ih w uh er
NAS	em en eng m n ng nx
LAT	el l
RHO	r er
RAD	hh hv
SIL	bcl dcl epi gcl h kcl pau pcl q tcl

6.4 Proposed Method

First, the DNN is trained using the training set to estimate the features as described in Section 6.1. Second, the layers for estimation of phonetic states from the features is trained using the training set. This training is carried out in the way explained in Section 6.2. There is no iterative re-alignment performed here, although we have found that realignment brings further improvement to the system.

Testing is carried out over the test set. The two neural networks – for feature estimation and for phonetic state estimation – are cascaded together. The decoding is performed using DNN-HMM system described in Section 6.2.

6.5 Baseline methods

The performance of feature-based adaptation scheme is compared with a number of other popular schemes given below.

6.5.1 GMM-HMM

A GMM-HMM system is used for phoneme recognition task. The Kaldi TIMIT-s5 recipe is used for implementing monophone tri-state models. The input is MFCCs with delta and delta-delta coefficients.

6.5.2 DNN-HMM

A conventional DNN-HMM is trained for phoneme recognition. It has four hidden layers consisting of 500, 500, 200 and 500 neurons. Notably, its architecture is

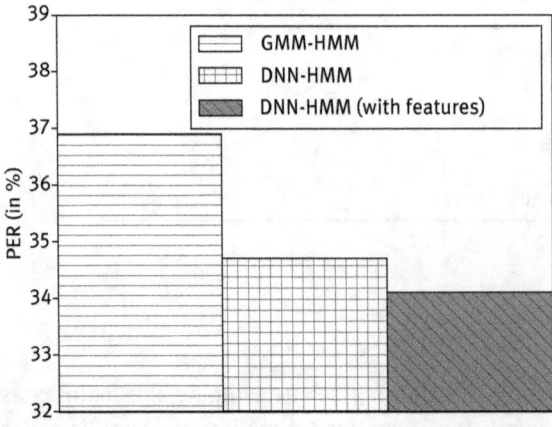

Figure 6: Phoneme Error Rate (PER), in %ge, over TIMIT test set.

the same as the cascaded DNN system in the proposed scheme, sans the layer of features. The input to the DNN and the decoding scheme is the same as that for the proposed method described in Sections 6.1 and 6.2. This method forms the baseline of how well a conventional DNN-HMM system performs.

6.6 Experiments

In order to evaluate the capability of features for faithfully capturing the acoustic information, experiments have been performed for phoneme recognition over the test set. The feature extraction as well as the phoneme recogniser layers are trained using the training set. For training feature estimation, all 61 phonemes of TIMIT are used; but for training and evaluation for phoneme recognition, they are reduced to 48 and 39 phonemes, respectively. The phoneme error rates obtained with different methods are presented in Figure 6.

As expected, the DNN-HMM system outperforms the GMM-HMM system. The advantage of using features is clearly visible. The improvement here may not be statistically significant but the main advantage here is that we get a phonologically meaningful way of implementing ASR, and yet perform on par with those without features. This is a very desirable property (Tan et al., 2015).

7 Conclusion

Modern ASR systems are mostly data-driven. Although being able to use large amounts of data, they are mostly opaque and uninterpretable. This chapter presents phonological feature based ASR systems which perform at par with other ASR systems, but provide an interpretable handle to the acoustic model.

There are many current problems which can be dealt with very efficiently by using this phonological feature based acoustic model. ASR for under-resourced languages and non-native language learning are some of such problems we are currently working on. Linguistic interpretability of low-levels units, like phonological features, can contribute to the problem of transferring acoustic knowledge from one language to another. Since these are the 'building blocks' of a sound system that resembles human's mental representation of sounds, universally across languages, they provide a common platform for knowledge transfer from resource-rich languages (in terms of annotated training data) to languages with scarce training data. Also, the well structured nature of phonological features, from the perspective of production as well as perception, makes them very useful for computer-assisted language learning tools – for detecting mispronunciations as well as providing feedback to the learners of a foreign language.

References

Behera, L. & Kar, I. (2010). *Intelligent systems and control: principles and applications*. Oxford: Oxford University Press.
Boersma, P. & Weenink, D. (2001). Praat, a system for doing phonetics by computer. Version 5.4.06 from http://www.praat.org.
Chiba, T. & Kajiyama, M. (1958). *The vowel: Its nature and structure*. Tokyo-Kaiseikan Pub. Co., Ltd. Tokyo.
Fant, G. (1960). *Acoustic theory of speech production*. The Hague: Mouton.
Garofalo, J. S., Lamel, L. F., Fisher, W. M., Fiscus, J. G., Pallett, D. S. & Dahlgren, N. L. (1990). The DARPA TIMIT acoustic-phonetic continuous speech corpus CD-ROM. *National Institute of Standards and Technology*.
Jakobson, R., Fant, G. & Halle, M. (1951). *Preliminaries to Speech Analysis: The Distinctive Features and their Correlates*. Cambridge, Mass: MIT Press.
Jansen, A. & Niyogi, P. (2009). Point process models for spotting keywords in continuous speech. *IEEE Transactions on Audio, Speech and Language Processing*, 17(8):1457–1470.
Johnson, K. (2005). Speaker normalization in speech perception. In Pisoni, D. B. & Remez, R. (eds). The Handbook of Speech Perception. Oxford: Blackwell, 363–389.
Jongman, A. (1989). Duration of frication noise required for identification of English fricatives. *The Journal of the Acoustical Society of America*, 85(4):1718–1725.
King, S. & Taylor, P. (2000). Detection of phonological features in continuous speech using neural networks. *Computer Speech and Language*, 14(4):333–353.
Klatt, D. H. (1977). Review of the ARPA speech understanding project. *The Journal of the Acoustical Society of America*, 62(6):1345–1366.
Koenig, W., Dunn, H. & Lacy, L. (1946). The sound spectrograph. *The Journal of the Acoustical Society of America*, 18(1):19–49.
Lahiri, A. & Reetz, H. (2010). Distinctive features: Phonological underspecification in representation and processing. *Journal of Phonetics*, 38(1):44–59.
Leonard, R. G. & Doddington, G. (1993). TIDIGITS LDC93S10. *Linguistic Data Consortium*, Philadelphia.
Lowerre, B. T. (1976). *The Harpy Speech Recognition System*. PhD thesis, Carnegie-Mellon University.
Markel, J. D. & Gray, A. J. (1976). *Linear prediction of speech*. Berlin: Springer.
Mitra, V., Sivaraman, G., Nam, H., Espy-Wilson, C. & Saltzman, E. (2014). Articulatory features from deep neural networks and their role in speech recognition. In *IEEE International Conference on Acoustics, Speech and Signal Processing (ICASSP)*, 3041–3045.
Newell, A. (1978). Harpy, production systems and human cognition. *Technical Report*, Carnegie Mellon University.
O'Shaughnessy, D. (2013). Acoustic analysis for automatic speech recognition. *Proceedings of the IEEE*, 101(5):1038–1053.

Povey, D., Ghoshal, A., Boulianne, G., Burget, L., Glembek, O., Goel, N., Hannemann, M., Motlicek, P., Qian, Y., Schwarz, P., Silovsky, J., Stemmer, G. & Vesely, K. (2011). The Kaldi speech recognition toolkit. In *IEEE 2011 Workshop on Automatic Speech Recognition and Understanding*. IEEE Signal Processing Society.

Scanlon, P., Ellis, D. P. W. & Reilly, R. B. (2007). Using broad phonetic group experts for improved speech recognition. *IEEE Transactions on Audio, Speech and Language Processing*, 15(3):803–812.

Stevens, K. N. (2002). Toward a model for lexical access based on acoustic landmarks and distinctive features. *The Journal of the Acoustical Society of America*, 111(4):1872–1891.

Tan, S., Sim, K. C. & Gales, M. (2015). Improving the interpretability of deep neural networks with stimulated learning. In *IEEE Workshop on Automatic Speech Recognition and Understanding*, 617–623.

Yu, D. & Deng, L. (2014). *Automatic Speech Recognition: A Deep Learning Approach*. Berlin: Springer.

Eiling Yee
Fluid semantics: Semantic knowledge is experience-based and dynamic

Abstract: Is our internal notion of, e.g., the object *lemon*, static? That is, do we have stable semantic representations that remain constant across time? Most semantic memory researchers still (at least tacitly) take a static perspective, assuming that only effects that can be demonstrated across a variety of tasks and contexts should be considered informative about the architecture of the semantic system. This chapter challenges this perspective by highlighting studies showing that the cognitive and neural representations of object concepts are fluid, changing as a consequence of the context that each individual brings with them (e.g., via current goals, recent experience, long-term experience, or neural degeneration). These findings support models of semantic memory in which rather than being static, conceptual representations are dynamic and shaped by experience, whether that experience extends over the lifetime, the task, or the moment.

Introduction

Lemon. We can consider its shape, approximate size, color, taste, texture, weight, etc. How is this information organized in the semantic/conceptual system? How does information about one concept relate to information about other concepts? How does an object concept's representation map onto the corresponding real world object? And what are some of the ways in which representations might change over time?

At first glance, conceptual representations (such as our internal notion of the object *lemon*) seem static. That is, we have the impression that there is something that lemon means (a sour, yellow, rugby ball-shaped, citrus fruit) and that this meaning does not vary. Research in semantic memory traditionally takes this

---

Eiling Yee, Department of Psychological Sciences, University of Connecticut; Basque Center on Cognition, Brain & Language

static perspective. Yet, according to more recent accounts of semantic/conceptual knowledge, knowledge of object properties (e. g., color, shape and smell) is distributed (in part) across brain regions that underlie sensory and motor processing (e. g. Allport, 1985; Barsalou, 1999; Damasio, 1989), and concepts are multi-dimensional representations across those substrates. Thus, according to these "sensorimotor-based" distributed accounts, the "meaning" of a lemon is not an indivisible whole, but is distributed across a range of featural dimensions (cf. McRae, de Sa & Seidenberg, 1997; Rogers & McClelland, 2004; Tyler & Moss, 2001; Vigliocco, Vinson, Levis & Garrett, 2004).

In this chapter, we focus on some of the things that such distributed, sensorimotor-based accounts of semantic representations allow for. For example, sensorimotor-based models predict that sensory and motor features are among those that make up semantic representations, and they make predictions about the organization of semantic representations. Specifically, if a brain area that perceives a given feature is the same region that represents it, then if two concepts share a perceptual feature, their representations must overlap in that brain region. Also, if representations are distributed, this means that an entire concept would not have to be activated at once – its various semantic features (e. g., its shape, or the purpose for which it is used) could be activated at different rates or, be more activated in some circumstances than others. Furthermore, if representations are sensorimotor-based, then disrupting or interfering with a sensorimotor brain area could interfere with conceptual access.

Although some of the predictions that sensorimotor-based distributed models make about how we represent and access semantic knowledge may seem, on the surface, surprising, in the sections that follow, we describe evidence supporting these predictions. In section one, we suggest that the semantic features over which objects are represented can include not only more "abstract" features, but also sensory and motor features. We also argue that different features may have different time courses of activation. In section two, we describe evidence that semantic representations of object concepts can overlap in sensorimotor and multimodal cortices. In the third section, we argue that for object concepts, sensorimotor activity is part of (rather than peripheral to) their semantic representations. In the fourth and fifth sections, we suggest that prior experience and individual abilities modulate semantic access. Finally, we conclude that semantic representations are much more fluid than they may seem at first glance.

1 Which semantic features are included in object representations, and what is the time course over which these features are activated?

Since distributed models of semantic memory assume that concepts that share features have overlapping patterns of representation, activating a particular concept should also partially activate other concepts that share its features. The semantic priming effect, wherein identifying a target word is facilitated when it is preceded by a (conceptually) related prime word (e. g., Meyer & Schvaneveldt, 1971), can therefore be interpreted as support for distributed models. However, semantically related objects are often category coordinates, which are related in multiple ways, e. g., *crayon* and *pencil* are both thin, oblong, used for marking paper, and grasped with the thumb and the second and third fingers (cf. Kellenbach, Wijers & Mulder, 2000). As a result, unless the features of overlap are examined separately, it is not clear which are responsible for the facilitation.

Identifying which features are responsible for the facilitation has implications for theories of semantic memory. Specifically, if words (referring to concepts) that are related via *sensorimotor* features partially activate each other, this would suggest that such features constitute part of the representation of concepts. An increasing number of semantic priming studies have explicitly manipulated the semantic relationship between primes and targets. For example, in an auditory semantic priming paradigm, Myung, Blumstein & Sedivy (2006) observed that lexical decisions on target words were speeded if the prime was an object that was manipulated similarly for use (e. g., *key* primes *screwdriver* because using each involves twisting the wrist; we discuss this study further in section 3).

Other semantic priming studies have explored whether semantic priming is obtained when primes and targets have the same shape (e. g., coin-button), or are related via a more abstract dimension similar to function/purpose of use (e. g., apple-banana, or stapler-paperclip). Broadly speaking, priming has been observed for both shape similarity (Schreuder, Flores d'Arcais & Glazenborg, 1984; Flores d'Arcais, Schreuder & Glazenbor, 1985; Pecher, Zeelenberg & Raaijmakers, 1998; Taylor, 2005) and function similarity (Schreuder et al., 1984; Flores d'Arcais et al., 1985; Taylor, 2005). However, findings across experiments have been varied, and one explanation put forth for the differences is that different features may become active at different times during semantic activation (Schreuder et al., 1984). Below we describe studies using the "visual world" eyetracking paradigm (Cooper, 1974;

Tanenhaus, Spivey-Knowlton, Eberhard & Sedivy, 1995) that suggest that this is indeed the case.

For instance, we have found evidence that during visual object identification, information about the form of an object (e. g., that knives are oblong) becomes available sooner than information about its function (e. g., that they are used for cutting; Yee, Huffstetler & Thompson-Schill, 2011). Specifically, in a visual world eyetracking study we found that when participants were briefly exposed (for 1 second) to an array of four objects and asked to click on the object corresponding to a heard word, they were sensitive to the fact that one of the other objects in the display was similar in shape (at the conceptual level) to that of the named object. For example, when they heard the target word "Frisbee", they looked at a slice of pizza (another object that can be round). Importantly, shape similarity was not apparent in the visual depictions (e. g., a slice of pizza is triangular, a shape that a Frisbee cannot take, see Figure 1); hence, preferential fixations on the shape-related object were attributable to activation of conceptual shape information (and not to the current input to the senses).

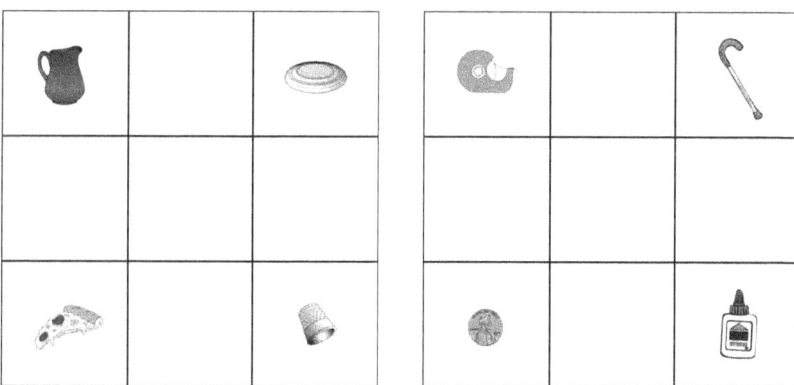

Figure 1: Shape (left panel) and function (right panel) related pairs form Yee et al. (2011).

However with the same 1-second exposure to the array, we found no preferential fixations on objects related in function to the named object. For example, when participants heard the word "tape", they did not preferentially fixate on a bottle of glue. Yet when exposure to the array was lengthened to 2 seconds, we observed the opposite pattern – participants preferentially fixated on the function-related object, but not the shape-related object. Thus, these findings suggest that semantic activation during visual object recognition is a dynamically unfolding process in which function follows form.

Other studies using the visual world paradigm have also found that function information becomes active after other, arguably more perceptually grounded, aspects of conceptual knowledge. For instance, knowledge about the thematic relationships that an object can participate in (i. e., the knowledge that a broom is often paired with/seen with a dustpan, or that a steak is paired/seen with a knife), and knowledge about an object's structural characteristics (its shape, size and volume) appear to become available more rapidly and more transiently than information about its function (see Kalénine, Mirman, Middleton & Buxbaum 2012 for thematic relationships and Lee, Middleton, Mirman, Kalénine & Buxbaum 2013 for structural relationships).

Future work will be needed to learn the cause(s) of this chronology – in which not only does the activation of function information follow the activation of form, but form information seems to be more transiently activated.[1] With respect to function information becoming active later, one possibility is that because information about the purpose for which an object is used is not directly available via the senses, accessing this information requires more processing (and hence more time) than accessing perceptual information. Another possibility is that in the studies reviewed above, perceptual information has special status because the visual world paradigm task – essentially a visual search task – *requires* attending to perceptual information. A third (compatible) possibility is that presenting stimuli in the visual modality (regardless of whether the task is visual search) places emphasis on visual information.

Studies using written words provide a hint that the modality of the stimulus, rather than the visual search task *per se*, contributes to the earlier activation of perceptual information. For example, when reading sentences referring to objects (e. g., a calculator), information that is directly available from perceiving the object (e. g., the grasp that one would use to pick up a calculator to move it) becomes less active over time, while information that requires more abstract knowledge about the purpose of the object (e. g., the finger poke that one would use to operate a calculator) becomes more active over time (Bub & Masson, 2010).

Along the same lines, the semantic priming studies referred to at the beginning of this section that did obtain evidence of shape priming all used written words (Flores d'Arcais, et al., 1985; Schreuder et al., 1984; Pecher et al., 1998: Experiments 4 and 6). Moreover, as alluded to earlier, they also found evidence that priming based on function emerges more reliably at long, rather than short

---

[1] One might speculate that form information rapidly decays (or is inhibited) in favor of function information because although form is needed for object recognition, once the object is recognized, other attributes, such as what it is used for, are typically more relevant.

interstimulus intervals, whereas priming based on shape relatedness was larger at short than long interstimulus intervals (Flores d'Arcais et al., 1985; Schreuder et al., 1984). In other words, the chronology parallels what has been found in the visual world paradigm, even for a task that does not require visual search.

Although these findings rule out visual search *per se* as the sole reason that perceptual features become active earlier than more abstract features, is it possible that perceptual information becomes active early because both written words and visual objects place emphasis on the visual modality? Or does perceptual information become active first during conceptual activation, regardless of context? As we describe next, when stimuli are not visually presented, perceptual information does not always become active first, suggesting that stimulus modality (e. g., visual vs. auditory) does indeed affect the dynamics of featural activation.

In a cross-modal semantic priming study in which primes were auditory words (targets were written), priming for visually related targets was observed, but it was delayed in time relative to priming for targets related to the typical use of the prime[2] (Moss, McCormick & Tyler, 1997). Another study that presented object names auditorily obtained analogous results: Information that is directly available from viewing the object (here, information about how one grasps an object to move it) became active later (and for a shorter duration) than information about how an object is manipulated in order to use it – i. e., its function (Bub & Masson, 2012). Thus, in contrast to when primes are visual, when the primes (or the sole presented words) are auditory, activation of perceptual information can appear later than functional information (see Garcea & Mahon, 2012 for related work).

Hence, the ebb and flow of different features seems to be influenced by the relationship between the modality of the stimulus and the specific feature: When the stimulus is presented visually, visual features may become active earlier than more abstract knowledge. In contrast, when the stimulus is presented auditorily, the reverse pattern is observed.[3] The dynamics of featural activation during

---

[2] Perceptually related targets were primarily visible parts of the prime or what the prime is typically made of (e. g., *blouse-button* or *sandal-leather*), while use-related targets typically denoted the primary purpose of the prime or the location in which the prime is used (e. g., *blouse-wear; satchel-school; radio-music*).

[3] Task may also interact with which features become available when: Rogers and Patterson (2007) have shown that when the task is categorization (e. g., judging whether the word "canary" [or on other trials, "bird", or "animal"] correctly identifies a picture of a canary), information that can distinguish among objects in the same semantic neighborhood (e. g., the property "yellow" distinguishes canaries from robins) becomes available later than more general information (information that does not help in distinguishing amount objects in the same neighborhood; e. g., the property "can fly" is shared by most birds).

semantic activation, therefore, appear to depend upon the modality (i.e., the context) in which the concept is presented, and may also depend on which features are typically most relevant. Importantly, the fact that some types of featural information become active earlier than others during semantic activation is consistent with distributed models of semantic representation because in these models different features can be differentially activated.

With respect to the "sensorimotor-based" claim of sensorimotor-based distributed models, it is important to note that priming has been observed for both perceptual (e.g., shape) and motor (e.g., manipulation) features, *as well as* more abstract features (e.g., function). While perceptual overlap is clearly predicted on sensorimotor models, such models do not require overlap on more abstract features (such as an object's function/purpose of use), as these cannot be directly perceived via any individual sensory modality. As a result, a *purely* sensorimotor-based model would not be sufficient to accommodate these patterns. Instead, a model is required in which higher order similarity can be represented – perhaps by abstracting across similarity in the contexts in which things are used. We will return to this idea in the next section.

In sum, the results described in this section are consistent with distributed semantic representations that are at least partially sensorimotor-based, but that also include higher-order information, such as the purpose for which an object is used.

2 In which brain regions does representational overlap occur?

The semantic relatedness effects described in the prior section suggest that *somewhere* in the brain, the representations of objects overlap such that they can partially activate one another, but they do not address the nature of this neural representation (e.g., *where* in the brain the representations overlap). In this section we turn to studies using functional magnetic resonance imaging (fMRI) to address this question.

A large body of fMRI studies have indicated that the different components of semantic knowledge about an object (e.g., its color, action or sound) activate neural systems that are close to, or overlap with those involved in perceiving those sensory features, or producing those actions (e.g., for color: Martin, Haxby, Lalonde, Wiggs & Ungerleider, 1995; Simmons et al., 2007 and Hsu, Kraemer, Oliver, Schlichting & Thompson-Schill, 2011; for action: Chao & Martin, 2000; for sounds: Kiefer, Sim, Herrnberger, Grothe & Hoenig, 2008).

Findings like these provide support for sensorimotor-based models because they are consistent with the idea that the brain regions that are active when we *perceive and interact with* an object are the same ones that represent it. And recall that, because of this, sensorimotor-based models predict that when two objects share a sensory feature such as shape, their representations would overlap in brain regions involved in perceiving shape. Similarly, if objects are manipulated similarly (e. g., *key* and *screwdriver*) their representations should overlap in brain regions involved in performing object-related actions (i. e., in the "dorsal stream"). In two fMRI studies, we examined the neural encoding of two sensorimotor-based features (shape and manipulation) as well as a more abstract feature (function).

The paradigm we used takes advantage of the fact that repeated presentation of the same visual or verbal stimulus results in reduced fMRI signal levels in brain regions that process that stimulus, either because of neuronal "fatigue" (e. g., firing-rate adaptation) or because the initial activation of a stimulus' representation is less neurally efficient than its subsequent activation (see Grill-Spector, Henson & Martin, 2006 for a review). In a typical fMRI-adaptation experiment, stimuli are presented which are either identical (which produces an adaptation/reduced hemodynamic response) or completely different (producing a recovery response). However, using stimuli pairs that are semantically related, rather than identical, also produces an adaptation effect (e. g., Kotz, Cappa, von Cramon & Friederici, 2002; Rissman, Eliassen & Blumstein, 2003; Matsumoto, Iidaka, Haneda, Okada & Sadato, 2005; Bedny, McGill & Thompson-Schill, 2008). Hence, the paradigm's sensitivity to similarity means that it can be used to detect which brain regions encode different conceptual features.

In our studies, we used an fMRI-adaptation paradigm to obtain a neural metric of similarity between objects. We found that in regions involved in guiding actions (i. e., premotor cortex and intraparietal sulcus), the degree of fMRI-adaptation to a pair of objects is correlated with the degree of similarity in the actions we use to interact with them. For example, a key and a screwdriver (which we use with similar hand and wrist motions) have similar representations in action regions, just as they should if representations are sensorimotor based. We also found several regions in which degree of adaptation is correlated with similarity in function. Two of these regions (medial temporal lobe and posterior middle temporal gyrus) are thought to be involved in integrating information; the activation in these regions is consistent with the idea that encoding more abstract information (such as an object's function) requires integrating information from multiple modalities (Yee, Drucker & Thomson-Schill, 2010). Unexpectedly, we found no evidence at all of representational overlap based on shape similarity, even when performing exploratory analyses that did not use stringent corrections for multiple statistical comparisons.

Recalling that semantic priming and eye-trakcing studies suggest that the activation of information about an object's form may be transient, we hypothesized that our null effect for shape similarity could be due to the timing of the presentation of stimuli. In particular, we speculated that shape information about the prime was no longer active by the time the target appeared. We therefore conducted a second fMRI-adaptation study using a shorter interstimulus interval (ISI). However, even with an ISI similar to that used in the semantic priming studies that did observe a priming effect for shape, we found no evidence of adaptation for shape, anywhere in the brain (Yee, Musz & Thompson-Schill, 2012). Nor did we observe behavioral priming for shape-related pairs (we did observe behavioral priming for manipulation-related pairs). One possible reason for this null result is that the task (concreteness judgment)[4] focused attention away from shape information.

The fact that we did not observe an adaptation or priming effect for shape suggests an interesting potential difference between shape and manipulation information. Although neither shape *nor* manipulation information is required to perform a concreteness judgment, we observed evidence that manipulation knowledge was accessed, and no evidence that shape knowledge was. This may suggest that (at least for the objects that we tested) manipulation is a more routinely, or more strongly accessed feature of conceptual knowledge than is shape. One possibility is that this difference exists because shape is more context-dependent than manipulation; for example, the shape in which a book appears depends on whether, in a given instance, you are looking at it from the top or the side, and it's shape can change depending upon whether it is open or closed. In contrast, how one manipulates an object for use tends to be more stable. The difference also highlights that different features can be activated independently, which provides more evidence that different features are separable components of distributed semantic knowledge.

These fMRI findings converge with the studies described in the first section to suggest that objects that are manipulated similarly, or that have similar functions have overlapping representations. Moreover, they provide information about *where* in the brain the representational overlap occurs. Specifically, objects that are manipulated similarly have overlapping representations in action regions, and objects that have similar functions have representational overlap in regions involved in integrating information. These findings suggest that semantic knowledge consists of both sensorimotor (e. g., manipulation) *and* abstract

---

[4] Note that that in the behavioral studies described above, shape priming was most robust when the task was naming (Pecher et al., 1998).

(e. g., function) knowledge. Therefore although semantic memory may have sensorimotor information at its base, it must also incorporate a way for more abstract knowledge to be represented.

3 Is sensorimotor activity part of conceptual knowledge?

As described above, there is good evidence that semantic knowledge about object concepts is distributed across multimodal and sensorimotor brain regions. However, a frequently raised question that the studies described above do not address is whether the neural activity that is observed in sensorimotor regions during semantic access is *part* of the semantic knowledge being accessed, or rather, is incidental to it. That is, on some theoretical models, sensorimotor activity could, in principle, be incidental to the activation of an amodal (or 'disembodied') concept, rather than part of the concept (for discussion see Mahon & Caramazza, 2008; Anderson & Spivey, 2009; Chatterjee, 2010).

One often-cited fact that has been pointed to as evidence that such activations are only incidental is that there exist patients with motor or sensory deficits who, despite having difficulty performing, e. g., object-related actions, can retain the ability to name, and may also be able to describe the use of objects with strongly associated actions. These abilities have been taken as evidence that such individuals have intact conceptual knowledge and thus, that sensory or motor information is not part of conceptual knowledge (see Negri et al., 2007).

However, distributed models of semantic memory posit that conceptual representations include many different components (e. g., visual, auditory, and olfactory as well as action-oriented and multi-modal) that are distributed across cortex. Moreover, there is evidence that conceptual information is represented at multiple levels of abstraction, and consequently, depending upon the context, conceptual activation may involve the activation of some levels more than others (for discussion, see Thompson-Schill, 2003; Binder & Desai, 2011). For instance, in an fMRI study, Hsu, et al. (2011) asked participants to judge which of two objects a third object most resembled in color. When the three objects were all from the same color category (e. g., butter, egg yolk, and school bus – all are yellow), and so the task context required retrieving detailed color knowledge, the neural response overlapped more with brain regions involved in color perception than when two of the three objects were from different color categories (e. g., one red and two yellow objects) and therefore less detailed color knowledge was necessary. This finding implies that a task that requires a high degree of perceptual resolution involves perceptual areas more than a task that can be performed on the basis of more categorical (or abstracted) knowledge.

For these reasons (as we and others – e. g., Taylor & Zwaan 2009 – have argued previously), having difficulty accessing part of a representation would not be expected to result in catastrophic conceptual loss (although depending upon the task, some impairment may be detectable). In other words, "brain damage leading to problems performing an action with a particular object does not entail difficulty recognizing that object ... the object may be recognizable on the basis of other aspects of its representation (and the extent to which there are other aspects to rely upon may vary across individuals)" (Yee, Chrysikou, Hoffman & Thompson-Schill, 2013; 917–918).

In fact, not only may object recognition (e. g., of a typewriter) remain successful for an individual who has an impairment in e. g., accessing knowledge about object-directed action, but even access to information that *is* specifically related to the affected modality may not be *entirely* lost (e. g., access to knowledge about how one moves one's fingers to press the keys of a typewriter may be delayed, but not lost). To illustrate, we have examined participants with ideomotor apraxia, which is a neurological impairment, typically caused by stroke that causes difficulty performing object-related actions. Our starting point was the finding that unimpaired participants exhibit priming for objects that are manipulated similarly – both standard auditory word priming (as described in section 1), as well as manipulation relatedness effects in the visual world paradigm (Myung, Blumstein & Sedivy, 2006). When we examined apraxic participants, we found that they had abnormally delayed access to manipulation information about objects (Myung et al., 2010), and moreover, the amount of delay was correlated with *how much* difficulty they had performing object related actions (see also Lee, Mirman & Buxbaum, 2014). This finding shows that damage to a brain region supporting object-related action can hinder access knowledge about how objects are manipulated, even if that information is not entirely lost.

However, while our study with apraxic individuals demonstrated that problems performing object related actions can cause problems accessing manipulation knowledge about an object, it was not designed to test whether such manipulation knowledge is *part of* an object's semantic representation. To answer the latter question, it is necessary to determine whether problems accessing manipulation knowledge about an object can interfere with thinking about that object more generally, e. g., even when access to manipulation information about it is not required. This is what we asked in a subsequent study. Specifically, we asked whether performing a concurrent manual task that is incompatible with how a given object is acted upon can interfere with thinking about that object. We found evidence that it can: If, while naming pictures, participants had to concurrently perform an unrelated sequence of hand motions, picture naming was more disrupted for objects that are typically interacted with manually than objects that are less frequently interacted with manually (e. g., there was relatively more interference for pencils vs. tigers; Yee et al., 2013; see also Witt, Kemmerer, Linkenauger & Culham, 2010).

Thus, the context of a concurrent manual task interfered with people's ability to think about objects that are frequently manipulated. This demonstrates that 1) manipulation information is part of the representation of frequently manipulated objects, and 2) that our ability to think about a given object depends on the match between our mental representation of that object's meaning and what we are doing at the moment.

Moreover, because activity in motor areas influences semantic retrieval, findings such as this one suggest that motor area activity is *more than a* "peripheral" part of conceptual knowledge – it is *part* of conceptual knowledge. More broadly, these findings from unimpaired participants converge with patient and fMRI work in supporting the idea that activity in sensorimotor brain regions can be part of an object's concept.

4 Can what we have recently been doing affect semantic activation?

The findings described above also have another implication: They suggest that our ability to access semantic representations is dynamic in the sense that it can change depending on what exactly we may be doing at the moment. This raises a question. Can what we have *recently* been doing also affect how we access semantic knowledge?

We addressed this question using a different approach than in our studies examining manipulation knowledge. Rather than testing whether accessing a particular semantic feature can be made more difficult (e. g., via brain damage or a concurrent incompatible task), we instead asked whether it is possible to *enhance* our ability to access a concept (or, a particular aspect of a concept) through a recent activity. We used the semantic feature of color as a test case (Yee, Ahmed & Thomson-Schill, 2012). Color is particularly interesting: In the visual object recognition literature, a point of contention has been whether color is, or is not a part of an object's representation (Biederman & Ju, 1988). There is evidence that color only becomes part of the representation of objects for which it is both consistent (e. g., lemons are normally yellow) *and* for which it is important for distinguishability (e. g., color is necessary for distinguishing lemons from limes; Tanaka & Presnell,

1999). The idea that consistency is important is clearly compatible with sensorimotor-based models – the more consistently associated a color is with an object, the more frequently it will be experienced in that color, and it is those experiences that cause color to become a part of the object's representation. Moreover, if distinguishability is also important, this suggests that *attention* can influence the extent to which color becomes a part of an object's representation – the idea being that the more important color is for distinguishing an object, the more that attention will be focused on color when that object is experienced, which will strengthen color's involvement in its representation. An intriguing extension of this idea is that, for objects for which color is already part of the representation, attention may play a role in the extent to which color information is activated in a given episode.

Our examination of color suggests that its activation is indeed modulated by attention: We found that recent experience can influence the activation of color as a semantic feature in a subsequent, unrelated task. Specifically, we have found that although lemons and daffodils, for example, overlap on the dimension of color (both are yellow), and might therefore be expected to partially activate one another, the word "lemon" does not ordinarily activate, or prime, "daffodil". However, it can prime "daffodil" if participants' attention has been focused on color in a prior task involving unrelated items (e. g., color words in a Stroop task; Yee Ahmed & Thompson-Schill, 2012). Similar findings have been reported in other modalities. For example, Pecher, and colleagues (1998) observed shape priming (e. g., the word "coin" priming the word "button") only when, prior to the priming experiment, participants made shape judgments about the objects to which the words referred. Thus, recent experience can linger long enough to affect conceptual activation in a subsequent, unrelated task.

Additional evidence that recent experience affects semantic activation comes from van Dantzig and colleagues (2008), who have shown that the modality to which attention is directed immediately prior to thinking about objects can affect conceptual activation: Between trials that required participants to make truefalse judgments on sentences referring to object properties (e. g., *broccoli is green* or *soup is hot*), participants responded to either a visual light, an auditory noise, or a tactile vibration; property judgments were faster when the modality to which the sentence referred was the same as the preceding perceptual stimulus.

Along similar lines, but using a more implicit measure of conceptual activation, Bermeitinger, Wentura & Frings (2011) found that when an independent task directing attention to shape was interspersed with a semantic priming task, priming for words referring to natural kinds (for which shape is known to be a particularly important feature) was greater than priming for artifacts. In contrast, priming was greater for artifacts (for which action is known to be a particularly important feature) than for natural kinds when the interspersed task directed attention to action. By inserting a task that directs attention to one modality or another, these two studies converge with our color-priming study (Yee et al., 2012) to show that directing attention to a particular modality changes subsequent conceptual activation such that information related to that modality is activated more easily. Several other behavioral studies have reported compatible results (e. g., Martens, Ansorge & Kiefer, 2011; Van Dam, Rueschemeyer, Lindemann & Bekkering, 2010), and neural activation patterns are also consistent with this kind of attentionally modulated flexibility in semantic activation (Hoenig, Sim, Bochev, Herrnberger & Kiefer, 2008; Mummery, Patterson, Hodges & Price, 1998; Phillips, Noppeney, Humphreys & Price 2002; Thompson-Schill, Aguirre, D'Esposito & Farah, 1999; Rogers, Hocking, Mechelli, Patterson & Price, 2005; Van Dam, van Dijk, Bekkering & Rueschemeyer 2012; for review, see Willems & Francken 2012).

5 Is your lemon different from mine?

So far, we have described evidence supporting distributed, sensorimotor-based semantic representations. However, we have not yet considered (1) whether factors intrinsic to the individual, such as individual differences in cognitive abilities, might impact an individual's semantic processing in general, or (2) whether such factors might impact the extent to which a given individual's semantic activation is affected by what they are doing at the moment or what they have been recently doing. In this section, we speculate about some individual factors that we hypothesize may affect both semantic processing and the influence of concurrent and recent experience on such processing.

First, individual differences in processing preferences may impact conceptual activation: In the color-priming study described in the prior section, in which lemon only primed daffodil if participants' attention had been focused on color in a prior, ostensibly unrelated Stroop task, we also observed that individual differences in the ability to selectively focus on color in the Stroop task predicted the amount of priming (see Figure 2). This relationship could reflect differences in the degrees to which people attend to or perceive color (as in Hsu et al., 2011): Individuals who attend to color more would more strongly associate conceptual color with both color words in the Stroop task (e. g., green) and with the names of objects in the priming task (e. g., cucumber).

However, another compatible possibility relates to selective attention: The general ability to selectively attend to one dimension at the expense of others (e. g., to focus on a word's font color while ignoring its meaning) is an aspect of cognitive control (Posner & Snyder, 1975) and varies across individuals. Thus, a high capacity for selective attention could manifest as enhanced selective attention to the features most relevant for the current task (in this case, judging animal status), and hence as less activation of other features (e. g., color).

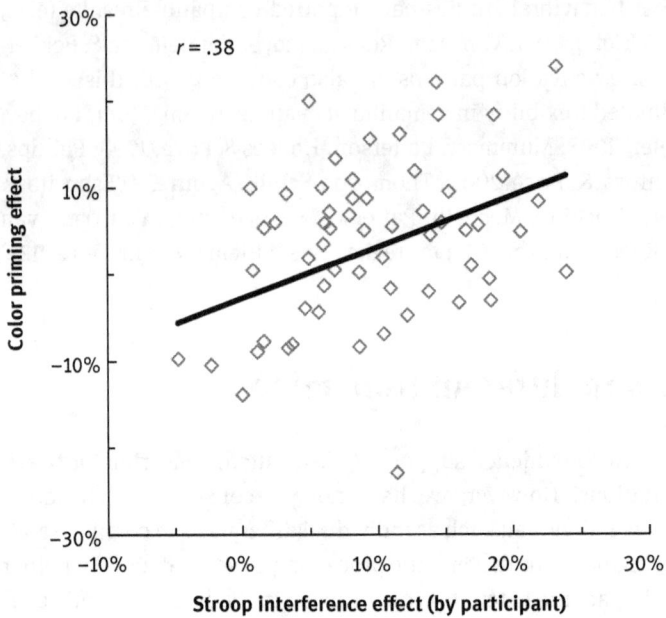

Figure 2: Scatter plot showing correlation between Stroop interference effect and color-priming effect (Yee et al., 2012).

This account is particularly interesting because it is consistent with the proposal that cognitive control regulates the ability to selectively attend to the task-relevant features of a concept in general (see Kan & Thompson-Schill, 2004a; Thompson-Schill, Bedny & Goldberg, 2005). Evidence consistent with this account has come from a recent study demonstrating that inhibitory electrical stimulation over left prefrontal cortex (a brain region that supports cognitive control) interferes with the ability to categorize objects according to a specific attribute (e. g., "round or red things") relative to categorizing objects at a more general level (e. g., "things that hold water"; Lupyan, Mirman, Hamilton & Thompson-Schill, 2012; for related work, see also Chrysikou et al., 2013; Kan & Thompson-Schill, 2004b; Lupyan & Mirman, 2013).

If individual processing preferences or cognitive control abilities indeed affect the extent to which semantic activation is affected by context, this suggests that "meaning" must vary, not only from one context to another, but also within a given context, from one person to another. Yet if this is true, then how is it that, in the face of different experiences, individuals are able to understand each other when they use conventionalized labels? In other words, if what is retrieved from semantic memory is so variable across time and individuals, then shouldn't communication be even more difficult than it is? Fortunately, there are significant commonalities in human experience (and especially within a given culture) that would lead different individuals' representations (and their labels) to be similar enough for most practical purposes. Moreover, often communication does not require that the interlocutors be activating the exact same conceptual representations (for further consideration of this point, see Casasanto & Lupyan, 2015; Connell & Lynott, 2014; Taylor & Zwaan, 2009), and in cases in which greater precision is desirable, communication often requires clarification ("no, no, no ... that's not kale, it's chard!").

Conclusions

Collectively, the studies reviewed above suggest that semantic knowledge about objects is instantiated as patterns of activation that are distributed across both sensorimotor and abstract features, with relationships between concepts captured by overlap in these patterns. Perhaps more surprisingly, they also suggest that semantic knowledge is fluid, changing not only as a function of our individual experiences with objects but, even more surprisingly, as a function of what we have recently been doing, and even as the process of object recognition unfolds. Thus, semantic memory is not static.

This fluidity highlights that semantic representations, like the word forms that refer to them, are highly context dependent. That is, just as the sequence of sounds that we produce to refer to something depends upon our long-term experiences (e. g., language, accent, whether we are toddlers or adults), short-term goals (e. g., register, emphasis) and the current articulatory context (e. g., surrounding words), so does the representation that is activated by those sounds.

That this kind of malleability exists in the mature semantic system has an important implication. It suggests that the same architecture that, in infancy, permits the semantic system to develop through interactions with the world,[5]

---

[5] See Yee & Thompson-Schill (2016) for a discussion of one such architecture – an emergentist approach to cognitive development (e. g., Elman et al., 1996) in which context effects are a natural consequence of how concepts are acquired and represented in the first place, and in which change over time is naturally accommodated.

also allows the mature semantic system to be sensitive to, and change as a consequence of, the ever-richer contexts in which we, as humans, continue to develop. Thus, while semantics are fluid, there may be continuity across the lifespan in the underlying mechanisms of the system that allows for this fluidity.

References

Allport, D. A. (1985). Distributed memory, modular subsystems and dysphasia. In S. K. Newman & R. Epstein (Eds.), *Current Perspectives in Dysphasia* (pp. 207–244). Edinburgh: Churchill Livingstone.
Anderson, S. E. & Spivey, M. J. (2009). The enactment of language: Decades of interactions between linguistic and motor processes. *Language and Cognition*, *1*, 87–111.
Barsalou, L. W. (1999). Perceptual symbol systems. *Behavioral Brain Science*, *22*, 577–660.
Bedny, M., McGill, M. & Thompson-Schill, S. L. 2008. Semantic adaptation and competition during word comprehension. *Cerebral Cortex 18*(11), 2574–2585.
Bermeitinger, C., Wentura, D. & Frings, C. (2011). How to switch on and switch off semantic priming effects: Activation processes in category memory depend on focusing specific feature dimensions. *Psychonomic Bulletin & Review*, *18*, 579–585.
Biederman, I. & Ju, G. (1988). Surface versus edge-based determinants of visual recognition. *Cognitive psychology*, *20*(1), 38–64.
Binder, J. R. & Desai, R. H. (2011). The neurobiology of semantic memory. *Trends in Cognitive Sciences*, *15*, 527–536.
Bub, D. N. & Masson, M. E. J. (2010). On the nature of hand-action representations evoked during written sentence comprehension. *Cognition*, *116*, 394–408.
Bub, D. N. & Masson, M. E. J. (2012). On the dynamics of action representations evoked by names of manipulable objects. *Journal of Experimental Psychology: General*, *141*, 502–517.
Casasanto, D. & Lupyan, G. (2015). All concepts are ad hoc concepts. In E. Margolis & S. Laurence (Eds.), *The conceptual mind: New directions in the study of concepts* (pp. 543–566). Cambridge: MIT Press.
Chao, L.L. & Martin, A. (2000). Representation of manipulable man-made objects in the dorsal stream. *NeuroImage*, *12*, 478–484.
Chatterjee, A. (2010). Disembodying cognition. *Language and Cognition*, *2*, 79–116.
Chrysikou, E. G., Hamilton, R. H., Coslett, H. B., Datta, A., Bikson, M. & Thompson-Schill, S. L. (2013). Non-invasive transcranial direct current stimulation over the left prefrontal cortex facilitates cognitive flexibility in tool use. *Cognitive Neuroscience*, *4*, 81–89.
Connell, L. & Lynott, D. (2014). I see/hear what you mean: semantic activation in visual word recognition depends on perceptual attention. *Journal of Experimental Psychology: General*. *143*(2), p. 527–533.
Cooper, R. M. (1974). The control of eye fixation by the meaning of spoken language: A new methodology for the real-time investigation of speech perception, memory, and language processing. *Cognitive Psychology*, *6*, 84–107
Damasio, A. R. (1989). The brain binds entities and events by multiregional activation from convergence zones. *Neural Computation*, *1*, 123–132.

Elman, J. L., Bates, E. A., Johnson, M. H., Karmiloff-Smith, A., Parisi, D. & Plunkett, K. (1996). *Rethinking innateness: A connectionist perspective on development.* Cambridge, MA: MIT Press, Bradford Books.

Flores d'Arcais, G. & Schreuder, R. & Glazenborg, G. (1985). Semantic activation during recognition or referential words. *Psychological Research 47,* 39–49.

Garcea, F. E. & Mahon, B. Z. (2012). What is in a tool concept? Dissociating manipulation knowledge from function knowledge. *Memory & cognition, 40*(8), 1303–1313.

Grill-Spector, K., Henson, R. & Martin, A., 2006. Repetition and the brain: neural models of stimulus-specific effects, *Trends in Cognitive Sciences 10*(1), 14–23.

Hoenig, K., Sim, E.-J., Bochev, V., Herrnberger, B. & Kiefer, M. (2008). Conceptual flexibility in the human brain: Dynamic recruitment of semantic maps from visual, motion and motor-related areas. *Journal of Cognitive Neuroscience, 20*(10), 1799–1814.

Hsu, N.S., Kraemer, D.J.M., Oliver, R.T., Schlichting, M.L. & Thompson-Schill, S.L. (2011). Color, Context, and Cognitive Style: Variations in Color Knowledge Retrieval as a Function of Task and Subject Variables. *Journal of Cognitive Neuroscience, 29*(3), 2544–2557.

Kalénine, S., Mirman, D., Middleton, E. L. & Buxbaum, L. J. (2012). Temporal dynamics of activation of thematic and functional knowledge during conceptual processing of manipulable artifacts. *Journal of Experimental Psychology: Learning, Memory, and Cognition, 38*(5), 1274–1295. DOI: 10.1037/a0027626.

Kan, I. P. & Thompson-Schill, S. L. (2004a). Selection from perceptual and conceptual representations. Cognitive, *Affective & Behavioral Neuroscience, 4,* 466–482. PMID: 15849891.

Kan I. P. & Thompson-Schill, S. L. (2004b). Effect of name agreement on prefrontal activity during overt and covert picture naming. *Cognitive, Affective & Behavioral Neuroscience, 4,* 43–57.

Kellenbach, M. L., Wijers, A. A. & Mulder, G. (2000). Visual semantic features are activated during the processing of concrete words: Event- related potential evidence for perceptual semantic priming. *Cognitive Brain Research, 10,* 67–75.

Kiefer, M., Sim, E.-J., Herrnberger, B., Grothe, J. & Hoenig, K. (2008). The sound of concepts for markers for a link between auditory and conceptual brain systems. *The Journal of Neuroscience, 28,* 12224–12230.

Kotz, S.A., Cappa, S.F., von Cramon, D.Y. & Friederici, A.D., 2002. Modulation of the lexical-semantic network by auditory semantic priming: *An event-related functional MRI study.* NeuroImage 17, 1761–1772.

Lee, C.-L., Middleton, E. L., Mirman, D., Kalénine, S., and Buxbaum, L. J. (2013). Incidental and context-responsive activation of structure- and function-based action features during object identification. *Journal of Experimental Psychology: Human Perception and Performance, 39*(1), 257–270. DOI: 10.1037/a0027533.

Lee, C.-L., Mirman, D. & Buxbaum, L.J. (2014). Abnormal dynamics of activation of object use information in apraxia: Evidence from eyetracking. *Neuropsychologia, 59,* 13–26. DOI: 10.1016/j.neuropsychologia.2014.04.004.

Lupyan, G. & Mirman, D. (2013). Linking language and categorization: Evidence from aphasia. *Cortex, 49*(5), 1187–1194. DOI: 10.1016/j.cortex.2012.06.006.

Lupyan, G., Mirman, D., Hamilton, R. & Thompson-Schill, S. L. (2012). Categorization is modulated by transcranial direct current stimulation over left prefrontal cortex. *Cognition, 124*(1), 36–49.

Mahon, B. Z. & Caramazza, A. (2008). A Critical Look at the Embodied Cognition Hypothesis & a New Proposal for Grounding Conceptual Content. *Journal of Physiology – Paris, 102,* 59–70.

Martens, U., Ansorge, U. & Kiefer, M. (2011). Controlling the unconscious: Attentional task sets modulate subliminal semantic and visuo-motor processes differentially. *Psychological Science, 22*, 282–291.

Martin, A., Haxby, J.V., Lalonde, F. M., Wiggs, C. L. & Ungerleider, L. G. (1995). Discrete cortical regions associated with knowledge of color and knowledge of action. *Science, 270*, 102–105.

Matsumoto, A., Iidaka, T., Haneda, K., Okada, T. & Sadato, N., 2005. Linking semantic priming effect in functional MRI and event-related potentials. *NeuroImage 24*(3), 624–634.

McRae, K., de Sa, V. R. & Seidenberg, M. S. (1997). On the nature and scope of featural representations of word meaning. *Journal of Experimental Psychology: General, 126*, 99–130.

Meyer, D.E. & Schvaneveldt, R.W. (1971). Facilitation in recognizing pairs of words: Evidence of a dependence between retrieval operations. *Journal of Experimental Psychology, 90*, 227–234.

Moss, H.E., McCormick, S.F. & Tyler, L.K. (1997). The time course of activation of semantic information during spoken word recognition. *Language and Cognitive Processes, 12*, 695–731.

Mummery, C. J., Patterson, K., Hodges, J. R. & Price, C. J. (1998). Functional neuroanatomy of the semantic system: Divisible by what? *Journal of Cognitive Neuroscience, 10*, 766–777.

Myung, J. Y., Blumstein, S. E. & Sedivy, J. C. (2006). Playing on the typewriter, typing on the piano: manipulation knowledge of objects. *Cognition, 98*(3), 223–243.

Myung, J., Blumstein, S. E., Yee, E., Sedivy, J. C., Thompson-Schill, S. L. & Buxbaum, L. J. (2010). Impaired access to manipulation features in apraxia: Evidence from eyetracking and semantic judgment tasks. *Brain and Language, 112*, 101–112.

Negri, G. A. L., Rumiati, R. I., Zadini, A., Ukmar, M., Mahon, B. Z. & Caramazza, A. (2007). What is the role of motor simulation in action and object recognition? Evidence from apraxia. *Cognitive Neuropsychology, 24*, 795–816.

Pecher, D., Zeelenberg, R. & Raaijmakers, J. G. W. (1998). Does pizza prime coin? Perceptual priming in lexical decision and pronunciation. *Journal of Memory and Language, 38*, 401–418. doi:10.1006/ jmla.1997.2557

Phillips J. A., Noppeney U., Humphreys G. W., Price C. J. (2002.) Can segregation within the semantic system account for category specific deficits? *Brain. 125*, 2067–2080.

Posner, M. I. & Snyder, C. R. R. (1975). Attention and cognitive control. In R. L. Solso (Ed.), *Information processing and cognition: The Loyola symposium* (pp. 55–85). Hillsdale: Lawrence Erlbaum Associates.

Rissman, J., Eliassen, J. C. & Blumstein, S. E., 2003. An event-related FMRI investigation of implicit semantic priming. *Journal of Cognitive Neuroscience 15*(8), 1160–1175.

Rogers, T. T. & McClelland, J. L. (2004). *Semantic cognition: A parallel distributed processing approach*. Cambridge, MA: MIT Press

Rogers, T. T. & Patterson, K. (2007). Object categorization: Reversals and explanations of the basic-level advantage. *Journal of Experimental Psychology: General, 136*, 451–469.

Rogers, T. T., Hocking, J., Mechelli, A., Patterson, K. & Price, C. (2005). Fusiform activation to animals is driven by the process, not the stimulus. *Journal of Cognitive Neuroscience, 17*, 434–445.

Schreuder, R., Flores d'Arcais, G. B. & Glazenborg, G. (1984). Effects of perceptual and conceptual similarity in semantic priming. *Psychological Research, 45*(4), 339–354.

Simmons, W., Ramjee, V., Beauchamp, M., McRae, K., Martin, A. & Barsalou, L. (2007). A common neural substrate for perceiving and knowing about color. *Neuropsychologia, 45*, 2802–2810.

Tanaka, J. M. & Presnell, L. M. (1999). *Perception & Psychophysics*, *61*, 1140–1153.

Tanenhaus, M. K., Spivey-Knowlton, M. J., Eberhard, K. M. & Sedivy, J. C. (1995). Integration of visual and linguistic information in spoken language comprehension. *Science*, *268*, 1632–1634.

Taylor, J. R. (2005). On The Perceptual Basis of Semantic Memory: Representation, process and attentional control revealed by behavior and event-related brain potentials. Unpublished Doctoral Dissertation.

Taylor, L. J. & Zwaan, R. A. (2009). Action in cognition: The case of language. *Language and Cognition*, *1*, 45–58.

Thompson-Schill, S. (2003). Neuroimaging studies of semantic memory: Inferring how from where. *Neuropsychologia*, *41*, 280–292.

Thompson-Schill, S. L, Aguirre, G. K., D'Esposito, M. & Farah, M. J. (1999). A neural basis for category and modality specificity of semantic knowledge. *Neuropsychologia*, *37*, 671–676.

Thompson-Schill, S. L., Bedny, M. & Goldberg, R.F. (2005). The frontal lobes and the regulation of mental activity. *Current Opinion in Neurobiology*, *15*, 219–224.

Tyler, L. K. & Moss, H. E. (2001). Towards a distributed account of conceptual knowledge. *Trends in Cognitive Sciences*, *5*, 244–252.

Van Dam, W. O., Rueschemeyer, S.-A., Lindemann, O. & Bekkering, H. (2010). Context effects in embodied lexical- semantic processing. *Frontiers in Psychology*, *1*, 150.

van Dam, W. O., van Dijk, M., Bekkering, H. & Rueschemeyer, S.-A. (2012). Flexibility in embodied lexical-semantic representations. *Human Brain Mapping*, *33*, 2322–2333.

van Dantzig, S., Pecher, D., Zeelenberg, R. & Barsalou, L. W. (2008). Perceptual processing affects conceptual processing. *Cognitive Science*, *32*, 579–590.

Vigliocco, G., Vinson, D. P., Lewis, W. & Garrett, M. F. (2004). Representing the meanings of object and action words: The featural and unitary semantic space hypothesis. *Cognitive Psychology*, *48*, 422–488.

Willems, R. M. & Francken, J. C. (2012). Embodied Cognition: Taking the next step. *Frontiers in Psychology*, *3*, 582.

Witt, J. K., Kemmerer, D., Linkenauger, S. A. & Culham, J. (2010). A functional role for motor simulation in naming tools. *Psychological Science*, *21*, 1215–1219.

Yee, E., Ahmed, S. & Thompson-Schill, S. L. (2012). Colorless green ideas (can) prime furiously. *Psychological Science*, *23*(4), 364–369.

Yee, E., Chrysikou, E., Hoffman, E. & Thompson-Schill, S. L. (2013). Manual Experience Shapes Object Representation. *Psychological Science*, *24* (6), 909–919.

Yee, E., Drucker, D. M. & Thompson-Schill, S. L. (2010). fMRI-adaptation evidence of overlapping neural representations for objects related in function or manipulation. *NeuroImage*, *50*(2), 753–763. doi:10.1016/j.neuroimage.2009.12.036

Yee, E., Huffstetler, S. & Thompson-Schill, S. L. (2011). Function follows form: Activation of shape and function features during object identification. *Journal of Experimental Psychology: General*, *140*, 348–363. doi: 10.1037/a0022840

Yee, E., Musz, E. & Thompson-Schill, S. L. Mapping the Similarity Space of Concepts in Sensorimotor Cortex. *Poster presented at the Neurobiology of Language Conference*, San Sebastian. October, 2012.

Yee, E. & Thompson-Schill, S. L. (2016). Putting concepts into context. *Psychonomic Bulletin and Review*, *23*(4), 1015–1027.

Subject index

acoustic invariance 1, 8, 11, 13, 18, 23, 24, 27, 28, 32, 38, 46–48, 78
adaptation 10, 12, 14, 17, 72–76, 78, 79, 83, 84, 108, 118, 126, 156, 168–172, 174, 178–180, 184, 185, 191, 232, 243, 244
adaptive plasticity 155, 156, 167–174, 176, 178, 181
adverse listening 180, 183
apraxia of speech 187, 190, 192
artificial neural network 154, 220
auditory word recognition 4, 16, 17, 47, 179
automatic speech recognition 211–213, 234, 235

C-CuRE model 38
category learning 52, 66, 75, 79, 82, 128, 193
cerebellum 168, 170–172, 175, 178–181, 183–186
compensation 28, 29, 32–35, 42, 46, 190, 192
competitors 16
concepts 213, 236–238, 245, 251
conceptual knowledge 240, 244, 245, 247
consolidation 68, 70, 71, 79, 80
context effects 31, 50, 159, 163, 167, 176, 181, 251
coronal 87–98, 100, 101, 104, 217, 219
critical period hypothesis 197, 198, 209
cue integration 32, 50, 172, 174

deep learning 211, 235
deep neural networks 211, 213, 224, 234, 235
degraded speech 79, 159, 164–166, 168, 171, 175, 179, 181, 183, 185
distinctive feature 5, 104

EEG 93, 96, 101, 102, 157, 174, 180
episodic 3, 8, 18, 48, 106, 107, 120, 124–127
episodic models 124
exemplar models 27, 28, 35
expectation-driven processing 39, 46
external sources of information 169

features 1–9, 13–20, 24, 25, 31, 33, 40, 47–50, 58, 69, 70, 71, 78, 86–94, 96–98, 101, 105, 109, 113, 117, 176, 187, 211, 213, 216–226, 228–231, 233–235, 237, 238, 241–244, 250, 251
feature extraction 218, 219, 229, 230, 233
feature representation 4, 104
fMRI 2, 10, 13, 15, 17–20, 64, 65, 73, 81–83, 157, 160–162, 165, 168, 170, 176, 179–181, 183–186, 189, 190, 196, 210, 242–245, 247
foreign accent syndrome 187, 192
fricative 13, 14, 17, 20–22, 29–37, 40, 42, 43, 46, 47, 50, 87, 88, 115, 117, 118, 127, 138, 140, 154, 191, 216
FUL 85–87, 89, 90, 92, 94–98, 213, 217, 218, 220
functional neuroimaging 4, 155, 157, 161, 171, 177, 179, 183
fundamental frequency 109, 111, 126, 130, 152, 188, 195

geminates 100, 102, 103, 106
gestural 7, 8, 22, 26, 29, 33, 39, 53, 56, 78
Great English Vowel Shift 5
Grimm's Law 5

individual variability 66
inferior frontal gyrus (IFG) 10, 11, 161
internally generated predictions 156, 168–170, 173
invariance 1–4, 6–9, 11–14, 17–28, 31, 32, 34, 38, 45–48, 50, 52, 53, 70, 78, 82, 108, 113, 123, 183

language change 4, 5, 86, 103
lexical access 2, 4, 9, 12, 15–19, 26, 47–49, 126, 166, 235
lexical density 15, 16
lexical representation 8, 12, 86, 87, 89, 101, 220
lexical specificity 121
lexical tone 83, 129–131, 143, 144, 146, 147, 149–154, 209, 210

Subject index — 257

Mandarin tone 129, 130, 134, 135, 137, 139, 144–147, 152, 153, 195, 210
manner of articulation 1, 5, 7, 13, 14, 22, 25, 28, 191
MMN 94, 96–98, 101, 103, 105, 106
motor theory 18, 24, 48, 49, 80, 81
music perception 153

N400 93, 96, 101–103, 182
nasal vowels 98, 101
natural classes 5, 9, 17, 211
neighborhood density 15, 16
non-native 3, 20, 52, 54–59, 61–67, 70–80, 71, 72, 73, 74, 75, 76, 77, 78, 79, 80, 82, 83, 121–123, 125–127, 129, 131, 133–138, 143, 152, 154, 167, 172, 179, 184, 194–196, 205, 208–210, 233
normalization 20, 27, 28, 141, 142, 144, 146, 147, 153, 154, 234

parsing 29, 33, 34, 38, 39, 46, 48
perceptual learning 58, 72–74, 79–83, 111, 115–118, 126, 127, 167, 174, 175, 178–180, 182, 183, 185, 196, 208, 210
phoneme recognition 211, 213, 230, 232, 233
phonetic category 2, 4, 7–12, 14, 17–19, 52, 56, 59, 63–66, 72–75, 82, 111, 112, 114, 115, 126–128, 172, 183, 193
phonetic features 4, 7–9, 18, 19, 24, 31, 47, 50, 69, 70
phonetics 18, 46–50, 78, 82, 88, 104–106, 126, 152–154, 184, 190, 192, 200, 209, 212, 234
phonological features 3, 4, 13, 14, 17, 92, 96, 211, 216–220, 222–224, 226, 229, 233, 234
phonological processing 1, 15, 19, 98, 166–168
phonology 1, 17, 19, 22, 49, 71, 80, 87, 88, 104–106, 187, 190, 211–213, 229
place features 86, 87, 92, 96
processing asymmetry 91, 100, 101

representations 4, 5, 8, 12, 15–17, 19, 20, 25, 40, 75, 77, 81, 85, 86, 91–94, 96, 98, 103–108, 118, 119, 126, 129, 159, 162, 172, 177, 180, 182, 184, 194, 196, 197, 215, 236–238, 242–245, 247, 249, 251

second language acquisition 81, 181, 197, 198, 209
segments 3, 4, 5, 9, 14, 15–17, 22, 88, 100, 106, 119, 153, 154, 192
semantic features 237, 238
semantic memory 236, 238, 245, 251
semantic priming 93, 95, 101–103, 238, 240, 241, 244, 248
semantic representations 162, 236, 237, 242, 247, 249, 251
semantic-perceptual interactions 162, 163
sleep 52, 58, 66–71, 76–80
speech perception 8, 9, 11, 17–24, 28, 35, 37, 39, 46–50, 53, 56, 58, 64, 76, 78, 80, 81, 83, 104, 105, 107, 108, 111, 123, 124, 126, 127, 129, 130, 135, 138, 154–159, 161, 162, 164–185, 193, 208, 209, 220, 234
spoken word production 4, 16, 17, 18, 20
stop consonants 1, 5, 6, 7, 10, 13, 14, 16–18, 20, 47–50, 73, 78, 80, 83, 109, 189, 209, 217
superior temporal gyrus (STG) 10, 157
suprasegmentals 188, 198

Taiwanese 142, 143, 147, 149
talker specificity 3, 104, 120

underspecification 48, 85, 87, 93–96, 100–103, 105, 234

variability 3, 6–9, 11, 12, 17, 19–22, 26, 28, 33, 34, 42, 45, 48–50, 52, 53, 54, 66, 72, 74–76, 81–83, 100, 104, 108, 110–115, 117, 118, 120, 123, 126, 127, 129–131, 133–135, 137–139, 142, 152, 154, 182, 187, 189, 196, 198, 199, 205, 208, 210, 211
voice-onset time (VOT) 10, 80
voice recognition 108, 121–123, 126, 127
voicing 5, 13, 14, 16, 17, 20, 21, 25, 29, 31, 40–47, 49, 50, 57, 75, 78, 82, 83, 109, 114, 127, 128, 191, 209, 217
vowel height 97, 98, 191

www.ingramcontent.com/pod-product-compliance
Lightning Source LLC
Chambersburg PA
CBHW070303240426
43661CB00057B/2633